Contagion

In the age of HIV, antibiotic-resistant bacteria, the Ebola virus and BSE, the metaphors and experience of contagion are a central concern of government, biomedicine and popular culture.

Contagion explores cultural responses to infectious diseases and their biomedical management over the nineteenth and twentieth centuries. It also investigates the use of 'contagion' as a concept in postmodern rethinking of embodied subjectivity.

These essays are written from within the fields of cultural studies, biomedical history and critical sociology. The contributors examine the geographies, policies and identities which have been produced in the massive social effort to contain diseases. They explore both social responses to infectious diseases in the past, and contemporary theoretical and biomedical sites for the study of contagion.

Alison Bashford is Chair of the Department of Gender Studies at the University of Sydney. She writes on the cultural history of medicine in the nineteenth and twentieth centuries. In 1998 she published *Purity and Pollution: Gender, Embodiment and Victorian Medicine* (St Martin's Press/ Macmillan) and is currently completing *Public Health and the Imagining of Australia, 1880–1940*.

Claire Hooker is a research associate with the History and Material Culture of Public Health in Australia Project, Department of Gender Studies, University of Sydney, in collaboration with the Powerhouse Museum, Sydney. Her book *Not a Job in the Ordinary Sense: Women and Science in Australia* is forthcoming (Melbourne University Press).

Routledge studies in the social history of medicine
Edited by Bernard Harris
Department of Sociology and Social Policy, University of Southampton, UK

The Society for the Social History of Medicine was founded in 1969, and exists to promote research into all aspects of the field, without regard to limitations of either time or place. In addition to this book series, the Society also organises a regular programme of conferences, and publishes an internationally recognised journal, *Social History of Medicine*. The Society offers a range of benefits, including reduced-price admission to conferences and discounts on SSHM books, to its members. Individuals wishing to learn more about the Society are invited to contact the series editor through the publisher.

The Society took the decision to launch 'Studies in the social history of medicine', in association with Routledge, in 1989, in order to provide an outlet for some of the latest research in the field. Since that time, the series has expanded significantly under a number of series editors, and now includes both edited collections and monographs. Individuals wishing to submit proposals are invited to contact the series editor in the first instance.

1 **Nutrition in Britain**
Science, scientists and politics in the twentieth century
Edited by David F. Smith

2 **Migrants, Minorities and Health**
Historical and contemporary studies
Edited by Lara Marks and Michael Worboys

3 **From Idiocy to Mental Deficiency**
Historical perspectives on people with learning disabilities
Edited by David Wright and Anne Digby

4 **Midwives, Society and Childbirth**
Debates and controversies in the modern period
Edited by Hilary Marland and Anne Marie Rafferty

5 **Illness and Healing Alternatives in Western Europe**
Edited by Marijke Gijswit-Hofstra, Hilary Marland and Hans de Waardt

6 **Health Care and Poor Relief in Protestant Europe, 1500–1700**
Edited by Ole Peter Grell and Andrew Cunningham

7 **The Locus of Care**
Families, communities, institutions and provision of welfare since antiquity
Edited by Peregrine Horden and Richard Smith

8 **Race, Science and Medicine, 1700–1960**
Edited by Waltraud Ernst and Bernard Harris

9 **Insanity, Institutions and Society, 1800–1914**
Edited by Bill Forsythe and Joseph Melling

10 **Food, Science, Policy and Regulation in the Twentieth Century**
International and comparative perspectives
Edited by David F. Smith and Jim Phillips

11 **Sex, Sin and Suffering**
Venereal diseases and European society since 1870
Edited by Roger Davidson and Lesley A. Hall

12 **The Spanish Flu Pandemic of 1918**
New perspectives
Edited by Howard Phillips and David Killingray

13 **Plural Medicine**
Waltraud Ernst

14 **Innovation in Twentieth-Century Medicine and Health**
Diffusion and resistance in international perspective
Jenny Stanton

15 **Contagion**
Historical and cultural studies
Edited by Alison Bashford and Claire Hooker

Contagion
Historical and cultural studies

**Edited by Alison Bashford
and Claire Hooker**

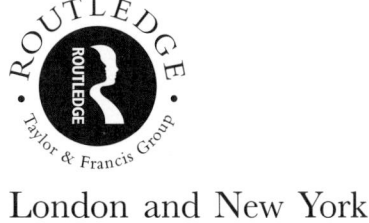

London and New York

RA 643 .C664 2001

Contagion

First published 2001 by Routledge
11 New Fetter Lane, London EC4P 4EE

Simultaneously published in the USA and Canada
by Routledge
29 West 35th Street, New York, NY 10001

Routledge is an imprint of the Taylor & Francis Group

© 2001 Editorial material and selection, Alison Bashford and
Claire Hooker, individual chapters, the authors

Typeset in Baskerville by
Florence Production Ltd, Stoodleigh, Devon
Printed and bound in Great Britain
by University Press, Cambridge

All rights reserved. No part of this book may be reprinted
or reproduced or utilised in any form or by any electronic,
mechanical, or other means, now known or hereafter invented,
including photocopying and recording, or in any information
storage or retrieval system, without permission in writing
from the publishers.

British Library Cataloguing in Publication Data
A catalogue record for this book is available from the British Library.

Library of Congress Cataloging in Publication Data
Contagion: historical and cultural studies / edited by Alison
   Bashford and Claire Hooker.
      p. cm.
   Includes bibliographical references and index.
   1. Communicable diseases—Social aspects.   2. Communicable
diseases—History—19th century.   3. Communicable diseases
—History—20th century.   4. Social medicine.   I. Bashford,
Alison, 1963– .   II. Hooker, Claire, 1971–
   [DNLM: 1. Communicable diseases—Essays.   2. Culture—
Essays. 3. History of Medicine, 19th Cent.—Essays.   4. History
of Medicine, 20th Cent.—Essays.   5. Infection—Essays.
6. Public Health—History—Essays. WC 9 C759 2001]
RA634.C715 2001
616.9′09–dc21   00–065338

ISBN 0–415–24671–7

Contents

List of illustrations vii
List of contributors viii
Acknowledgements xi
Abbreviations xiii

Introduction: contagion, modernity and postmodernity 1
ALISON BASHFORD AND CLAIRE HOOKER

PART 1
Contagion and cultural histories of the modern world

1 **The meaning of contagion: reproduction, medicine and metaphor** 15
   MARGARET PELLING

2 **Foreign bodies: vaccination, contagion and colonialism in the nineteenth century** 39
   ALISON BASHFORD

3 **Moral contagion and the will: the crisis of masculinity in *fin-de-siècle* France** 61
   CHRISTOPHER E. FORTH

4 **Excremental colonialism: public health and the poetics of pollution** 76
   WARWICK ANDERSON

5 **Leprosy and the management of race, sexuality and nation in tropical Australia** 106
   ALISON BASHFORD AND MARIA NUGENT

6 Sanitary failure and risk: pasteurisation, immunisation and the logics of prevention 129
CLAIRE HOOKER

PART 2
Contaminating capacities in postmodernity

7 Vulnerable bodies and ontological contamination 153
MARGRIT SHILDRICK

8 A pig's tale: porcine viruses and species boundaries 168
MARSHA ROSENGARTEN

9 Taking the HIV test: self-surveillance and the making of heterosexuality 183
LISA ADKINS

10 The promiscuous placenta: crossing over 201
JANE-MAREE MAHER

11 Carrier – becoming symborg 217
MELINDA RACKHAM

Select bibliography 227
Index 232

Illustrations

Figures

Figure 2.1	'Start Planning Your Overseas Trip Here'. Courtesy, SmithKline Beecham Biologicals.	47
Figure 2.2	From J. Ashburton Thompson, *A Report to the President of the Board of Health: containing photographs of a person suffering from variola discreta, and accounts of the case*, Sydney, Government Printer, 1886. Copy in author's possession.	49
Figure 7.1	Karl Grimes, *Still Life*, 1997, chromogenic print, 72 × 48 in. Courtesy of the artist and Gallery of Photography, Dublin.	154

Table

Table 5.1	Nationality of recorded cases of leprosy in Australia Source: J. H. L. Cumpston, 'Health and Disease in Australia: A History', unpublished typescript, vol. 1, 1928, p. 318. Courtesy, Burkitt–Ford Library, University of Sydney.	111

Contributors

Lisa Adkins is a Lecturer in Sociology at the University of Manchester. Her research interests are in the areas of social theory, feminist theory, sexuality, gender and economy. Publications include *Gendered Work* (1995), *Sexualising the Social* (1996) and *Sex, Sensibility and the Gendered Body* (1996). Recent articles have been published in *Theory, Culture and Society* and *Economy and Society*. She is currently completing a book called 'Revisions: Towards a Feminist Sociology of Late Modernity' which considers theories of identity transformation in relation to gender and sexuality, to be published by Open University Press.

Warwick Anderson is the Director of the History of the Health Sciences Program in the Department of Anthropology, History and Social Medicine at the University of California, San Francisco, and has appointments at the University of California at Berkeley and the University of Melbourne. Until recently he was the Director of the Centre for the Study of Health and Society at the University of Melbourne. Dr Anderson's research interests include the development of public health and health promotion policy. An article examining the politics of harm reduction measures in New York City appeared in the *American Journal of Public Health* and was reprinted in *AIDS and Contemporary History* (1994). He has published widely in international journals, including *Victorian Studies, Critical Inquiry, Positions*, the *American Historical Review*, and *Social Studies of Science*.

Alison Bashford is senior lecturer in the School of Philosophy, Gender, History and Ancient World Studies at the University of Sydney. She writes critical and cultural medical history of the nineteenth and twentieth centuries. In 1998 she published *Purity and Pollution: Gender, Embodiment and Victorian Medicine* and is currently completing a book, 'Public Health and the Imagining of Australia'. Her next project is a history of world health organisations in the twentieth century and the concept of 'population'.

Christopher E. Forth teaches European intellectual and cultural history at the Australian National University. He is the author of *Zarathustra in Paris: The Nietzsche Vogue in France, 1891–1918*, and is currently preparing a study of masculinity and the male body in France during the Dreyfus Affair.

Claire Hooker is a research associate with the History and Material Culture of Public Health in Australia Project, Department of Gender Studies, University of Sydney. Her interests are in nineteenth- and twentieth-century histories of health and medicine, and in history and feminist studies of science. Her recent articles concern diphtheria and immunisation in developing public health instrumentalities.

Jane-Maree Maher is a lecturer in women's studies at Monash University in Melbourne. She writes on embodiment, pregnancy and Virginia Woolf. She completed her doctoral research in 1999 and is currently working on a book provisionally entitled 'The Promiscuous Placenta: Toward a New Spectacle of the Pregnant Body'.

Maria Nugent is a public historian. Her doctoral research explored new ways of writing histories of sites of colonial encounter.

Margaret Pelling is Reader in the Social History of Medicine in the Modern History Faculty of the University of Oxford. She is Consultant Editor for Medicine, 1500–2000, for the *New Dictionary of National Biography*. Her recent publications include a volume of her essays, *The Common Lot: Sickness, Medical Occupations and the Urban Poor in Early Modern England* (1998). She is currently completing a monograph on 'irregular' medical practitioners in early modern London.

Melinda Rackham is an artist and writer who has been constructing imaginal and hypertextual net.art since 1995. She is currently undertaking a Ph.D. in Virtual Media at COFA, University of New South Wales, has presented and published theoretical and poetic texts in Australia and internationally, and recently won the Faulding Award for Multimedia. Her sites have been included in Beyond Interface, Arco Electronico, Arts_Edge, Perspecta99, Maid in Cyberspace, Transmediale2000 and Art Entertainment Network.

Marsha Rosengarten is a research fellow at the National Centre in HIV Social Research at the University of New South Wales. Her current research is on the workings of pharmacology in shaping the HIV epidemic at this time. She has a continuing interest in the subject of organ transplantation, particularly as it unsettles presumptions of bodily identity, including national identity, and has published on this topic as well as on the matter of blood in relation to female identity.

Margrit Shildrick is SURI Research Fellow at Staffordshire University and an Honorary Research Fellow at the University of Liverpool. She has written extensively on the body and on feminist theory, and has recently completed a new book entitled *Touching the Monster: Encounters with the Vulnerable Self*. Her previous books are *Leaky Bodies and Boundaries: Feminism, (Bio)ethics and Postmodernism* (1997), and two edited collections with Janet Price, *Vital Signs: Feminist Reconfigurations of the Bio/logical Body* (1998), and *Feminist Theory and the Body: A Reader* (1999).

Acknowledgements

This book has been a genuinely collaborative effort, and we would like to thank the contributors for their hard work and stimulating discussion. The project began in 1999 as the Contagion conference, and so we thank participants and contributors to that event as well. The book has been immeasurably enriched by pleasurable daily conversation between ourselves and our 'shadow editors': conversation between Alison and Carolyn Strange, and between Claire and Martha Sear. We are deeply grateful for the amount of reading and incisive commentary offered by Carolyn. Martha Sear and Megan Hicks have been working with us on a related public health history project, and we are indebted to them, and to the Powerhouse Museum, Sydney, for stimulating explorations of public health from many different points of view. Several research assistants have participated, contributing knowledge and expertise far exceeding the mundane work asked of them: thanks to Michelle Arrow, Maria Nugent, Megan Jones. We are grateful to the Department of Gender Studies – Pat Davies, Gail Mason, Elspeth Probyn, Linnell Secomb, Nikki Whipps – for their collegiality and support. Other friends and colleagues have read chapters and we are grateful for their input, in particular Glenda Sluga, Stephen Garton, Roy Macleod, Catriona Elder and Jill Levenberg. Claire would like to thank her family, and Alison the various generations and extensions of hers.

This project has been partly funded by the Australian Research Council in a collaborative project with the Powerhouse Museum and by a Wellcome Trust Travel Grant. Alison is grateful to the Institute for Advanced Studies in the Humanities, University of Edinburgh, where she was a Visiting Fellow in 1999, for resources and support.

We are grateful to the University of Chicago Press for permission to reprint Warwick Anderson's article, and to Kluwer Academic/Plenum, for permission to reprint a version of Margrit Shildrick's essay. Thanks also to Routledge, W. F. Bynam and Roy Porter for permission to reprint a version of Margaret Pelling's essay. We are extremely grateful to Karl Grimes for permission to reproduce from his exhibition *Still Life*, and to SmithKline Biologicals for permission to reproduce their poster, 'Start Planning Your Overseas Trip Here'.

Chapter 1 is a revised version of M. Pelling, 'Contagion/Germ Theory/Specificity' in W. F. Bynum and R. Porter (eds), *Companion Encyclopedia of the History of Medicine*, 2 vols, London, Routledge, 1993, vol. 1, pp. 309–34.

Chapter 4 was previously published in *Critical Inquiry*, vol. 21, 1995, pp. 640–69.

Chapter 7 is a revised version of 'Becoming Vulnerable: Contagious Encounters and the Ethics of Risk', *Journal of Medical Humanities* (forthcoming).

Abbreviations

AIDS	Acquired Immune Deficiency Syndrome
BMJ	*British Medical Journal*
CPEDERF	Centre Parisien d'Études et de Documentation pour l'Enseignement et le Rayonnement du Français
HAR	Hyper Acute Rejection
HIV	Human Immuno-deficiency Virus
MJA	*Medical Journal of Australia*
NH&MRC	National Health and Medical Research Council
NSW	New South Wales
QDHHAR	Queensland Department of Health and Home Affairs Records
QHSO	Queensland Home Secretary's Office
QPWD	Queensland Public Works Department
QSA	Queensland State Archive
USNA	United States National Archive
WHO	World Health Organization

Introduction
Contagion, modernity and postmodernity

Alison Bashford and Claire Hooker

In 1998 the US Department of State held a forum on Emerging Infectious Diseases. Participants were welcomed and warned in the same breath:

> I trust that everyone washed their hands before they entered the conference today. Unfortunately, I'm only half-joking. Infectious diseases once thought to be controlled are re-emerging worldwide. They endanger the health of Americans and our national security interests. These diseases are the silent enemies of economic growth, national well-being and stability around the globe, as infectious diseases know no borders.[1]

As this statement indicates, contagion has a powerful reach. Defying fantasies of control, corroding internal integrity, and ignoring the borders that define and defend identity, contagion is considered a threat to individual, national and global security. The fear of contagion in this case was met by powerful institutions of globalisation: World Health meets the World Bank meets US foreign policy meets the UN Security Council. Merging metaphor and public policy, contagion here intertwines personal conduct with the management of populations, nations and economies.

In the age of HIV/AIDS, antibiotic-resistant bacteria, the Ebola virus and mad cows, the metaphors and corporeal experience of contagion, resistance and immunity greatly exercise the spheres of government, biomedicine and popular culture, as well as post-structuralist theory and history. The essays in this book are written from within the fields of cultural studies, biomedical history and critical sociology. We explore historical and cultural responses to infectious diseases and their biomedical management over the nineteenth and twentieth centuries, in conjunction with the use of 'contagion' as a concept in postmodern reconceptualisations of embodied subjectivity. We are interested in the geographies, policies and identities which have been produced in the massive social effort to contain diseases – that extensive culture of hygiene which we know as public health but which we might also call 'the dream of hygienic containment'.[2] The essays here are best considered as a critical elaboration on the history and present of this dream.

The uncontrollability and unknowability of contagion, its surprise appearance in other bodies, in other places, in other creatures, invites systems of control and knowledge: hence the huge scientific and bureaucratic machine of public health, touching on so many levels of conduct and social organisation, from the personal and local to the national and international. Many of the essays explore critically the various lines of hygiene drawn to contain the circulating dangers represented as contagion, and to render particular subjects or spaces safe or immune. They also elaborate on the ways in which these cultural, political and social efforts so often fail. This fantasy of controlling contagion, this 'dream of hygienic containment', has strongly marked modern western history and culture. The control of contagion is a 'dream' in two senses. It describes the wish for contagion-free selves and societies, articulated above by the US government. There are, of course, very real reasons for this dream of containment and prevention, and reasons more valid than the imperative of 'national security' and 'economic productivity' driving the Emerging Infectious Diseases Program – the pain of disease as well as treatment, the unpredictability of epidemics, the deaths, the social dislocation. The success in controlling some diseases – notably smallpox – has been significant and of profound social consequence. Yet 'dream' also suggests the very impossibility of total hygienic containment, for contagion always exceeds measures for prevention. It is this capacity for excess that sustains the fascination of contagion in the cultural imagination of the west.

The first part, 'Contagion and Cultural Histories of the Modern World', deals with the complex history of the concept of contagion and the related term infection. Here, cultural historians explore a range of contagion-anxieties which emerged from the nineteenth to the mid-twentieth centuries in the European and colonial world. The second part, 'Contaminating Capacities in Postmodernity' offers readings of contemporary biomedicine, with a focus on the possibilities (and limitations) of rethinking 'contagion' as an idea. Contagion's capacity for excess has interested rather than frightened some in postmodernity, and has encouraged some exploration in 'giving up the dream'. Several essays in the second section of this book, then, explore contagion as capacity, rather than incapacity. Together, the essays examine the changing contexts in which practices of hygiene have been imagined and implemented, as well as the social imperatives driving the demand for, and modes of, control. Our contributors are interested in the social effects of contagion and resulting hygienic practices: the identities, civic, personal, colonial or national, which are thus constituted; the drawing and redrawing of individual and communal boundaries; the creation of communities and geographies marked as clean or unclean. The essays examine the ways in which such practices and identities have been, and are, inflected through specific cultures and histories of fitness, citizenship, gender, race, and sexuality. In the governance of 'health and hygiene', we examine what else is governed, what created and what obscured.

The historical essays in this volume are interested in how contagion, infection, contamination, colonisation, reproduction and pollution were precisely, and differently, understood in the past and the corollaries of these technical meanings in terms of policy and practice. Conceptualisations of both the processes and agents of contagion have been highly contested and are historically specific. It is only through careful research that the real complexity of contagion and hygiene may be unpacked. We open the book with Margaret Pelling's chapter which historicises 'contagion' with great care and detail. She alerts us to the changing meanings of contagion in the west, meanings constituted in, and in part shaping, larger shifts in thinking about bodies, illness, disease aetiologies and philosophical systems of knowledge and reasoning. Beginning with pre-modern and early modern ideas, Pelling works carefully through the crucial changes over the nineteenth century, a very complicated field, still well served by her early *Cholera, Fever and English Medicine*.[3] She reflects on the renditions of 'contagionist', 'anti-contagionist' and 'germ' theories which have been created within medical historiography, and the effects of these delineations in masking as well as clarifying more complicated histories. As an intellectual history, her essay shows also how 'contagion' worked through social, symbolic, moral and technical meanings which were often inseparable, even at the level of the strictest aetiological theory.

As well as making the past comprehensible in more complex and critically informed ways, we understand that a fundamental purpose of history is to make the present strange. We place historical and cultural studies together very deliberately, and put each scholarly tradition hard at work in relation to the other, in pursuit of new ways of understanding contagion and its control as embodied social and personal experience. While the two parts of the book are separated chronologically, similar ideas richly infect both sections. Thus, where Bashford discusses nineteenth-century anxieties about cross-species contagion through vaccine matter in an era which obsessively separated the social and natural categories, Rosengarten retheorises anxiety over species boundaries in the arena of late twentieth-century pig–human organ transplantation. Where Hooker charts conceptualisations of 'carriers' in the social framework of early and mid-twentieth-century public health, Rackham provides a juxtaposition in her intensely interior reworking of the lived notion of the carrier. Where Shildrick and Maher discuss the contamination of the normative idea of the autonomous subject, in the context of current moral and biomedical reactions to the disabled and of the physico-metaphoric function of the placenta respectively, Forth's essay demonstrates the processes through which this construction was produced in one setting, late nineteenth-century France.

Throughout the book the metaphoric aspects of contagion are made central to our understanding of biomedicine and embodied subjectivity. The potent web of signifiers with which contagion is connected – resistance, immunity, colonisation, hygiene, blood, plague, hysteria – are concepts deployed poetically, theoretically, politically and scientifically. Despite the complex history of contagion which Pelling alerts us to it is possible to generalise about reasons for this powerful metaphoric reach. First, contagion is always about contact. Thus through most of the nineteenth century 'contagious diseases' meant sexually transmitted diseases – transmission through the closest and most problematised contact of all. However, both the nature of what we now think of as contagious material, and understandings of the means and modes by which it is transferred and multiplies, have been contested in the post-Enlightenment period. For example, while we now equate contagion with infection, the two ideas were historically distinguished through consideration of the means by which the 'matter' (however constituted) was passed: that is, contagion generally implied direct contact, and infection implied indirect or mediated contact. In its capacity to spread by contact, contagion invites uneasy consideration of connections between things – people, animals, organic objects, inanimate objects – things with which humans do not know, or always wish to know they are connected. In carefully dissecting the meaning of contagion as an 1883 dictionary entry, the authoritative English public health bureaucrat, John Simon, wrote that in addition to spreading through undesirable contact between people, contagion connects 'living bodies' with the 'not living': 'contagiousness of disease is a fact not only for man, but apparently for all living nature.'[4] Contagion reaches over domains of nature and culture which we often want to understand, or have an investment in understanding, as separate.

Contagion requires contact, but it always implies more than this: it implies absorption, invasion, vulnerability, the breaking of a boundary imagined as secure, in which the other becomes part of the self. Contagion connotes both a *process* of contact and transmission, and a substantive, self-replicating *agent*, and is centrally concerned with the growth and multiplication of this agent. From the middle of the nineteenth century onwards, this began to be conceptualised in terms of *self*-multiplication, not of inanimate matter, but of matter which was alive, organic and capable of exponential self-replication. This uncontrolled and exponential aspect of the various early germ theories was deeply unsettling. John Simon wrote in 1883: 'each of the diseases propagates itself in its own form as an exact identity, as if it were a species in zoology or botany; and in each such repetition of the disease there is a multiplication – always large and sometimes an inconceivably immense multiplication, of material which has the same infective property.'[5]

The notion of contact and uncontrolled spread which is crystallised in the term 'contagion' remains powerfully in operation in our own time.

The disconcerting idea of the self-multiplication of contagia, the existence of minute self-willed life-forms beyond human control, has exercised popular as well as expert western culture and has appeared as standard fodder in twentieth-century science fiction, from *Alien* to *Virus* to the *X-Files*. But contagia are not always 'alive': consider the computer virus which self-multiplies exponentially. Nor are contagia always 'actual': witness recent work on emotional contagion, the infectiousness of affect, the 'Elvis Contagion', copy-cat murders as contagious, war as an infectious state, hysterical epidemics, gossip as a form of epidemic communication.[6] And the most common recent media use of 'contagion' is in the financial sphere, the so-called 'Asian Contagion'. The authors of one recent publication on the Asian monetary crisis write of 'vulnerability' and 'spillover', of unpredictable mental states, of panic, of out-of-control excess, all of which reminds us most of Forth's exploration of the crisis of masculine control and the infectious diseases of the will in late nineteenth-century France (discussed below).[7]

We are deeply interested in the metaphoric reach of contagion, but our analyses focus specifically on the field of origin as it were: biomedicine and embodiment. As scholars in cultural history and cultural studies, the authors in this collection think of biomedicine *as* culture, in which language constitutes the very possibilities of conceptualisation and experience. The terms of contagion were and are never purely technical, but are always thought through culture. The capacity of 'contagion' to simultaneously function as deeply resonant metaphor for the circulation of social, moral or political dangers through a population, *and* as visceral, horrible infection, drives the contributors' and editors' interest. This capacity for 'contagion' to be so intensely both metaphor and flesh explains its cultural resonance, but it also *requires* explanation. Broadly characterised as post-structuralists, many of the contributors to this volume are interested in bodies (people) as the location where ideas become flesh, and flesh becomes ideas. This book deals with fleshliness as the *matter* of identity and works from the knowledge that our metaphorical resourcing is drawn from our visceral bodies, our always-embodied identity.[8]

Exploring the transmission of ideas across the mythical boundary between modernity and postmodernity is central to our objective. The structure of the book is not simply chronological; it is, rather, essential to our analysis. We evoke a sense of shifts and contrasts between modern and postmodern approaches to, and effects of, contagion and hygienic control. Rather than a triumphant story of increasing sanitation and disease control, the cultural historians see in the modern world all kinds of anxious practices in which selves and societies sought (vainly) to secure clear boundaries. Some contributors in Part 2, by contrast, welcome the crossing and dissolving of these boundaries as they think about and embody contagion in new ways. Yet we do not propose a new triumphal story in which our enlightenment, as postmodern scholars, stands in opposition to the obtuse fear and smug, hypocritical hubris of our modern predecessors. There is no cordon sanitaire dividing modernity from postmodernity. The concerns of modernity continue to circulate in current public health just as the conceptual tools of postmodernism have colonised our vision of the history of health and medicine. The 'dream of hygienic containment' recurs, as fully justified fears of new viruses, antibiotic-resistant bacteria, inter-species mutations or biological warfare find expression, albeit in often unjustifiable ways: as homophobia, or as racist restriction of immigration, for example. And, we might agree with Donna Haraway that stress management has replaced hygienic practice in the postmodern world.[9] Social and subjective anxiety continues to preoccupy all the contributors in Part 2, and what is different is their exploration of possible alternatives in our response.

The chronological and epistemological schema of modernity/postmodernity can (with care) be mapped onto colonialism/postcolonialism. It is no accident that the two centuries under interrogation in this collection of essays was the period both of an intense assertion and then dismantling of colonialism, as well as the assertion and subsequent deep questioning of scientific and biomedical authority. A number of the essays deal squarely with the nexus of modernity, biomedicine and colonialism, while the exploration of these issues in the contemporary context will be left for another volume. To study infectious disease historically is also to question and make visible the processes and concept of colonisation, for like contagion, colonisation is about 'contact', self-multiplication and, not infrequently, destruction. The three-way travel of terminology between imperial/national governance, infectious disease and laboratory medicine is just one indicator of the entwined histories of biomedicine and imperialism: the 'colony' of bacteria on the petri-dish; the appearance of leper or epileptic 'colonies' in the nineteenth and early twentieth centuries; the defence of the immune self and of the 'immune' community or nation from external invasion; the notion of 'diplomatic' immunity; the 'resistance' of colonised people and the resistance of the individual embodied subject to 'invading' disease.[10] The global distribution of hegemonic practices of western biomedicine as well as this cross-over of concepts situates the very notion of 'contagion' inside a history of imperialism and colonial discourse, as well as a history of biomedicine.

Anderson's study of American colonialism in early twentieth-century Philippines, 'Excremental Colonialism', reveals the imperative of health to be an effective way of constructing and maintaining boundaries between colonisers and colonised; a way of creating the 'otherness' of colonised territory and people. He details the process by which contagion and its management created American colonial identity through the regulation of conduct, producing and sustaining wider social relations. Precariously placed as wielders of colonial power, American physicians and public health experts installed a culture of hygiene and sanitary inspection of indigenous Filipinos at the turn of the century. Anderson details the effects of this culture in terms of creating an American colonial identity of cleanliness, which implied greater security and safety, in contrast to a Filipino identity of contamination in which ceaseless regulation of social life and personal conduct was apparently required. The role of government in creating public health practices which served to distinguish the colonised from the colonisers is discussed by Bashford and Nugent in their study of leprosy management. Their essay shows how implicated public health was in the work of colonisation as well as nationalism in early and mid-twentieth-century tropical Australia. The governance of colonial populations through public health was often racialised: that is, health governance often doubled as, and was inseparable from, racial governance. Showing the centrality of colonialism, metaphorical and literal, to ideas of contagion is also part of Bashford's purpose in 'Foreign Bodies'. She suggests that nineteenth-century smallpox vaccination was partly shaped by orientalist and colonial discourse, and that this persists in the historiography through which we are asked to understand the history of vaccination.

Government of the healthy self has become, over the nineteenth and twentieth centuries, not only an imperative of western and colonial states, but a deeply internalised expression and assertion of subjectivity. Now a pivotal object of analysis in cultural studies, subjectivity was taken up significantly by Michel Foucault in terms of practices and techniques, what he called 'care of the self'.[11] The essays in this book explore questions about the shaping of identity through biomedical practices. We look at the relation between individual embodied subjectivity and other self-defining social bodies, for example communities and nations, as well as analysing the mechanisms by which individuals form their own sense of self by differentiating from others. Most importantly, we ask how infectious disease and its management, in conjunction with the poetic use of contagion and its web of signifiers, is implicated in the formation and subversion of selfhood. How, why, and with what effect does the question of identity *imply* the question of contagion? Writers in the sociological, philosophical and historical traditions have all noted in various ways that a primary (possibly in the modern period the supreme) mode for understanding and asserting the individual self has been through ideas of cleanliness and containment – what Julia Kristeva has termed 'the clean and proper body'.[12] Conversely, ill-health implies loss of self into some sort of other and these processes of loss of self have often been conceptualised through metaphors of infection. Rosengarten's essay on xenotransplantation – organ transplantation between humans and animals, in this case pigs – speaks eloquently to the question of what constitutes human identity as clean and proper in the current moment. Her essay draws attention to the cultural and scientific effort devoted to the creation and maintenance of a (nonetheless fluctuating) species divide. Practices like xenotransplantation, and the threat of porcine viruses in the human population, throws the human need for such a species divide into sharp relief. She explores the processes of identification and differentiation through which sense is made of transplantation, a practice in which part of the other becomes integated into the self, indeed becomes literally necessary viable functioning.

If the notion that practices shape identity has rightly become central in cultural studies, it is rather less so in history and is more or less absent in the subfield of medical history. These historical studies offer detailed information about very specific practices and activities (hence subjectivities) produced by contagion-anxieties. 'Practice' is approached in this book as necessarily and simultaneously involving individual subjectivities (as in 'care of the self'), health policies, modes of education and instruction, and expert biomedical knowledges. Practices of hygiene have never been simply about the avoidance of contagious disease. Rather, as Anderson demonstrates, they constitute a positive identity, often a morally inflected identity, although what 'moral' means is one of the most difficult, and certainly historically contingent, ideas to be pursued. In many cases, the mediation of identity through public health instrumentalities renders 'morality' in terms of citizenship.

Recent theory suggests that contemporary public health relies on a new form of civic identity, produced through complex statistical instruments: the morally inflected concept of the prudential citizen. Adkins speaks to these theories by taking up the notion of risk and its relation to biomedical practices productive of identity, in this case the relation between HIV testing and heterosexuality. Critiquing the notion that HIV testing constitutes a social drive to identify the homosexual, and also figures heterosexuality in terms of either immunity or boundary maintenance in regard to sexuality, Adkins argues that testing makes available a technique of the self through which heterosexuality is performed as self regulating and responsible. Hooker also addresses the notion of risk, historicising its introduction in public health practices. Her work on the history of hygienic practices, bureaucratised and implemented as national public health, is intertwined with the development of centralised states and the production and management of 'populations' suitable for industrial and capitalist economies. Hooker argues that the twentieth-century public health policies of pasteurisation and mass immunisation were among the earliest preventive procedures based on a logic of risk reduction at the levels of population and economy. They thus differed starkly from the logic of prior preventive practices based in sanitation, or on the equally unreliable location of 'dangerous individuals', 'carriers', for example. However, as state-deployed mass prophylactic policies, pasteurisation and immunisation are also fundamentally different from the techniques of recent risk-based public health, which *are*, as Adkins suggests, invested in prudential practices. In indicating a mid-twentieth-century transition in health management, Hooker's essay suggests the importance of rigorous, local historicising of schematic sociologies of risk and of the processes by which the shift from modernity to postmodernity occurred.

Identity is only one of the boundaries paradoxically made visible through its crossing in the process of contagion. The management of contagion has always involved the establishment of cordons sanitaire in one form or another, the drawing of lines and zones of hygiene.[13] The social management of contagion involves processes of differentiation and identification which are often conceived spatially: as quarantine, as isolation, or as containment within one's bounded body where skin is the protective barrier and the movement of bodily fluids through that barrier needs heavy regulation. Bashford and Nugent explore one of the most extreme examples of social and spatial quarantine in the modern period: the controversial compulsory isolation of lepers which returned as a largely colonial practice in the late nineteenth century, after centuries of virtual abeyance in Europe. However, part of their objective is to demonstrate how very complicated the seemingly clear cordon sanitaire of leprosy was: for lines of hygiene were not only drawn around the lepers, in this case banished to islands, but also as racialised 'interior frontiers' in mainland society which worked to keep races apart, ostensibly in the pursuit of public health. In 'Foreign Bodies', Bashford argues that the circulation of the 'foreign body' of the smallpox vaccine within nineteenth-century populations worked through a logic of contagion (the transgression of hygienic boundaries), rather than through the familiar public health logic of quarantine (the assertion of hygienic boundaries).

Whereas the constant, anxious attempts to secure and re-secure lines of hygiene make up the primary story of public health in Part 1, the essays in Part 2 find the fracturing of boundaries in postmodernity interesting, necessary, and even politically productive. Postmodernity is marked by intellectual and artistic expressions of transgression of such lines of hygiene. Shildrick recognises the deep sense of human vulnerability which makes contagion so culturally resonant, yet rather than avoiding this, she seeks to revalue it. She asks questions about the capacity of the disabled embodied subject to profitably 'contaminate' the normative idea of the 'clean and proper body,' so central to identity in the west. She seeks to refigure bodily vulnerability not as something to be disavowed and to be 'covered over' with attempts to secure boundaries, but rather as something necessary, inevitable and positive; vulnerability to invasion or infection or disability might entail 'the very possibility of becoming'. Similarly, Maher focuses specifically on the placenta, arguing that its existence as part of (at least) two embodied subjects simultaneously, refuses western masculinist notions of the bounded self with its instrumentalised body. Thinking of the placenta as a fleshly expression of contagion – the point of contact, merging, transfer and transmission – makes its possibilities as a theoretical figure both rewarding and challenging. Theirs is a different dream of ways of being which does not depend on the possession of a 'clean and proper body'.

It is in comparison with Forth's historical work that the difference in ways of being is illuminated. Forth discusses the notion of 'moral contagion' in relation to bourgeois masculine subjectivity in *fin-de-siècle* France. He explores the construction of a normative masculinity figured in terms of strength of will and the absence of the feminising quality of weakness and vulnerability to suggestion, influence or the sensual urgings of a man's own body. He shows how the obsessive repetitions of willpower advocated at the time were in themselves a tacit acknowledgement of the fragility of masculinity. Forth's detailed examination of the practices through which manly willpower was cultivated and a masculine self constantly performed reveal the processes through which the normative notion of personal autonomy came to be constituted.

As Donna Haraway has written, the late twentieth century is characterised by 'implosions of subjects and objects and of the natural and the artificial'.[14] Thus she famously pursues the figure of the cyborg, in which boundaries between organism and technology are impossible to perceive, and, for some, are no longer desired. Instead, what is at issue is the communication of information across a variety of domains: in the postmodern world of texts, the play of signifiers, cybernetics and system management, contagion becomes a frequently non-threatening form of information replication, and immunity a dynamic of communication.[15] The implosion (or what might be refigured as the mutual infection) of the natural and the artificial, the human and non-human is explored specifically in Rackham's beautiful visual essay 'carrier'. Based on her website,[16] she seeks to reposition her own viral infection not as a war over bodily boundaries between the virus and the self, but, in her words, 'as positive biological merging with the flesh – a love story with an intelligent being'. Playing over and with the borders of physicality, virtuality and artificial intelligence, Rackham recasts the question of infected identity and the host–virus relationship. She makes communication and information a central mode of being; another way of thinking 'contagion', another way of being 'contagious'.

The essays reveal the multilevel imperative toward hygienic practices – personal, familial, communal, economic, national, colonial and global. Contagion connects civic with personal selves, nations and populations with individuals and bodies, local dialect with global metaphor. Contagion is powerful because it is one point at which health, hygiene and the human body transmits meaning and infects as metaphor and analogy, thinking about the nation-state, as well as transnationalism and globalisation. As in the nineteenth century, so are we still fascinated by what most threatens our security and identity. Contagion signifies the dangers circulating in social bodies and in populations – actual viruses and bacteria, 'contagious' morals and ideas, social dangers re-thought as bodily infectiveness. But it is not always and only about danger. It is telling that what used to be categorised as 'contagious' diseases are now most often categorised as 'communicable' diseases. Quite literally, according to its etymology ('con': together; 'tangere': to touch), contagion can put us in touch.[17]

Notes

1 W. R. Sherman, Department of State Counselor, 'Emerging Infectious Diseases are a National Security Challenge to the United States'. 25 March 1998. Online. Available http://www/state.gov/www/policy_remarks/1998/980325_sherman_diseases.html. Accessed 10 Jan. 2000.
2 The phrase is Margrit Shildrick's.
3 M. Pelling, *Cholera, Fever and English Medicine*, Oxford, Oxford University Press, 1978.
4 J. Simon, 'Contagion', *Dictionary of Medicine*, London, Longmans, Green, 1883, p. 286.
5 Ibid., p. 287.
6 R. S. Denisoff and G. Plasketes, *True Disbelievers: The Elvis Contagion*, New Brunswick, Can., Transactions, 1995; E. Hatfield, *Emotional Contagion*, Cambridge and New York, Cambridge University Press, 1994; A. Lynch, *Thought Contagion: How Belief Spreads Through Society*, London, Basic Books, 1999; Maria Angel and Belinda Wilson, 'Copycats and Deadly Simulacra: Is Murder Contagious?', paper delivered at the 'Contagion' conference, University of Sydney, April 1999; Anna Gibbs, 'Contagious Feelings: The Epidemiology of Affect', paper delivered at the 'Contagion' conference, University of Sydney, April 1999; E. Showalter, *Hystories: Hysterical Epidemics and Modern Media*, New York, Columbia University Press, 1997; M. Guillaume, 'The Metamorphoses of Epidemia', in M. Feher (ed.), *Fragments for a History of the Human Body*, New York, Zone, 1989, pp. 59–69.
7 G. E. Perry and D. Lederman, *Financial Vulnerability, Spillover Effects, and Contagion: Lessons from the Asian Crises for Latin America*, World Bank, 1998; see also J. Lowell, D. Tong and C. R. Neu (eds), *Financial Crises and Contagion in Emerging Market Countries*, Rand, 1998; K. D. Jackson (ed.), *Asian Contagion: The Causes and Consequences of a Financial Crisis*, Boulder, Colo., Westview Press, 1998.
8 For studies of disease and metaphor, and further discussion of the other issues raised here, please consult the select bibliography in this volume. This bibliography is selected from a very wide field. We have chosen texts for their applicability across and between scholarly traditions: work which is interdisciplinary or which applies or uses methods of both historical and cultural inquiry to explore and explain contagion.
9 D. Haraway, 'The Biopolitics of Postmodern Bodies: Constructions of Self in Immune System Discourse', in *Simians, Cyborgs and Women: The Reinvention of Nature*, New York, Routledge, 1991, p. 209.
10 Mutually constitutive understandings of bodily immunity and resistance and political/national defence and militarism have been well explored. See e.g. E. Martin, 'Toward an Anthropology of Immunology: The Body as Nation-State', *Medical Anthropology Quarterly*, 1990, vol. 4, pp. 410–26; E. Martin, *Flexible Bodies: The Role of Immunity in American Culture from the Days of Polio to the Age of AIDS*, Boston, Mass., Beacon Press, 1994; S. L. Montgomery, 'Codes and Combat in Biomedical Discourse', *Science as Culture*, 1991, vol. 2, pp. 341–90.
11 M. Foucault, *The Care of the Self: Volume Three of the History of Sexuality*, New York, Vintage, 1986.
12 J. Kristeva, *Powers of Horror: An Essay on Abjection*, New York and London,

Columbia University Press, 1992. The literature which develops the idea of selfhood and cleanliness is vast, and is partially covered in the select bibliography at the end of this book. In each of these traditions, however, we might single out: C. Waldby, *AIDS and the Body Politic: Biomedicine and Sexual Difference*, London and New York, Routledge, 1996; D. Armstrong, 'Public Health Spaces and the Fabrication of Identity', *Sociology*, vol. 27, 1993, pp. 393–410; D. Lupton, *The Imperative of Health: Public Health and the Regulated Body*, Sage, London, 1995; A. Petersen and D. Lupton, *The New Public Health: Health and Self in the Age of Risk*, Sage, London, 1996; S. Gilman, *Health and Illness: Images of Difference*, London, Reaktion Books, 1995.
13 Armstrong, 'Public Health Spaces and the Fabrication of Identity', pp. 393–410.
14 D. Haraway, *Modest_Witness@Second_Millennium*, New York and London, Routledge, 1997, p. 12.
15 Haraway, 'Biopolitics of Postmodern Bodies', pp. 204–30.
16 M. Rackham, 'carrier'. Online. Available http://www.subtle.net./carrier.
17 *Oxford English Dictionary*, compact edn, Oxford, Oxford University Press, 1971, vol. 1, p. 533.

Part 1
Contagion and cultural histories of the modern world

1 The meaning of contagion
Reproduction, medicine and metaphor

Margaret Pelling

Contagion, it seems, is spreading again.[1] This is owing in part to the social, political and moral climate induced by the recrudescence, in the later twentieth century, of significant infectious disease. Migrations, revolutions in means of communication, and other changes bringing proximity where before there was distance, have also encouraged commentators to plunder the concept. As an idea, particularly a negative idea expressing a sense of threat, crowding, or contamination, contagion has proved remarkably persistent in western culture, and present usage probably owes more than it would admit to this tradition.[2] As a source of analogies relating to means of influence, it has a particular attraction for cultural historians as well as social psychologists. Analogical reasoning, heavily criticised but never eliminated by dominant traditions in western natural philosophy from the seventeenth century onwards, is intrinsic to the history of the concept of contagion, and is increasingly favoured by historians. The present chapter will focus on theories of disease in the nineteenth century, when popular notions of contagion, as it would appear, finally became 'scientific'. A crucial point to make at the outset is that this does not necessarily involve narrowing the terms of discussion. The structure of reasoning about contagion and disease causation included within itself as broad a frame of reference as a cultural historian could desire. That this has been lost sight of is due partly to a failure to understand the terms of contemporary discussions, partly to our own conditioning as beneficiaries of twentieth-century biomedicine, and partly to anglophone neglect of the history of ideas. In addition, the figures inviting discussion – Sydenham, Cullen, Liebig, Farr, Pasteur – were all, in different ways, able to reach wide international as well as national audiences.

The terms contagion and infection, although vague, convey a relatively straightforward meaning to the modern lay person. They refer primarily to the fact that certain diseases, caused by living organisms, are passed from one person to another. It would generally be assumed that contagion is direct, by contact; infection indirect, through the medium of water, air, or contaminated articles. Both are comprehended in the apparently simple question, 'is it catching?' However, as recent attempts at health education in respect of AIDS have shown, this question is not simple at all. Moreover 'infection' is commonly applied in a more general sense, for example for clean wounds that 'go bad'. Each concept has a long and complex history which was temporarily simplified by the triumphs of bacteriology in the later nineteenth century. The twentieth century inherited a story involving a striking contrast, between the germ theorists (scientific, laboratory-based, objective), and the sanitarians (bureaucratic, unscientific, politically motivated, bringing about improvement as it were by accident), who were miasmatists and believed that smells caused disease. This story, based primarily upon the two main phases of the British public health movement, was reinforced by older medical historians searching for early believers in germ theory who could be portrayed as lonely pioneers in a struggle between opposite points of view.[3]

This retrospective account had many attractive features. It implied that the decline of infectious diseases was brought about by scientific progress in the field of medicine.[4] It laid stress on the importance of instrumentation, especially microscopy. Interest in germ theory appeared to have burgeoned with the renewed scientific spirit first of the Renaissance and then of the seventeenth and nineteenth centuries.[5] However there were also many problems. One was that the classical world, in spite of laying the groundwork for modern science, did not appear to have evolved a concept of contagion.[6] A second was that the status of the contributions of the early pioneers proved difficult to determine from the positivist point of view. Most importantly, detailed analysis tended to show that even 'germ theorists' used the concepts of contagion, infection and miasm as if they were difficult to distinguish, overlapping, or even interchangeable.

If there is a single explanation for these difficulties, it lies in the need for precise definition according to historical context. As in the case of other long-lived and related concepts, for example 'germ', 'species', 'virus', and 'spontaneous generation', the concepts of contagion, infection and miasm accumulated layers of connotation over time, and effectively became not single concepts but many. Each period added its own attempts at definition, but was inevitably affected by the previous history of the concept. Interestingly, attempts to replace traditional terminology for the sake of clarity usually failed.[7] It should be stressed that the historian's difficulty in arriving at workable definitions even within a specific historical context is often a reflection of contemporary lack of precision. For a number of reasons this area of debate was particularly subject to confusion and ambiguity. In addition, many writers deliberately exploited this confusion, using over-simplification either to discredit ideas, or to force their acceptance. One obvious way of doing this was not to distinguish between the new version of the concept, and the old.[8]

The first point of definition that needs to be made is that it is historically inadequate to regard these concepts as purely medical. They have had a wide currency in a range of areas of thought and practice, which is reflected in an accretion of metaphor and analogy. Most of these analogies were not irrelevant to, but were part of, the argument. Contagion and infection are intimately bound up with basic concepts of matter and purpose in the natural world, and at one level can be seen as part of elite culture. However, they are also closely related to (*a*) folk belief and practice, (*b*) practical experience in agriculture, horticulture, animal husbandry and technologies such as dyeing and wine-making, (*c*) modes and metaphors of reproduction, in the immaterial as well as the material world, (*d*) different crises of epidemic disease and shifts in the prevalence of endemic diseases at different periods, and (*e*) political, economic and epistemological conditions at a given time influencing the relationship both between 'theory' and 'practice', and between the individual and the state. Ideas of contagion are inseparable from notions of individual morality, social responsibility, and collective action. This is shown most strikingly in respect of measures of isolation and quarantine, and the public health movements subsequent to industrialisation.

The 'person to person' emphasis of the post-bacteriological period might lead us to see concepts of contagion as dependent upon high-density living or urbanisation. This is however too narrow: it is more accurate to see contagion as reflecting the relationship between things in the world, as well as the influence upon the human being of factors in close and remote spheres of his/her environment. In analysing humanity's situation the classical period adopted a structure of causation which was elaborated in subsequent periods, and which continues to be relevant, although often going unrecognised. The history of the concept of contagion cannot be understood without reference to this traditional multifactorial structure of natural and supernatural causation. This structure was briefly obscured, not invalidated, by the bacteriological period and by advocates of laboratory medicine. Laboratory science was successful in severely restricting, and hence manipulating, the number of factors involved in causing the phenomenon under investigation. Modern western medical science has proceeded not by supplying full explanations, but by a process of specialisation in which some categories of cause have been ignored, or eliminated. In the later twentieth century, with the decline of most infectious diseases in the developed world, and the transition to chronic and degenerative diseases as dominant causes of death, there began a gradual return to multifactorial explanations of disease more in accordance with traditional concepts. This 'exclusivity' of bacteriology was challenged by clinicians and epidemiologists from as early as the turn of the twentieth century.[9] It is arguable however that many medical scientists are still inclined to reductionist habits of thought which have also persuaded the layperson to expect both single-factor causes of disease, and their corollary, 'magic bullets' as specific cures for such diseases.

This artificial simplicity in the explanation of disease is well represented for present purposes by the aphorism of John Snow (1813–58), a major

English epidemiologist: 'to be of the human species, and to receive the morbid poison in a suitable manner, is most likely all that is required.'[10] This formula seems inspired as well as straightforward in its attribution of cause and effect. However, even this statement is not as simple as it appears. What did it mean to receive the poison in a suitable manner? Why, if effect simply followed cause, was not everyone affected by disease who was exposed to it? To his contemporaries, there was a range of additional questions which Snow was simply choosing to ignore. Why did diseases prevail in some places and not others? Why did epidemics – or pandemics – rise and then decline, and affect the world at some times and not at others? Does disease consist of stimuli affecting the body, or the body's reaction to these stimuli? By the nineteenth century these were long-established questions, which could be made to correspond to the traditional structure of causation. As in Snow's own case, conflicting views were often an effect of concentrating upon one among the possible range of causes at the expense of the others.

Classical philosophy and epistemology made available to medicine an elaborate structure of explanation involving a hierarchy of causes.[11] First, primary, or remote causes were cosmological or divine (for example the influence of stars and planets, the wrath of god or gods) and were more obviously subject to religious controversy. The refusal to consider primary causes is usually seen as an aspect of secularisation and is identified with periods of particular conflict in western thought between religion and science, but as a strategy it dates back to the classical period. Remote causes related to the state of the atmosphere, or influences (such as volcanic action or the weather) broad enough in scope to bring about the rise and fall of epidemics. The 'epidemic constitution' of Thomas Sydenham (1624–89) is an example.[12] Exciting, efficient or immediate causes related primarily to the more local environment or experiences of the diseased person, and were generally congruent with the 'non-naturals'.[13] They could include factors such as diet, emotion (stress) or exposure to weather, but also injury, poisons, or other more specific agents of disease. Predisposing causes could overlap with this category but were also invoked to cover characteristics of the individual's life or heredity which might render him or her unusually liable to a given disease. Proximate causes came closest to defining the diseased state or process occurring in the diseased body.[14] Different periods are perhaps distinguished less by their answers to these questions, than by the questions that were selected as the most important. The first bacteriological explanations of disease in the nineteenth century tended to ignore proximate and predisposing causes, as well as primary causes, a strategy of which contemporaries were well aware, and which fuelled both resistance and reaction.

It follows that to compare a belief in epidemic constitutions with a belief in germ theory is not necessarily to compare like with like. Similarly, 'miasm' would tend to describe a more general level of cause, relating to locality, compared with contagion, which could best be seen as an exciting cause. Infection might be seen as bridging these two levels of cause. It should be stressed that an agent in one category of cause could be seen as also belonging to, or changing into, another category, as a result of a given set of circumstances. Causes could act singly or in concert in any given instance of disease. This traditional, inclusive form of analysis was often used tacitly or imperfectly, but was remarkably persistent. It helps to explain why in historical terms contagion and miasm have been more readily seen by theorists as alternative or complementary, rather than contradictory, factors in disease.

The notion of contagion also involved the question of how properties or qualities were transferred or propagated at the level of the ultimate constituents of matter. Contagion described an event in which an influence was 'increased' in some way. Historians of medicine looking for precursors of the germ theory tended to identify this increase as a crucial feature and one which should have suggested a form of reproduction peculiar to living organisms. It is however anachronistic to look at older ideas in this manner. The properties of living organisms were constantly being redefined and the boundaries between living and nonliving entities constantly shifting. In the seventeenth century for example, minerals were thought to grow in the earth, which could itself be seen as animate; magnets apparently possessed some of the properties of life. Reproduction was not definitively biological; the term 'biology' was itself not introduced until the late eighteenth century.[15] The enormous variety of complex phenomena involving such lower organisms as insects, parasites and worms meant that different versions of the concept of spontaneous generation survived into the twentieth century.[16] Thus one form of life could dissolve by putrefaction only to give rise to other forms by spontaneous generation. Moreover, reproduction did not need to be a material process. A range of concepts was available to describe phenomena involving the propagation of influence by 'action at a distance': the eye for example could transmit occult qualities affecting another individual.[17]

It is consequently not too grandiose to relate views on contagion to classical philosophies regarded as basic to western science. Natural philosophers of later periods theorised in the knowledge of alternatives stemming from Epicureanism and from Aristotelianism, alternatives summarised by Darlington, a twentieth-century geneticist deploring the divorce between science and philosophy, as the choice between 'purpose and particles'. Aristotelianism is identified with biological models, Epicureanism or Greek atomism with physics. For Darlington, modern science represented a paradox: Aristotelianism and therefore teleology had been far more fruitful in the development of science, but modern scientific achievements, based on the atom, the molecule, the gene, and the organism, had endorsed instead the principles of Epicurus (341–270 BC) and Lucretius (c.99–c.55 BC).[18] In spite of its reference to the as-yet mysterious activities of living organisms, bacteriology came ultimately to be associated with this materialist, atomistic view of nature, and with the reification of different forms of social interaction. Some of those who theorised about contagion at different periods naturally gravitated towards views involving particles. For others, however, the myriad particles which might best explain the phenomena of infectious disease were most analogous to swarms of insects or other lower organisms, which had independent powers of movement and increase.[19]

Certain analogies recur in the history of contagion which derive from almost-universal experience. One example is that of rotting fruit: the observation that decay spread from one part of a fruit to another, and from one fruit to the next if they were in contact. Another persistent and even more important point of reference was the process of fermentation, especially of wine. Different interpretations of fermentation and putrefaction have been fundamental to theories of epidemic disease, although these processes belong primarily to a wider cycle of reference connecting reproduction and decay. Analogies were detected inside as well as outside the body. In each case familiar everyday events repeatedly demonstrated how a part could inform or affect the whole. Other analogies were found in the spread of odours, or the effects of the vapours of marshes, caves and mines – what would now be ascribed to the laws of diffusion of gases. Odours, it may be pointed out, are still little understood either in themselves or in terms of their effects on the body, though some are clearly of considerable potency, giving scope to the persistence of cultural attitudes as well as aromatherapy.[20] Similar properties could be attributed to the animal breath. A final source of analogy, important in the classical period but not irrelevant to homoeopathic ideas, was the effect of dyes in water, in which a small amount of material transmitted its main property to the whole mass. Not surprisingly, parallels were also constantly drawn between the spread of disease and the effects of poisons, where again an often tiny dose was able to affect the whole body, or, for example, to poison a well. The historical reference to poisons, including animal poisons such as the venom of snakes, is reflected in the co-option into the present day of the term 'virus'.[21]

The classical contribution to concepts of contagion and infection thus related less to the individual than to the environment. The term 'infection' has a root meaning 'to put or dip into something', leading to *inficere* and *infectio*, staining or dyeing. This is a further reminder that 'an infection is basically a pollution'. The same is true not only of 'contagion', but also of the noun 'miasma', which derives from the Greek verb *miaino*, a counterpart to the Latin *inficere*. Impurity is therefore a basic element in all three concepts.[22] These derivations hark back to empirical observation but also evoke the broad spectrum of religious and moral ideas clustering around notions of pollution and taboo. Pollution is concerned not only with time and place, propriety and order, the material and the immaterial, but with the individual's sense of separateness from his or her environment and how this separateness is to be maintained or regulated.[23]

The themes of shame, guilt and pollution were continued under Christianity with the idea of disease as having followed the Fall. This did not of course mean that all disease was sinful; 'naturalistic' explanations were also common.[24] The Christian was also expected to welcome trial by suffering, as well as earning grace by relieving the suffering of others. Sin itself could be seen as contagious: one individual could mislead others, a false idea could spread, or the erring body could contaminate the soul. New forms of communication have given fresh impetus to secularised versions of these ideas.[25] Conversely, sin could, or should, produce visible stigmata corresponding to itself, an idea very much alive as late as Oscar Wilde's *Picture of Dorian Gray* (1890). Infectious diseases affecting the surface of the body were traditionally of considerable moral significance. The institutional isolation of lepers became the privilege and responsibility of the Church. It is worth noting that lazar-houses were sometimes also used to confine the mentally ill. Leprosy, like syphilis later, differed from acute infectious diseases like plague and smallpox by being gradual and lifelong; both leprosy and syphilis embodied forms of exemplary suffering.[26] From its first epidemic effusion in the sixteenth century, syphilis inspired a vocabulary of labels reflecting national stereotypes, anti-clericalism, moral reformism, gender conflict, and differential diagnosis according to social status.[27] Plague had a major effect on Europe and its empires from the fourteenth to the early twentieth centuries and prompted administrative provisions affecting relations between towns, ports and countries as well as individuals.[28] Measures based on isolation were probably from the beginning also used as a political and economic weapon. Having invented quarantine, initially as a barrier between east and west, Italy also originated public health practices aimed at the control of disease inland and in towns.[29] Plague also initiated a special class of ethical literature about infectious disease, the so-called plague tractates, which contained medical and spiritual advice and discussed rights and duties in times of pestilence; such issues are of course still current. Syphilis and plague, like cholera and fever later, both have a history in terms of the perceived threat posed by their concentration among the poor.

In the above discussion, it will be seen that attention readily shifts between agency and process in disease. This reflects another major difficulty in distinguishing concepts of contagion, infection and miasm. Confusion arises from the failure to distinguish between the *material or influence* (living or non-living) which is transmitted between persons or environments, and the *process* of transmission or affection, direct or indirect. Historically there has been a tendency for contagion to imply the former, and infection the latter, but there has been considerable freedom of usage which has blurred this seemingly straightforward distinction.

An intimately connected concept, which has also had a long history subject to oversimplification, is specificity.[30] Because animals and plants are said to belong to species, specificity in disease is readily seen simply as a function of causation by living organisms. The effect of the principles for the isolation of disease agents known as 'Koch's postulates' (after the bacteriologist Robert Koch, 1843–1910) is for the presence of a given disease to be defined by the presence of a given bacterial or viral organism.[31] The layperson tends now to see it as inappropriate to apply the concept of specificity to congenital, developmental, or degenerative diseases, or to disease states of even less integrity such as 'syndromes'. Nonetheless, in historical terms the idea of specificity has had a broader meaning, within which the infectious diseases appear simply as a special case. For older medical historians, the discovery of diseases which were the result of the invasion of the body by independent organisms represented a climax in the development of the modern, 'ontological' theory of disease. Ontology is concerned with essences of things and with individuality. The ontological view of disease is one which stresses the realities of disease entities and therefore the constancy of any given disease from patient to patient. This contrasts with holistic interpretations stressing instead the individuality of the *patient* and the uniqueness of his or her experience of disease. The ontological view chimes well with the idea of disease as invading the body from without, and implies that disease is characterised primarily by local effects, rather than affecting the whole body. By the nineteenth century however it was possible to transpose the ontological idea to the cellular level, so that disease could be seen as invasive within the interior environment of the body.[32]

The rise of the ontological theory of disease has been associated with the challenge to Galenic humoralism mounted in the sixteenth and seventeenth centuries, particularly by the religio-medical philosophies of Paracelsianism and Helmontianism.[33] It has also been identified with Baconian methods of observation and the compiling of case histories in order to arrive at a consistent picture of a particular disease.[34] Case histories stressed not only signs and symptoms but the course followed by a case of a given disease over time. The infectious diseases seemed to show periodicity not only in the individual but in their epidemic rise and fall. However the recognition of specific diseases, or at least of specific disease states, was a feature of Arabic medicine and probably of ancient civilisations. The pitfalls of retrospective diagnosis from textual descriptions make this area a very difficult one for historians, who frequently cannot agree, in principle at least, whether such diagnosis should be attempted at all.[35] What is certain is that descriptions should not be isolated from the overall framework of interpretation of disease as it can be reconstructed for any given society. However it is equally unsound to assume *a priori* that past societies lacked either the will or the ability to describe distinct diseases, or that each society had only one way of looking at disease.[36]

Specificity and the analogy with species of animals and plants came together in the work of Thomas Sydenham, the 'English Hippocrates'. That Sydenham was so described is perhaps a reflection of the fact that he was initially more influential on the Continent, especially in Germany, than he was in England.[37] Sydenham's view that diseases, though they might be ephemeral, had a character as constant as the immutable species of the organic world was deployed in the eighteenth century to create elaborate classifications of diseases analogous to the classifications of plants and animals.[38] However, the 'natural history' approach to disease, rather than leading directly to bacteriology, was taken to its logical conclusion in the early nineteenth century by exponents of *Naturphilosophie*, who saw diseases not only holistically but *in toto* as organisms, which grew and lived and died over long periods of time, parasitic upon a world which was itself living. However, for most nineteenth-century medical practitioners, specificity was a pragmatic concept, increasingly based on a mixture of clinical observation, quantification and pathological anatomy.[39] Paradoxically, the identification of the (efficient) causes of major diseases as independent living organisms coincided with Darwinism and evolutionary theory which stressed the mutability of species.[40] The relationship between disease theory and evolution is one requiring much further investigation.[41] It is not clear, for example, how ideas about the ascent if not the perfectibility of man, especially man as a social animal, were reconciled with the increasing conviction that the highest of organisms could be arbitrarily destroyed by the lowest. There is no doubt that for some, bacteriology conveyed the gloomiest of messages, a kind of biological determinism subversive of human society, and that the lifting of this gloom was one reason for welcoming the findings of immunology, which stressed the human body's natural defences against disease.[42]

By the later eighteenth century there was an awareness of a spectrum of specific infectious diseases stretching from smallpox (highly infectious person to person irrespective of locality) at one end, to malaria or ague (not infectious person to person, but caught in particular localities) at the other.[43] These diseases appeared to have as their common denominator the generic disease process known as fever, in which the whole body was affected. Most of these diseases seemed also to be characterised by local effects, such as the pustules in smallpox. The disease process was still most commonly explained in terms of a febrile crisis within the body involving a 'coction' of peccant matter, which was resolved by excretion of this matter through the body's pores or orifices. According to Sydenham's 'Hippocratic' view of disease, this process occurred naturally, and it was the practitioner's task to enable and support it, not hinder it. This interpretation encouraged the already strengthening view that such diseases had a 'life of their own' in that they followed a specific course in the patient which ought not to be cut short or diverted. However for Sydenham each case of disease, and each epidemic, remained a unique experience determined by a given set of circumstances.[44]

The infectious diseases came to illustrate major debates revolving around fever and inflammation: general and local phenomena respectively which seemed to constitute primary disease, or the body's first reaction to abnormal stimuli. The disease classifications produced in the eighteenth century by de Sauvages, Linnaeus and others were simplified and distilled for teaching purposes in the Scottish medical schools and their diasporas by the chemist and physician William Cullen (1710–90). Cullen placed most of the diseases now regarded as infectious in the category of *Pyrexiae* or febrile diseases, differentiated by local inflammations. Within the *Pyrexiae*, diseases spreading by contact and well defined, such as smallpox, were attributed to specific contagions (and were also known as 'strictly contagious' diseases). Between these and the diseases of locality at the other end of the spectrum (typified by ague or intermittent fever, associated with the vegetable putrefaction of marshes) lay the no-man's land of the 'doubtful' diseases, which seemed to partake of the character of both. Some of these diseases were attributed to 'common' contagions, a term reflecting two main ideas: first that, although definable, such diseases were modifiable by circumstances one into another; second, that such diseases were intimately related to the environment which could be responsible for the nature of their causes. According to a range of factors identified as affecting their behaviour and development, these diseases were, as repeatedly stressed, 'sometimes contagious and sometimes not' – a mutable character alien to bacteriological specificity but compatible with long-established observations, especially those stressing pollution and putrefaction as factors in disease, as well as innumerable 'negative instances' or 'caprice' in the spread of diseases now known to be transmitted indirectly or through vectors. The most ill-defined members of this group were the continued fevers, which were later distinguished mainly into typhus, enteric (typhoid) and relapsing fevers. Possessing some of the same characteristics were the diseases apparently most closely related to common animal putrefaction – the 'septic' diseases, pyaemia, gangrene, septicaemia, scarlet fever, diphtheria, erysipelas and puerperal fever.

For the nineteenth century, indigenous or endemic diseases (for example, continued fever, smallpox) were of major importance, as well as chronic diseases only gradually regarded as communicable, such as the many forms of tuberculosis. For the activists of the English sanitary movement, 'fever nests' and outbreaks of continued fever epitomised the preventable excesses of disease prejudicing the productivity of the labouring poor. Yet again, the poor were shown to suffer a greater burden of disease than other classes, which was associated with the insanitary conditions in which they were forced to live and which were to be seen as outside their control. It was therefore, according to utilitarian principles, the duty of government to intervene at this crucial (and vulnerable) point in the chain of causation of disease. In theory, a multifactorial view was preserved; in practice and over time, stress came to be placed almost solely on the products of environmental putrefaction, especially of substances of animal origin. In many respects, this approach was a natural extension of approaches evolved in the eighteenth century.[45] In other ways however it represented a departure which, at least in respect to some of its adherents, was described as 'anticontagionism'.

From the latter half of the seventeenth century to the first pandemic of cholera in the 1830s, exotic epidemics threatened western Europe but (with the exception of cattle plague) did not arrive. There was less of a role for primary or remote causes, and more emphasis on factors influencing local outbreaks. However the growth of intercontinental trade, as well as military and colonial activity, meant an enforced acquaintance with alien diseases such as yellow fever in their places of origin. Plague itself was increasingly seen as a disease of locality and lack of civilisation. A broad range of other trends influenced the development of environmental views, stressing in effect the intermediate range of causes, which tended to be overtly socio-political in their implications.[46] Isolationist and coercive measures against plague were increasingly seen as primitive; quarantine measures were denounced by advocates of *laissez faire* economics as politically suspect, inefficient, and obstructive to trade. Popular belief in contagion was seen as belonging to a primitive state of society, and as entailing a breakdown in social responsibility. English sanitarianism, which drew heavily upon the anticontagionism of the 1820s and 1830s, adopted less a causal than a correlative mode of reasoning. Its theorists, the most important of whom – notably the lawyer Edwin Chadwick (1800–90) and the physician Thomas Southwood Smith (1788–1861) – were also Benthamite utilitarians, sought to avoid speculation as to causes in a manner influenced indirectly by the sceptical philosophy of David Hume (1711–76).

The effect of such rationalist views on theories of disease was to push the 'doubtful' diseases such as plague, yellow fever, continued fever, influenza and cholera along the spectrum of infectiousness towards the intermittent fevers, which were related to certain localities. Many anticontagionists could claim experience of the doubtful diseases in the alleged countries of origin of these diseases. This was advantageous in Baconian terms, but made it less likely that these colonially-inspired insights would be acceptable to orthodox metropolitan opinion in Europe, which was required to accept parallels between societies it regarded as categorically different. Stress on locality as forming the character of disease also meant comparative disregard for disease specificity as defined by the consistent clinical and pathological criteria being established in the European hospital-based medical schools. The energetic campaigning of the anticontagionists caused them to be identified by contemporaries as a particular body of politicised opinion.[47] It was in the interests of the anticontagionists to suggest that only two extremes existed with respect to the contagiousness of a given disease. Like some later germ theorists, the anticontagionists insisted that a disease was either contagious or it was not. Although both the sick body and the environment could contribute to the conditions bringing about non-contagious disease, diseases could not be of mixed character, or 'contingently contagious'. Popular belief, and administrative orthodoxy, tended to assume an epidemic disease was contagious; for anticontagionists, this character had to be proved.

Most of their contemporaries, however, asserted that the notion of contagion opposed by the anticontagionists bore no resemblance to that currently held: rather, an antiquated view was deliberately being used so that controversial diseases like continued fever and cholera could be pushed into the non-contagious category. There was broad-based (if often inactive) agreement on the need for sanitary reform, and on the uselessness of quarantine; but the anticontagionists, although influential, were, like the contagionists, very much in the minority. Their influence was never greater than at the time it was first asserted, in the 1820s and 1830s. The bulk of contemporary opinion preferred to consider each disease in the 'epidemic, endemic and contagious' category individually and specifically, and to see the 'doubtful' diseases as contingently contagious.

The traditional multifactorial view was reinforced rather than otherwise by the characteristic nineteenth-century concern to make medicine more 'scientific'. A good example of this is the way in which statistical generalisation was applied according to the French *méthode numérique*. The reaction against eighteenth-century systems in medicine encouraged an *inclusive*, fact-gathering methodology which was friendly to the broad generalisations of sanitarianism, but hostile to its hardening into an *exclusive* system of explanation of infectious disease. This hardening was not due either to the elaboration of anticontagionist views or to their increased influence, but to political and administrative constraints and the need to produce propaganda. The complexity – and confusion – of debates about epidemic disease in the nineteenth century arises not from any simple clash of opposite views, or (as used to be claimed) the conflict of the unscientific with the scientific, but from the general epistemological context (the nineteenth-century idea of a 'fact', for example), the special relationship between science and politics in the context of disease control, frequent overlap between the actual views being espoused, and increasing professional investment in different parts of the structure of causation.

The attempt to be sceptically scientific (in contemporary terms) meant that medicine was prepared to draw heavily upon other developing sciences, especially organic chemistry and gas chemistry, and such phenomena as electricity. Ironically, this caused frequent resort to argument by analogy, a procedure just as frequently condemned by contemporaries as unscientific. This dilemma, as well as the inclusive methodology adopted by the majority, is well illustrated by the framework of explanation of the infectious diseases evolved for England and Wales by the Compiler of Abstracts in the new Registrar General's Department, William Farr (1807–83).[48] Farr was required to produce a classification of diseases for national statistical purposes, and a nomenclature which was later adopted internationally. Farr first grouped together as the 'epidemic, endemic and contagious' diseases all those which 'were of a specific nature, propagated in a peculiar manner and known by experience to become epidemic in unhealthy places and among the sickly classes, at greater or less intervals of time'. This group, the 'index to salubrity', was typified by smallpox but also included malaria.[49] A little later (in 1842) Farr redefined them as the 'zymotic' diseases, a term deliberately chosen to reflect an idea of the disease process as analogous to fermentation. As we have seen, fermentation was a traditional point of reference for explaining the 'extension of influence' – or reproduction – which seemed to characterise infectious disease as well as other bodily processes such as digestion.

Although stressing (English) precursors, and a particular admirer of Sydenham, Farr was chiefly dependent upon the enormously influential (and comprehensive) synthesis of the German chemist Justus von Liebig (1803–73). For his contemporaries in many countries Liebig's theories redefined the relationship between the organic and inorganic worlds; they had great popular success and were extremely important in such areas as agriculture. Liebig did not reduce the living to the non-living, but suggested a molecular basis of continuity by which they could interact. He paid particular attention to fermentation, putrefaction, and decay. His formulations were thus ideally suited to explain diseases involving a continuity between the body and its physical environment. Liebig's chemical explanation of catalysis could also explain the process of increase of morbid matter, either in the body or outside it.

Farr recognised specificity in infectious diseases in terms less of their causes than of their predictable, law-like behaviour both as epidemics and in the individual patient. On his own account he recognised a 'species' 'whenever important pathological states and phenomena were isolated or could be individualised'.[50] In this he was simply reflecting opinions typical of the 1830s and 1840s. On the one hand he sought to distance himself from some 'natural historical' accounts of disease, and on the other he was inclined to preserve for the infectious diseases the analogy Sydenham had drawn between them and plants and animals. However, his adaptation of Liebig also catered for specificity by proposing the existence in each case of a specific zyme, ferment, or 'exciter', an organic poison affecting the blood but also showing a special affinity with certain organs or tissues. Unlike the mode of action of poisons, the process of zymosis could explain how (though not why) a disease suddenly became epidemic, or was more contagious in some circumstances than in others. By the 1840s, enough was known of the properties of gases to rule them out as the direct agents of infectious disease, in spite of the fact that such agents were usually seen as entering the body via the lungs. It seemed clear that the *materies morbi* was unlikely to be a simple, volatile substance like a gas, but rather 'highly organised particles of fixed matter', possibly resembling the pollen of flowers.[51] Such matter was in a state of pathological transformation at the molecular level. For Farr, however, non-specific decomposing organic matter was either a predisposing cause only, or a link in a chain of causation dominated by a zymotic exciter. Nonetheless on epidemiological grounds he felt obliged to retain the possibility of spontaneous generation.

Chemically influenced ideas about the pathological process, referring ultimately to the activity and selective affinities of organic molecules, dominated disease theory in the middle of the nineteenth century and were taken up even by those regarded as prototypical germ theorists, such as John Snow, who produced a whole essay on 'contagious molecular action'. Within this broad framework, the association of, for example, some processes of fermentation with the multiplication of micro-organisms appeared not as a counter-instance but as a special case. Chemical theories also seemed better able to accommodate the possibility of spontaneous generation, detaching this concept from earlier versions of it seen by nineteenth-century writers as antique. However, enthusiasm for microscopical observation was also a feature of the second quarter of the century, and the emergence of cell theories coincided with a rash of claims for the role of organisms in skin diseases and diseases affecting lower animals and plants. Terms later used by bacteriologists, such as 'bacillus', and 'vibrio', were already current; 'bacterium' and 'spirochaete' were introduced at this time.[52]

'Fungi' were as characteristic a preoccupation of the nineteenth century as were animalcules of the seventeenth. Many of these observers were, like Louis Pasteur (1822–95), investigating 'blights' and other diseases of considerable economic importance. Because fungi were proved to affect food plants, the idea that such agents might be connected with epidemic diseases of the gut such as cholera continued to be attractive until late in the century. Well-known 'germ theorists', such as William Budd (1811–80) and Joseph Lister (1827–1912), were inclined to be 'fungi theorists' in the 1840s and 1850s. A selection of the observations of this period (for example that of Filippo Pacini (1812–83) of the cholera bacillus) are now regarded as having pre-dated the better-known bacteriological work of the 1870s and 1880s. To the earlier decades also belongs work uncovering the complicated life-cycles of some parasites and the puzzling phenomena of the 'alternation of generations', in which organic forms very dissimilar and appearing in unexpected locations were revealed to be related by unusual forms of reproduction. This not only increased scepticism about spontaneous generation but complicated the parasite analogy to which the germ theory (often to its disadvantage) was closely related.[53]

Between 1830 and the 1860s repeated onslaughts of cholera encouraged speculation about epidemic disease. As with plague earlier, it is not surprising to find that some of these speculators opted for *contagium vivum*. It was usually felt that this option needed added justification because as an idea it seemed to be dredged up from the dim past, was heavily dependent upon analogy, explained little or nothing about the disease process, and laid its author open to charges of being a vitalist. Moreover the microscopical observations of the same decades, however suggestive, also encouraged critics to demand 'ocular demonstration' when agents like 'fungus germs' were posited. In this they were partly invoking the parasite analogy, since parasites were regarded as causing ill effects primarily by the bulk of their physical presence. Thus it was held against the most prominent of these mid-century theorists, the pathologist and anatomist Jacob Henle (1809–85), that even he, an eminent microscopist, had been unable to demonstrate the existence of the 'epidemic infusoria'. Typically, Henle was given credit for 'ingenuity', a form of praise often implying marginalisation. Nonetheless, Henle reflected contemporary views in defining three categories of disease, the contagious, the miasmatic, and the miasmatic-contagious, of which the last, 'mixed' category was predictably the most problematic. Henle felt obliged also to accept that some development of the disease agent could take place outside the body.

Predictably, historians have tended to lay emphasis on terms used in the explanation of disease which seem to be biologically related – the two obvious examples being 'seed' and 'germ'. The impetus behind this could now perhaps be described as sociobiological rather than Whiggish, but the effect is the same. As already indicated, it is a matter of precise analysis of any given historical context (and of the appropriate language) to clarify whether these terms were being used so as to suggest the attributes of organisms in anything like the modern sense. The combination of bacteriology and popular belief has produced a simple equation between 'germ' and (fully developed) 'disease-causing organism'. Historically, however, 'germ' was borrowed from discussions to do with generation, growth, and differentiation. In the hands of nineteenth-century writers, it was applied to disease causation particularly in terms of the evolution of bodily products (including cells) into discrete entities capable of causing disease in a second person. In this context, 'germs' were by definition *not* fully developed organisms capable of causing disease. Instead, some process of 'germination' was required, often outside the body, and with it a range of other factors or causes, usually environmental, before disease could result.

For the mid-nineteenth century, therefore, the phrase 'germs of disease' would have conjured up, not the ingenious but self-sufficing hypotheses of theorists like Henle, but the beginnings of a disease outbreak, the onset of the pathological process, or a range of postulations suggesting the evolution of degenerate bodily products into agents of disease. Different versions of cell theory suggested how unorganised matter could take on form and differentiation; the ways in which organised matter broke down also attracted attention. Diseases in which decay seemed to begin in the living body were of special interest, as well as related bodily products such as pus. However other diseases apparently involved not disintegration, but a special kind of growth in the body, such as tuberculosis and cancer. The predominance of such concerns, which were related to major issues in biology, is evident when comparison is made with the peripheral position of a speculator like John Grove (1816–95), a true 'germ theorist' who suggested that the ova of parasites and the spores of fungi normally circulated in the blood. Grove's germ theory was only one of many which failed to gain general acceptance. Cellular and chemical pathology on the other hand had created a new microcosmic vision of the body in which its minute constituents themselves possessed many of the properties of independent life, exercised in an environment governed by the principles of chemical affinity and action at the molecular level.

These broader concerns also informed what was becoming known as 'sanitary science'. That cholera and typhoid were described simply as 'filth diseases' until late into the century demonstrates the success of sanitary propaganda, which used oversimplified equations but was justified by accumulated evidence of correlation. In addition the original utilitarian arguments for sanitary reform had been co-opted into a widely-held and holistic religious and moral framework which resisted reformulation. Nevertheless, by about 1860 the position on 'filth' had become relatively refined. Although all forms of putrefaction involved hazards, epidemic disease was thought most likely to arise from changes in organic material that had once been part of the animal body. This view was able to accommodate the findings of epidemiologists suggesting, for example, the specific role of choleraic or typhoid discharges in the water supply.

The wide popularity of Liebig's chemical explanations of pathology and physiology was a measure of the strength of contemporary feeling that medicine and biology should achieve the same dignity as physics and mathematics and should be found subject to the same natural laws. The success of Pasteur's germ theory of disease reveals the strength of feeling that this 'reductionism' could be taken too far, towards materialism and even atheism. In France, Pasteur's ideas were associated with anti-evolutionism, spiritualism, and conservative politics.[54] Pasteur had been committed since the 1840s to a programme of research in stereochemistry designed to separate 'the chemistry of non-living nature from the chemistry of living nature' – disconnecting where Liebig was seeking to connect.[55] From 1855 Pasteur's employment involved problem-solving in industrial contexts, in particular the production of wine, vinegar and beer. Pasteur's claim to originating 'pasteurisation' – preservation by heating in closed vessels – began with a patent of 1865 for preserving wine. Pasteur's conclusion that fermentations could not take place in the absence of specific living organisms was based on notions of fact and experiment which contemporaries also found persuasive. In addition Pasteur was a highly effective polemicist, able to simplify opposing views to striking rhetorical effect, and able also to represent his work as an issue affecting national self-respect. Although his and Liebig's views eventually emerged as being complementary, their debate remained competitive. Pasteur's explanation of varieties of fermentation offered a model for current preoccupations about disease, in suggesting the presence (varying with locality) of micro-organisms in the air; a specific, one-to-one relationship between the micro-organism and the type of fermentation; a similar specific dependency between the organism, its 'food', and other chemical features of the environment in which it multiplied; and methods by which the cause might be isolated and then made to reproduce the process for which it was responsible. In the early 1860s Pasteur presented a similar explanation for putrefaction, suggesting a cycle, rivalling that of the chemists, in which 'life stems from death and death from life'. Pasteur underlined his biological explanation of the paradigmatic processes of fermentation and putrefaction by similar experimental findings with respect to economically important diseases of animals, especially anthrax. Effectively, Pasteur 'revealed the enormous medical and economic potential of experimental biology'.[56] The work relevant to germ theory was intimately connected to implications for the control of disease, although Pasteur himself developed only one treatment (for rabies) directly applicable to human disease.

The political, economic and humanitarian potential of applying his ideas to specifically medical problems was obvious to Pasteur but as a chemist he was relatively reticent to tackle the medical profession on its own territory. The germ theory was established as an issue of immediate clinical relevance to medical practitioners by the antiseptic methods of surgery advocated by Joseph Lister from the 1860s.[57] As Pasteur himself realised, Listerism involved acceptance that those who healed also caused disease, a dilemma in social and professional attitudes which had earlier destroyed Ignaz Semmelweis (1818–65), who advocated hygienic procedures to reduce the incidence of puerperal fever.[58] Lister however was not promoting cleanliness, but practices which could prevent infection by Pasteurian germs even in the absence of cleanliness. He therefore met the same kind of opposition as those who proposed the use of deodorisers and disinfectants as a substitute for the removal of 'filth' and overcrowding. The debate over Listerism provides a focus of conflicting contemporary concepts of pollution as well as putrefaction. The moral absolute of purity was more compatible with the concept of asepsis, which rapidly followed Listerism and was ideologically more acceptable (although perhaps even more difficult to put into practice). Asepsis rather than antisepsis produced the stereotype of the masked surgeon in the bright white operating theatre. Asepsis was also more compatible with traditional multifactorial interpretations of disease.[59]

Pasteur's vision of specificity was based more on chemical process than on morphology. He was inattentive to problems of classification and to changing contemporary distinctions between microscopic animals and plants. Pasteur was perhaps thereby the better able to reject – by 1872 – persistent claims by many observers that they had seen organisms at this level change one into another, claims which were cited in support of evolution. Overall Pasteur tended to ignore rather than deny the implications of Darwinian evolution. He was strenuously opposing spontaneous generation from at least 1860, but even Pasteur's 'victories' in this wide-ranging debate were more apparent than real, leading to reformulation rather than elimination of questions about the origin of life. Pasteur's insistence on this issue undoubtedly helped to link disease specificity with the specificity of an invasive, disease-causing organism which reproduced itself consistently and showed 'normal' heredity. However Pasteur was relatively casual about whether his '*germes*' were in any given instance latent precursors, or fully developed 'adult' organisms. His use of 'germ' prefigured the generalised popular usage of that term. That micro-organisms 'bred true' and did not normally transform themselves was established not by Pasteur but by naturalists and botanists, in particular Ferdinand Cohn (1828–98) and Anton de Bary (1831–88), and in the context of disease causation primarily by the co-founder of modern bacteriology, Robert Koch.

Koch's first decisive contribution was published in 1876 and related to anthrax, an important disease of large animals and also of man which had been a focus of observation and experiment for some decades.[60] Koch's work demonstrated the existence of a resistant spore phase, which explained puzzling aspects of the disease's behaviour; undermined chemical analogies and emphasised the role of biological reproduction by showing that virulence persisted even after extreme degrees of dilution; introduced the use of solid media which facilitated pure cultures; and established the experimental model by which a specific disease could be repeatedly induced in a sequence of susceptible subjects. Although the criteria of 'Koch's postulates' were not fulfilled in each case, even by Koch himself, the technical model Koch provided set off a chain reaction of findings in the 1870s and 1880s which constitute the 'bacteriological revolution'. This revolution became international in scope but was mainly due to German investigators. As befitted his chemical background Pasteur had always laid stress on the conditions necessary for the activity of micro-organisms, and under his direction the French school concentrated its attention on extending the principles of vaccination.

Bacteriology created a new source of scientific authority for medicine, and made an enormous difference to its reputation for effectiveness in both prevention and cure. The historical reality behind these undoubted changes is inevitably more complex. Ironically bacteriology did much to create a schism, evident today, between the laboratory scientist and the clinical practitioner.[61] More generally, bacteriological extremism seemed to deny the feasibility of modern urban society. Safety for the individual seemed to lie in extreme isolation, and a similar estrangement was implied between practitioner and patient. As long as bacteriology appeared to entail a kind of biological determinism, it gave radical new meaning to concepts of infection and contagion, pollution and taboo. These extremes were however rapidly modified, not only by immunology but by one of its corollaries, a reversion to the group as opposed to the individual. This reversion also marked a return to a more multifactorial, less exclusive approach.[62]

What, finally, of the recent effusion of historical work deploying the concept of contagion? Partly by way of trying an established model on for size, and partly inspired by a renewed interest in national identity, major studies have extended the scope of discussion to a wide range of countries, uncovering national or regional styles of disease control. These studies have discovered afresh the interest of the relation between theory and practice in public health, and the effects of the imperative to action in controlling disease. In the context of new epidemic threats to human health, the perennial contest between individualism and absolutism seems even to mainstream historians to find its most pointed illustration in policies directed against disease, or persons seen as diseased.[63] For the most part, concepts of contagion have not been much elaborated in these accounts, whatever their other merits, and on occasion have been taken almost as a given.[64] This means that cultural dimensions, in particular those suggested by analogy, have been added on as a matter of historiographical principle, rather than recognised as intrinsic to the subject matter of contagion. Apart from underestimating the complexity of contemporary debates, this may mean that the cultural approach proves more ephemeral than it should. A reliable exception here must be gender, which has added a genuinely new dimension to recent debates.[65] Detailed investigations have nonetheless tended to confirm the general applicability of a more complete analysis which sees anticontagionists and germ theorists alike as exceptions, rather than the rule, and the opposition between them as more of a political than a theoretical construct. For the most part, anticontagionism is now located where it belongs, in the 1820s and 1830s.[66] Similarly, recent work has tended to concentrate on overlaps rather than differences between microbiological science and environmentalism, especially with regard to their applications in the practice of public health.[67] However the polarities of contagion and miasm, contagionist and anticontagionist, connected as they have been to two sharply contrasted styles of politics, continue to prove irresistible, even when their historical inadequacies are freely confessed.[68] The correlative schema sketched in bold outline by Ackerknecht[69] has had the highly desirable effect of persuading political and economic historians to venture into new territory, but at the expense of the equally vital task of elucidating the political, social and cultural content of science itself.

Notes

1 What follows is a revised version of 'Contagion/Germ Theory/Specificity', W. F. Bynum and R. Porter (eds), *Companion Encyclopedia of the History of Medicine*, 2 vols, London, Routledge, 1993, vol. 1, pp. 309–34. I am grateful to the editors and to the publisher for permission to reprint the bulk of this essay.
2 See e.g. A. M. Kraut, *Silent Travelers: Germs, Genes, and the 'Immigrant Menace'*, New York, Basic Books, 1994.
3 See e.g. C. Singer, quoted by M. Greenwood, 'Miasma and Contagion', in E. A. Underwood (ed.), *Science, Medicine and History*, 2 vols, London, Oxford University Press, 1953, vol. 2, p. 501.
4 In what follows, the term 'infectious' will be used generically to embrace the whole group of epidemic, endemic and contagious diseases caused by bacteria, viruses and some other parasitic organisms.
5 See R. H. Shryock, *The Development of Modern Medicine*, Madison, University of Wisconsin Press, 1979.
6 O. Temkin, 'An Historical Analysis of the Concept of Infection', in his *The Double Face of Janus*, Baltimore and London, Johns Hopkins University Press, 1977, pp. 456–71; V. Nutton, 'The Seeds of Disease: An Explanation of Contagion and Infection from the Greeks to the Renaissance', *Medical History*, 1983, vol. 27, pp. 1–34.
7 See e.g. (on 'species') J. Beatty, 'What's in a Word? Coming to Terms in the Darwinian Revolution', *Journal of the History of Biology*, 1982, vol. 15, pp. 215–39.
8 See e.g. M. Pelling, *Cholera, Fever and English Medicine 1825–1865*, Oxford, Oxford University Press, 1978, pp. 262–3, 284–6.
9 O. Rosenbach, *Physician versus Bacteriologist*, trans. A. Rose, New York and London, Funk & Wagnalls, 1904; I. Galdston, 'The Epidemic Constitution in Historic Perspective', *Bulletin of the New York Academy of Medicine*, 1942, 2nd ser., vol. 18, pp. 606–19.
10 Laid down (although with a qualifying footnote) in Snow's *On Continuous Molecular Changes* (1853), quoted in Pelling, *Cholera*, p. 206.
11 The ultimate reference is to Aristotle's analysis of causes into formal, final, material and efficient.
12 D. Bates, 'Sydenham, Thomas', *Dictionary of Scientific Biography*, vol. 13, p. 215; E. W. Goodall, 'The Epidemic Constitution', *Proceedings of the Royal Society of Medicine (Section of Epidemiology)*, 1927–8, vol. 21, pp. 119–28.
13 See C. R. Burns, 'The Non-Naturals: A Paradox in the Western Concept of Health', *Journal of Medicine and Philosophy*, 1976, vol. 1, pp. 202–11.
14 The terminology used here reflects nineteenth-century usage. For a historically-based exposition of aetiology aimed at twentieth-century medical students, see L. King, *Medical Thinking. A Historical Preface*, Princeton, NJ, Princeton University Press, 1982, ch. 10.
15 P. J. Weindling, *Darwinism and Social Darwinism in Imperial Germany: The Contribution of the Cell Biologist Oscar Hertwig*, Stuttgart and New York, Gustav Fischer Verlag, 1991, p. 29.
16 J. Farley, *The Spontaneous Generation Controversy from Descartes to Oparin*, Baltimore and London, Johns Hopkins University Press, 1977.
17 K. Hutchison, 'What Happened to Occult Qualities in the Scientific Revolution', *Isis*, 1982, vol. 73, pp. 233–53; J. Henry, 'Occult Qualities and the Experimental Philosophy: Active Principles in Pre-Newtonian Matter Theory', *History of Science*, 1986, vol. 24, pp. 335–81.
18 C. D. Darlington, 'Purpose and Particles in the Study of Heredity', in Underwood, *Science, Medicine and History*, vol. 2, pp. 472–81. On the 1860s as 'the era of the particle' see J. K. Crellin, 'The Dawn of the Germ Theory:

Particles, Infection and Biology', in F. N. L. Poynter (ed.), *Medicine and Science in the 1860s*, London, Wellcome Institute of the History of Medicine, 1968, pp. 57–76.
19 Pelling, *Cholera*, pp. 189–202; P. H. Futcher, 'Notes on Insect Contagion', *Bulletin of the Institute for the History of Medicine*, 1936, vol. 4, pp. 536–58.
20 A. Le Guérer, *Scent: The Mysterious and Essential Powers of Smell*, trans. R. Miller, London, Chatto and Windus, 1993; A. Corbin, *The Foul and the Fragrant: Odour and the Social Imagination*, trans. M. Koshan, London, Picador, 1994; C. Classen, D. Howes and A. Synnott, *Aroma: The Cultural History of Smell*, London, Routledge, 1994.
21 Pelling, *Cholera*, ch. 4.
22 Temkin, 'An Historical Analysis', esp. p. 457; R. Parker, *Miasma: Pollution and Purification in Early Greek Religion*, Oxford, Clarendon Press, 1990.
23 O. Temkin, review of E. R. Dodds, *The Greeks and the Irrational*, 1951, in *Isis*, 1952, vol. 43, pp. 375–7. The anthropological *locus classicus* is M. Douglas, *Purity and Danger: An Analysis of Concepts of Pollution and Taboo*, London, Routledge & Kegan Paul, 1974.
24 J. Kroll and B. Bachrach, 'Sin and the Etiology of Disease in Pre-Crusade Europe', *Journal of the History of Medicine*, 1986, vol. 41, pp. 395–414; C. Hamlin, 'Providence and Putrefaction: Victorian Sanitarians and the Natural Theology of Health and Disease', in P. Brantlinger (ed.), *Energy and Entropy: Science and Culture in Victorian Britain*, Bloomington and Indianapolis, Indiana University Press, 1989, pp. 93–123; C. J. Grimley Evans, 'Divine Providence and Epidemic Cholera: A Contribution to the Study of Secularisation of Thought in Nineteenth-Century England', Ph.D. thesis, Oxford Brookes University, 1995.
25 A. Siegfried, *Germs and Ideas: Routes of Epidemics and Ideologies*, trans. J. Henderson and M. Claraso, Edinburgh and London, Oliver and Boyd, 1965, especially part 4; J. M. Nuttin and A. Beckers, *The Illusion of Attitude Change: Towards a Response Contagion Theory of Persuasion*, London, Academic Press, 1975; A. Lynch, *Thought Contagion: How Belief Spreads through Society*, New York, Basic Books, 1996 (adopting the concept of meme introduced by the geneticist Richard Dawkins); B. Browning, *Infectious Rhythm: Metaphors of Contagion and the Spread of African Culture*, New York and London, Routledge, 1998; D. Woodward, *Contagion and Cure: Tackling the Crisis in Global Finance*, London, Catholic Institute for International Relations, 1999.
26 A. Weymouth, *Through the Leper Squint: A Study of Leprosy from Pre-Christian Times to the Present Day*, London, Selwyn and Blount, 1938; S. N. Brody, *The Disease of the Soul: Leprosy in Medieval Literature*, Ithaca, NY, and London, Cornell University Press, 1974.
27 C. Quétel, *History of Syphilis*, trans. J. Braddock and B. Pike, Cambridge, Polity Press, 1990.
28 M. Dols, 'The Comparative Communal Responses to the Black Death in Muslim and Christian Societies', *Viator*, 1974, vol. 5, pp. 269–97; N. E. Gallagher, *Medicine and Power in Tunisia 1780–1900*, Cambridge, Cambridge University Press, 1983; M. Harrison, *Public Health in British India*, Cambridge, Cambridge University Press, 1994.
29 For a view of contagion and hence quarantine as purely political constructs, see C. Maclean, *Evils of Quarantine Laws*, London, T. & G. Underwood, 1824. See also G. B. Rothenberg, 'The Austrian Sanitary Cordon and the Control of Bubonic Plague: 1710–1871', *Journal of the History of Medicine*, 1973, vol. 28, pp. 15–23.
30 Still authoritative is O. Temkin, 'The Scientific Approach to Disease: Specific Entity and Individual Sickness', *Double Face*, pp. 441–56.

31 See L. S. King, 'Dr Koch's Postulates', *Journal of the History of Medicine*, 1952, vol. 7, pp. 350–61; A. Evans, 'Causation and Disease: The Henle–Koch Postulates Revisited', *Yale Journal of Biology and Medicine*, 1976, vol. 49, pp. 175–95.
32 W. Pagel, 'The Speculative Basis of Modern Pathology. Jahn, Virchow, and the Philosophy of Pathology', *Bulletin of the History of Medicine*, 1945, vol. 18, pp. 1–43; cf. J. Bleker, 'Between Romantic and Scientific Medicine: Johann Lukas Schoenlein and the Natural History School 1825–1845', *Clio Medica*, 1983, vol. 18, pp. 191–201.
33 W. Pagel, 'Paracelsus', *Dictionary of Scientific Biography*, vol. 10; and in general, C. Webster, 'The Nineteenth-Century Afterlife of Paracelsus', in R. Cooter (ed.), *Studies in the History of Alternative Medicine*, London, Macmillan, 1988, pp. 79–88.
34 See K. Faber, *Nosography in Modern Internal Medicine*, London, Oxford University Press, 1923.
35 L. J. Jordanova, 'The Social Construction of Medical Knowledge', *Social History of Medicine*, 1995, vol. 8, pp. 361–81; C. E. Rosenberg, 'Framing Disease: Illness, Society and History', in his *Explaining Epidemics and Other Studies*, Cambridge, Cambridge University Press, 1992, pp. 305–18.
36 See O. Temkin, 'Health and Disease', *Double Face*, pp. 419–40.
37 F. N. L. Poynter, 'Sydenham's Influence Abroad', *Medical History*, 1973, vol. 17, pp. 223–34.
38 E. Goldschmid, 'Nosologia Naturalis', in Underwood, *Science, Medicine and History*, vol. 2, pp. 103–22.
39 G. A. Lindeboom, 'From the History of the Concept of Specificity', *Janus*, 1957, vol. 46, pp. 12–24; Pelling, *Cholera*, p. 73 ff. and *passim*.
40 W. Aitken, 'Darwin's Doctrine of Evolution in Explanation of the Coming into Being of Some Diseases', *Glasgow Medical Journal*, 1885, vol. 24, pp. 98–107, 161–72, 241–53, 354–68, 431–46, and 1886, vol. 25, pp. 1–20, 89–113; W. Collins, *Specificity and Evolution in Disease*, London, H. K. Lewis, 1884, argues for the obsolescence of specificity and for diseases being able to arise *de novo*.
41 Pelling, *Cholera*, pp. 254–6; W. F. Bynum, 'Darwin and the Doctors: Evolution, Diathesis and Germs in 19th-Century Britain', *Gesnerus*, 1983, vol. 40, pp. 43–53. See in general for the earlier period A. Desmond, *The Politics of Evolution: Morphology, Medicine and Reform in Radical London*, Chicago and London, University of Chicago Press, 1989.
42 See e.g. J. H. Baas, *Outlines of the History of Medicine*, trans. and enlarged by H. E. Handerson, 1889; 2 vols, Huntington, NY, Robert E. Krieger, 1971, vol. 2, pp. 1008–10.
43 For this and ensuing paragraphs, see Pelling, *Cholera*, with additional references as cited.
44 Temkin, 'Health and Disease', p. 427.
45 J. Pickstone, 'Dearth, Dirt and Fever Epidemics: Rewriting the History of British "Public Health", 1780–1850', in T. Ranger and P. Slack (eds), *Epidemics and Ideas*, Cambridge, Cambridge University Press, 1992, pp. 125–48.
46 L. J. Jordanova, 'Earth Science and Environmental Medicine: The Synthesis of the Late Enlightenment', in L. J. Jordanova and R. Porter (eds), *Images of the Earth*, Chalfont St Giles, UK, British Society for the History of Science, 1979, pp. 119–46; J. C. Riley, *The Eighteenth-Century Campaign to Avoid Disease*, Basingstoke, UK, Macmillan, 1987; C. Hamlin, 'Predisposing Causes and Public Health in Early Nineteenth-Century Medical Thought', *Social History of Medicine*, 1992, vol. 5, pp. 43–70.
47 For European anticontagionism of the 1820s and 1830s see E. Ackerknecht, 'Anticontagionism between 1821 and 1867', *Bulletin of the History of Medicine*, 1948, vol. 22, pp. 562–93.

48 On Farr, see Pelling, *Cholera*, esp. ch. 3; J. Eyler, *Victorian Social Medicine: The Ideas and Methods of William Farr*, Baltimore and London, Johns Hopkins University Press, 1979.
49 Pelling, *Cholera*, p. 93.
50 Ibid., p. 94.
51 Ibid., p. 107.
52 Baas, *Outlines*, vol. 2, p. 1003; W. Bulloch, *The History of Bacteriology*, London, Oxford University Press, 1960, ch. 8.
53 On the ambivalence of the parasite analogy see Pelling, *Cholera*, pp. 196 ff., 253–5, and *passim*; J. Farley, 'Parasites and the Germ Theory of Disease', *Milbank Quarterly*, suppl. I, 1989, vol. 67, pp. 50–68.
54 See G. L. Geison, 'Pasteur, Louis', *Dictionary of Scientific Biography*, vol. 10, pp. 350–416; G. L. Geison, *The Private Science of Louis Pasteur*, Princeton, NJ, Princeton University Press, 1995; J. F. Hutchinson, 'Tsarist Russia and the Bacteriological Revolution', *Journal of the History of Medicine*, 1985, vol. 40, pp. 420–39.
55 N. Roll-Hansen, 'Louis Pasteur – a Case against Reductionist Historiography', *British Journal of the Philosophy of Science*, 1972, vol. 23, p. 351.
56 Geison, 'Pasteur', pp. 364, 352.
57 See C. Dolman, 'Lister, Joseph', *Dictionary of Scientific Biography*, vol. 8, pp. 399–413; also D. Hamilton, 'The Nineteenth-Century Surgical Revolution – Antisepsis or Better Nutrition?', *Bulletin of the History of Medicine*, 1982, vol. 56, pp. 30–40. Shifts in Lister's pathological views in accordance with French and then German findings are detailed by C. Lawrence and R. Dixey, 'Practising on Principle: Joseph Lister and the Germ Theories of Disease', in C. Lawrence (ed.), *Medical Theory, Surgical Practice*, London, Routledge, 1992, pp. 153–215, focusing on the notion of 'laudable pus'.
58 The detailed work of K. Codell Carter is aimed at defending Semmelweis's contribution to modern science. See his *Childbed Fever: A Scientific Biography of Ignaz Semmelweis*, Westport, Conn., Greenwood Press, 1994. See also e.g. A. Rubinstein, 'Subtle Poison: The Puerperal Fever Controversy in Victorian Britain', *Historical Studies*, 1983, vol. 20, pp. 420–38, which adopts Ackerknecht's account of the mid-century.
59 N. J. Fox, 'Scientific Theory Choice and Social Structure: The Case of Joseph Lister's Antisepsis, Humoral Theory and Asepsis', *History of Science*, 1988, vol. 26, pp. 367–97.
60 C. E. Dolman, 'Koch, Robert', *Dictionary of Scientific Biography*, vol. 7, pp. 420–35.
61 R. Maulitz, 'Physician versus Bacteriologist: The Ideology of Science in Clinical Medicine', in M. Vogel and C. E. Rosenberg (eds), *The Therapeutic Revolution*, Philadelphia, University of Philadelphia Press, 1979, pp. 91–108.
62 I. Galdston, 'Social Medicine and the Epidemic Constitution', *Bulletin of the History of Medicine*, 1951, vol. 25, pp. 8–21; S. Kunitz, 'The Historical Roots and Ideological Functions of Disease Concepts in Three Primary Care Specialties', *Bulletin of the History of Medicine*, 1983, vol. 57, pp. 412–32.
63 Major studies not already cited include: R. J. Evans, *Death in Hamburg: Society and Politics in the Cholera Years, 1830–1910*, Oxford, Clarendon Press, 1987; F. M. Snowden, *Naples in the Time of Cholera, 1884–1911*, Cambridge, Cambridge University Press, 1995; A. R. Aisenberg, *Contagion: Disease, Government and the 'Social Question' in Nineteenth-Century France*, Stanford, Calif., Stanford University Press, 1999; P. Baldwin, *Contagion and the State in Europe, 1830–1930*, Cambridge, Cambridge University Press, 1999.
64 See e.g. C. J. Kudlick, *Cholera in Post-Revolutionary Paris: A Cultural History*, Berkeley, Calif., University of California Press, 1996. An obvious exception is F. Delaporte, *Disease and Civilisation: The Cholera in Paris, 1832*, trans. A. Goldhammer,

Cambridge, Mass., MIT Press, 1986, who repudiates Ackerknecht's interpretation in favour of a Foucauldian analysis of 'physiological medicine'.
65 See e.g. R. M. Morantz, 'Feminism, Professionalism and Germs: The Thought of Mary Putnam Jacobi and Elizabeth Blackwell', *American Quarterly*, 1982, vol. 34, pp. 459–78; A. Bashford, *Purity and Pollution: Gender, Embodiment and Victorian Medicine*, Basingstoke, UK, Macmillan, 1998.
66 E. Heaman, 'The Rise and Fall of Anticontagionism in France', *Canadian Bulletin of Medical History/Bulletin canadien d'histoire de la médecine*, 1995, vol. 12, pp. 3–25.
67 See e.g. the following very different approaches, Snowden, *Naples*; B. Latour, *The Pasteurization of France*, trans. A. Sheridan and J. Law, Cambridge, Mass., Harvard University Press, 1988.
68 Baldwin, *Contagion and the State*, pp. 15–16.
69 Ackerknecht, 'Anticontagionism'.

2 Foreign bodies

Vaccination, contagion and colonialism in the nineteenth century

Alison Bashford

Vaccination against smallpox is commonly understood as one of the most important public health innovations of the nineteenth century. But it has never been settled as an unambiguously beneficial practice: opposition to vaccination, variously configured, has always been, and remains, the constant historical companion to the practice itself. Struggles over the procedure occurred in most English-speaking and European countries and were visible, loud, influential and organised, if rarely uni-vocal. Even amongst those who were convinced of the benefits of vaccination, there was an extraordinary range of opinion and argument about the specific processes, the different types of vaccine or lymph as it was generally called, from where and how it should be created, secured and supplied. In analysing and explaining these (anti-)vaccination debates historians usually make some reference to the sense in which the vaccine matter was understood as a contaminant and the procedure itself contaminating: 'a compulsory pollution of our veins', as one anti-vaccinationist put it in 1882.[1] But this aspect of anti-vaccinationism is implicitly constructed in medical histories as almost incidental to the more pressing questions of compulsion, liberalism and the state's relation to citizens. While the latter were undeniably crucial to anti-vaccinationism over the century (and, in a less recognised way, to the development of liberal subjectivities), here I focus specifically on the discussion about poisoning, pollution, contamination, and impurity through which vaccination was opposed and, in less strident versions sometimes even theorised and supported.

Over the nineteenth century 'public health' came to mean the ordering of categories of clean and unclean, normal and pathological, healthy and unhealthy, self and other. This involved what I think of as 'quarantining' strategies, even if this stretches the technical sense of the term: strategies and technologies of isolation, containment, barriers, the policing of spaces. As many medical sociologists and historians have pointed out, such practices formed the most long-standing and familiar preventive response to epidemic disease in European cultures.[2] While vaccination is often understood similarly as a preventive measure in a (now) commonsense way, my suggestion is that in the nineteenth century, smallpox vaccination in fact fundamentally challenged established methods of disease prevention: it challenged medical and lay sensibilities because it did *not* separate clean and dirty, but rather involved the deliberate introduction of a foreign body into the individual, the incorporation of one person's body into another's; it involved the circulation of vaccine matter through the social body as a kind of contagion; it required acceptance of the counter-intuitive logic of getting sick in order to stay healthy.

In this chapter I take nineteenth-century commentators at their word and explore the ways in which vaccination worked rather more through a logic of contagion, than a logic of quarantine.[3] That is, far from working on a preventive model of separation and the maintenance of lines of hygiene, vaccination was precisely about contact, mixing and dissolving the foreign 'other' within the self. But in offering this argument, a range of rather more subtextual issues emerge which explain (anti-)vaccinationism in new ways. If vaccination was like a contagious disease in that it involved the introduction and 'spread' of a foreign body within an individual, it was also like a contagious disease in that it 'spread' through populations, both spatially and temporally, and was integrally related to local and global migrations and to a history of travel, orientalism and colonialism.

In the first section, 'Foreign bodies', I examine the specific ways in which vaccination-as-contagion confused self and other, the normal and the pathological, the clean and the dirty. The most common mechanism for the spread of the vaccine was known as the 'arm-to-arm' technique, in which children were infected with cowpox through direct contact with one another; a process which literally incorporated one child's body into another's. Not only was the vaccine matter itself a contagious foreign body – already a deeply problematical proposition – there was a real concern about vaccination as an illegitimate vehicle for other diseases, syphilis most importantly. Further, practices of (anti-)vaccination raised anxieties of human/animal species boundaries and the 'beastliness' of the procedure. As Catherine Waldby has written, with respect to HIV/AIDS, 'contagion is confusion of self and other; cleanliness is singularity/unity'.[4] But, unlike many sociologists and anthropologists of the body and medicine from Mary Douglas onwards who tend to formulate cultural anxieties about '(im)purity and danger' in terms of generic 'otherness', I get specific about just what the 'foreign' in foreign bodies meant in nineteenth-century British imperial culture; a culture thoroughly inflected by formations of class, race, gender and colonialism, and by anxious efforts (always failures) to keep these categories and social relations identifiable and intact.[5]

Both contagious disease and the preventive measure of vaccination need to be understood as part of modern histories of travel, colonialism, orientalism and migration, and once this is recognised it becomes clear how this connection has been unwittingly reproduced and sustained in the historiography.[6] In 'Connections', I trace these material and discursive similarities between 'contagion' and the technology of vaccination, in spatial terms. Like contagious disease, indeed *as* the contagious disease of cowpox, vaccine matter was spread locally from person to person, and globally through shifting populations. And like contagious diseases the technology of vaccination was spread around the globe in a colonising move, sometimes via the very ships which unconsciously contaminated populations with the disease itself. I also suggest that the conventional story of inoculation versus vaccination, including its more recent tellings in medical history, needs to be understood as a colonial story – specifically, an orientalist one. Vaccination was a 'home-grown' English idea in which people were infected with the cowpox rather than the smallpox virus. Inoculation, on the other hand, was a much older practice, and has been represented as a specifically 'eastern' practice, and, as I argue, as an implicitly feminised one. It involved the transmission of actual smallpox matter from the pustule of one inoculated person under the skin of another, usually with a scalpel or needle, or sometimes involved placing dried crusts of smallpox pustules in the nasal membranes. This rendition of inoculation with smallpox matter as old, eastern and 'folk' constructs vaccination with cowpox matter as modern, western and 'expert', although as I discuss at the end of this paper, the distinction between the practices has been questioned more or less since it was invented.

Finally, in 'Genealogies', I argue that vaccination and the discourses through which it was known and practised implied a temporal dimension which was related to this 'contagious' logic. Contagious disease and the discipline of epidemiology through which it has primarily been understood in the modern period, are organised not only spatially, but also through crucial temporal questions: moments of origin, 'natural history', viral mutations over time, incubation periods, fading immunities.[7] Just as epidemiologists insistently traced an epidemic to an originary moment, a 'case zero', so a genealogical imperative operated in the culture of nineteenth-century vaccination: concern about the genealogy of the vaccine matter itself, and the genealogy of the population through which it had passed. Obsessive questioning of the purity and impurity of particular strains of vaccine lymph were partly concerns about its human or animal genealogy/origins, but also compelled careful tracing of that vaccine's history and global movement over time and through populations of children named as desirable or undesirable according to both race and class.

I locate this argument within the British imperial world, using mainly English published medical and lay texts for and against vaccination, and material from the Australian colonies. I have relied considerably on the evidence presented to two New South Wales committees of enquiry on compulsory vaccination, one held in 1872 and the other in 1881, which offer unparalleled detail about the range of opinion on the matter and a certain perspective on the colonial politics shaping the vaccination question. In some respects Australian public health history is very specific. As I have argued elsewhere, it has been driven by a particular racial and nationalist politics, by the geography of a tropical island-nation with its own governmental/health investments in notions of immunity and quarantine, and by the development of strong welfarism.[8] However the argument I make in this chapter – that vaccination functioned discursively as a kind of contagion – is not a specific one, but seems to me to be generally applicable to other modern western cultures, at the very least to the British debates. Throughout the chapter I am interested not only in the discursive practices which took place in the nineteenth century, but also in the *representations* of these vaccination debates in more recent medical histories. Aspects of this 'vaccination as contagion' logic have been sustained, often as metaphor, and continue to organise our understandings of vaccination as a technology and of the history of the smallpox virus and its decline in the modern period.

Foreign bodies

Vaccine lymph was foreign matter introduced into the individual body in order to set up an illness – cowpox – to prevent another illness – smallpox. The point of cowpox was precisely that it was contagious; that it could be passed between humans by direct contact and thus circulated through the social body, creating not just individual but population immunity. Cowpox, or 'vaccinia' was an epidemic contagious disease in and of itself, and as such, involved an actual connection/infection between humans; the direct contact of 'arm-to-arm' vaccination, which was the favoured, if not the only method of vaccination through most of the nineteenth century. A group of children (and in epidemic times, adults) would be vaccinated, and were to return to the vaccinator on the seventh day; first, so that the local reaction could be assessed and measured as successful or unsuccessful and, second, in order that several children could be chosen to perpetuate the vaccine. A new batch of children would be brought in, a scratch made on the pustule of the first child's arm, several scratches on the arm of the unvaccinated child, and their arms would be connected. Sometimes, the lymph would be withdrawn and injected into the unvaccinated child with a needle. That group of children would return on the seventh day, and another arm-to-arm process would take place. Thus the vaccine matter was kept in circulation in an exponential way.[9] While the use of stored lymph from calves became more common around the turn of the century, most experts in the mid to late nineteenth century thought that the arm-to-arm method was preferable, that this process kept the lymph 'alive', 'active' and effective in a population of children.[10]

Thus, when anti-vaccinationists proclaimed about the 'contagion' and 'pollution' involved in the procedure, they were, in fact, stating the obvious: immunity *was* achieved through a process of infection. This contagious aspect of vaccination was agreed upon by both opponents and proponents of the procedure: the contagious mechanism was the way in which those who supported vaccination theorised its effect and efficacy in individuals and in populations. As one proponent explained: 'Vaccination means the setting up of a septic fever in a healthy infant – the contamination, however slightly, of a pure circulation by the introduction of a poisonous substance.'[11] Just how vaccination resulted in immunity from smallpox was certainly speculated upon, although most nineteenth-century practitioners were less concerned with physiological explanation than with empirically observable effect.

Donna Haraway has written of the immune system that it 'is a map drawn to guide recognition and misrecognition of self and other in the dialectics of western politics. That is, the immune system is a plan for meaningful action to construct and maintain the boundaries for what may count as self and other in the crucial realms of the normal and the pathological.' She is right to call the immune system 'pre-eminently a twentieth century object',[12] for the mechanism/system of 'immunity' only existed as a tentative and disputed concept in the nineteenth century. While we are now familiar with the idea of immunity involving an *internal* self/other (mis)recognition (of foreign bodies by anti-bodies), this was not available as a concept in the nineteenth century. *External* self/other recognition was, however. That is to say, vaccination involved the deliberate introduction of foreign/'other' matter into the integrated self/body. Sometimes mid to late nineteenth-century physicians understood immunity as a local reaction. Alfred Roberts, for example, understood vaccination to be not systemic, but local: 'I believe it is a local inflammation ... it is a concentration; any humours there may be are drawn to the vesicle.'[13] More often it was understood as a systemic process involving (usually) ideas about blood, but sometimes ideas about a lymphatic system. In 1883, Metchnicoff produced a new theory of immunity, one involving ideas of active defence mechanisms of the host and the principle of host resistance in the action of the phagocyte. Although Virchow and Pasteur supported this theory, Koch opposed it, and in general, argues the historian of immunology Alfred Tauber, 'Metchnicoff's thinking places him outside the thrust of nineteenth-century conceptions ... [he was] misunderstood or ignored.' The more successful theory at the end of the nineteenth century (but not into the twentieth) was Pasteur's: 'the invading organism exhausted an essential nutrient during the first infection and was thus unable to survive in a host depleted of the substance. Such passive theories were the model of immunity and rested upon an ancient metaphysical understanding of health and disease, the balance of humours and the organism's ability to restore its wholeness.'[14] It is also important to note that homoeopathy offered one model for understanding the mechanism and effect of vaccination in beneficial terms. Many homoeopaths were interested in vaccination because it seemed to work around the principle 'similia similibus curantur'.[15] J. Compton Burnett wrote: 'Vaccination is a homoeoprophylactic diseasing measure: one disease is given to prevent a like one

– vaccinia to prevent variola ... for in vaccinating a person we are *diseasing* him, we communicate vaccinosis to him.'[16]

Notwithstanding such possibilities for understanding vaccination positively, it is clear that anxiety about this contagious and foreign quality to the vaccine was voiced in anti-vaccinationism throughout the nineteenth and well into the twentieth centuries: 'millions of people have now a ruined constitution through having the loathsome filth in the blood.'[17] And as late as 1946 the Melbourne Branch of the British Union for Abolition of Vivisection pronounced that: 'Every vaccination ... [is] a poisonous injection.'[18] In a culture where it was lay and expert commonsense that 'dirt ... is matter in the wrong place' as the physician Elizabeth Blackwell put it, well and truly prefiguring the anthropologist Mary Douglas,[19] this production of health through disease seemed counter-intuitive for many. 'Can disease protect health?' was the question which structured but one set of exchanges in 1880.[20]

Those who proposed and supported vaccination asked other practitioners and the public to understand that 'health' or at least 'immunity' could be achieved through a process of infection and cross-infection across multiple boundaries, including, possibly most problematically, species boundaries. This inter-species exchange, the very idea of introducing a bit of *diseased* animal into the human frame, was sometimes religiously, sometimes popularly, sometimes expertly opposed. In this respect, anti-vivisectionism, anti-vaccinationism and vegetarianism have entwined histories. At the very least problematising the animal origin of the vaccine prompted arguments for maintaining the vaccine in the human population only, resisting the theory, discussed below that the matter needed to be strengthened by sending it back through the cow's system. But there were far stronger anxieties at work about the maintenance of proper inter-species boundaries, anxieties which resonate with our own Creutzfeldt-Jacob syndrome about inter-species feeding, about using animal hormones as human therapies, about transplanting animal organs. In the early and mid-nineteenth century a working-class British response to vaccination (at least as reported by anti-vaccinationists) was to describe animalistic features in recently vaccinated children. Thus mothers reported small horns growing in the heads of their infants, or that the voices of these children began to change to animalistic grunts. Vaccines were understood to produce unnatural hybrids.[21]

The sense in which vaccination was in some way 'against nature' continued in the more organised and theorised anti-vaccinationist/anti-vivisectionist responses of the later nineteenth century. The influential Sydney homoeopathic physician John le Gay Brereton argued that vaccine lymph 'might engender diseases which you might never get rid of ... you have diseases of animals to consider, which are more to be dreaded than those proper to man'.[22] He considered 'the pure vaccine disease' of cowpox itself dangerously virulent, rather than benign, but was also deeply concerned about the as-yet unknown results of unnaturally crossing diseases between species. A Melbourne doctor reported the method by which a cow was infected for the purposes of producing vaccine: the cow was wrapped in the blanket used by a person who had died of smallpox. 'From the crops of vesicles that formed on her udder, successful vaccinations were performed.'[23] The crossing and re-crossing of boundaries in this exercise was more than many nineteenth-century medical, lay and political sensibilities could tolerate or even imagine.

Notwithstanding anti-vaccinationists' concerns about inter-species crossings and animal diseases, it was human diseases that gave most cause for alarm and for this reason, calf lymph steadily replaced 'humanised' lymph both in England and in the Australian colonies, as governments increasingly regulated public health procedures.[24] Some states, for instance Germany in 1898, decided to use only animal vaccine.[25] In all of these cases, the shift toward calf lymph was largely a response to well-placed anxieties about the transmission of syphilis and some other diseases between children in the 'arm-to-arm' method. J. W. Beaney, a prominent Melbourne surgeon with interests and expertise in venereology wrote in 1870: '*what practitioner is able to determine the purity of the lymph?* It is often far beyond his power to know the constitution of the parent of the child from whom the lymph is taken, or the nurse by whom it has been suckled; hence the difficulties that lie in his way are insurmountable, setting aside the . . . latent germs that may lurk in the child ready to be transmitted through its lymph to others.'[26] While syphilis was the major concern, the possibility that vaccination was a conduit for the infection/inheritance of other diseases and conditions was also raised. For example, Mr John Marx, a hydropathic physician, who was examined by the 1872 Select Committee in New South Wales attributed his own 'weak eyes' to vaccination, not his own, but his mother's: 'My mother was vaccinated, and shortly after the vaccination the glands of the neck swelled up, and the disease flew to her eyes. She was bad until a few months after she got married. I was her first-born, and I inherited this complaint . . . I attribute my complaint indirectly to vaccination.'[27] His statements illustrate the intriguing nineteenth-century conflation of heredity and infection. Anti-vaccinationists also published material on 'Cancer: a result of vaccination',[28] and sometimes argued that leprosy was newly transmitted amongst Europeans in the tropical colonies because of the increase in smallpox vaccination.[29]

In contradistinction to increasingly intricate nineteenth-century public and private hygienic practices which separated out clean and dirty, smallpox vaccination was a process which crossed and dissolved boundaries between self and other, boundaries between species, and boundaries between individual embodied subjects and populations. The process of vaccination was one of a deliberate confusion of the normal and the pathological as a minute amount of a pathological foreign body became a normalised part of the self, and a bit of one's own transformed body became part of another. This dissolution was not a comfortable one in a culture otherwise anxious to secure clear, firm and stable boundaries.

Connections

Epidemics of contagious disease involve the movement and growth of microbes through spatially stable populations, but historically epidemics of contagious diseases have also been closely linked with the movement of people and populations, through trade and commerce, through immigration, through colonisation, through military campaigns, through systems of indentured labour and slavery. Public health, epidemiology and especially early twentieth-century tropical medicine have all been centrally concerned with global and local movement and displacement. These are disciplines of human connections in place and genealogies in time. Ironically, the last two centuries, characterised so profoundly by imperialism, colonisation and globalisation, have also been marked by anxieties that people were not in their 'proper' local and global locations, that people were illegitimately placed and displaced for one reason or another, and that this caused the escalation of epidemic disease.[30] To take some disparate examples, in popular culture and in expert epidemiology of the nineteenth century, Chinese immigrants and goldseekers brought smallpox and typhus fever to North America. In the early twentieth century leprosy was understood to spread through the white population in Australia because of 'illegitimate' sexual contact facilitated by inadequate containment and separation of the races.[31] And from another time and place, late twentieth-century refugee crises in Kosovo or Afghanistan or East Timor almost immediately become stories of imminent or actual disease outbreak. As Roy Porter has recently put it, 'the demands of international capitalism for migrant workforces, the opening up of borders, the ebb and flow of peoples due to war and persecution, the increased mobility of affluent air-travelling populations – all these factors mean that formerly contained diseases now have no fixed abode'.[32] Displacement, migration, colonisation, travel, health and contagion are linked.

But less familiar is the sense in which vaccination also has a history connected with travel and the movement of individuals and populations. When I was young I remember being proud of the vaccination scar on my left arm, for it was an immediately readable sign of having travelled. In the 1960s and early 1970s not many Australian schoolgirls had been to Europe, let alone Ceylon, Egypt, and Morocco, and my vaccination scar signified travel to places considered exotic and dangerous; places marked as such precisely because they required vaccination. A recent Australian poster (see Figure 2.1), designed to increase vaccination rates against the so-called 'travel diseases', is a late twentieth-century version of this cluster of signs and meanings. This kind of imperative toward vaccination is expressly orientalist, working as it does through a set of racialised

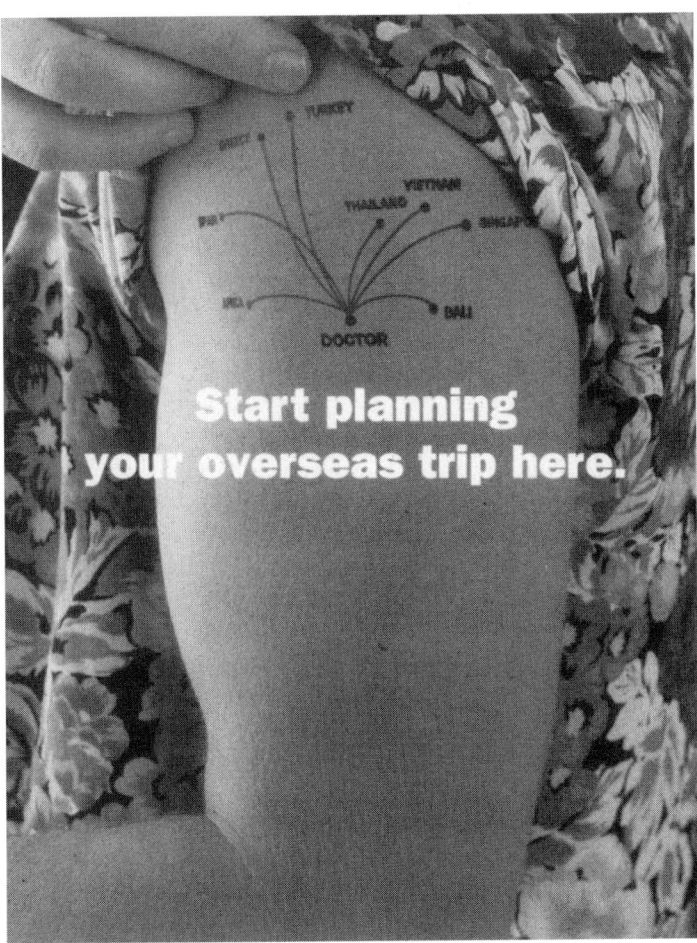

Figure 2.1 'Start Planning Your Overseas Trip Here'. Courtesy, SmithKline Beecham Biologicals.

assumptions about who needs protection in which 'exotic' places. The arm in this poster is ultra blonde, its white owner travelling to those dark places of disease and adventure which require the protection of vaccination. The countries for which vaccination is recommended are not only Vietnam, Thailand, Bali and India, but 'even' Spain and Greece, those liminally European, liminally Other nations. Although vaccination is no longer *required* by most nations, there is nonetheless still a sense in which vaccination scars often function as signs of travel and as passports which confer a biological if not a diplomatic immunity.[33]

If the vaccination scar in the late twentieth century functions as a kind of passport for safe ('immune') travel into dangerous places, in the nineteenth century it functioned much more literally as a passport into certain spaces, and sometimes as an immigration requirement into countries: it allowed crossings of clean and dirty lines of hygiene. For example, in the 1881 epidemic of smallpox in Sydney there was a quarantine measure established at the border between the colonies of New South Wales and Victoria. Passengers on the Sydney–Melbourne train would be examined at the border town of Albury. Only those with certificates of vaccination and a viable vaccination scar were permitted entry.[34] In 1913 smallpox appeared again in Sydney and the Commonwealth Government declared all of Sydney a quarantined space, with road blocks established in a circumference 15 miles from the GPO. Again, people were permitted over those barriers in either direction only if they could display a viable vaccination scar.[35]

The vaccination scar facilitated movement into and out of both 'clean' and 'contaminated' spaces: over borders and over lines of hygiene. But it could also get one safely into 'unclean' spaces (for example, a quarantine station or an infectious disease hospital to visit a relative in times of epidemic). If there was smallpox on an overseas ship which was quarantined, vaccinated people could possibly bypass the quarantine procedure and move into the colony as an immigrant or a traveller. Over time, and especially in the newly bureaucratised culture of the early twentieth century, vaccination was to be recorded on the body as a scar which *needed* to be visible to be viable and recognised, but also recorded by an emergent health and immigration machine. A 'Personal Detail Card' recorded the 'vaccine history' of an individual, not only if vaccination had taken place, but where, when, by whom, with what vaccine, and with what reaction (that is, size, colour, and discharge).[36]

Smallpox was the most visible of diseases, leaving its sufferers permanently marked as smallpox sufferers, permanently pock-marked. It was a disease which disfigured, giving any sufferer who survived the stigmata of the ill and the unclean (see Figure 2.2). But if the sufferer survived the disease, their very scars then marked that person as immune – pock-marks could be interpreted as multiple vaccination scars. In this logic, having no scar at all, being completely pure, if you like, was more suspect. This was the threat of an incubation period – one may well be diseased but not yet show the signs. To have one mark, the single pock mark of vaccination rendered the disease status of that person permanently knowable, conferring an immunity to disease and an immunity to travel over governmental lines of hygiene. Thus the bodily evidence of the deliberate introduction of the foreign body of the smallpox vaccine was the real marker of safety and security, if not quite cleanliness. In this scheme, purity itself becomes the danger.

This connection between contagious disease, vaccination and travel is apparent at another level in representations of the history of smallpox, inoculation and vaccination, which are orientalist in implicit and sometimes

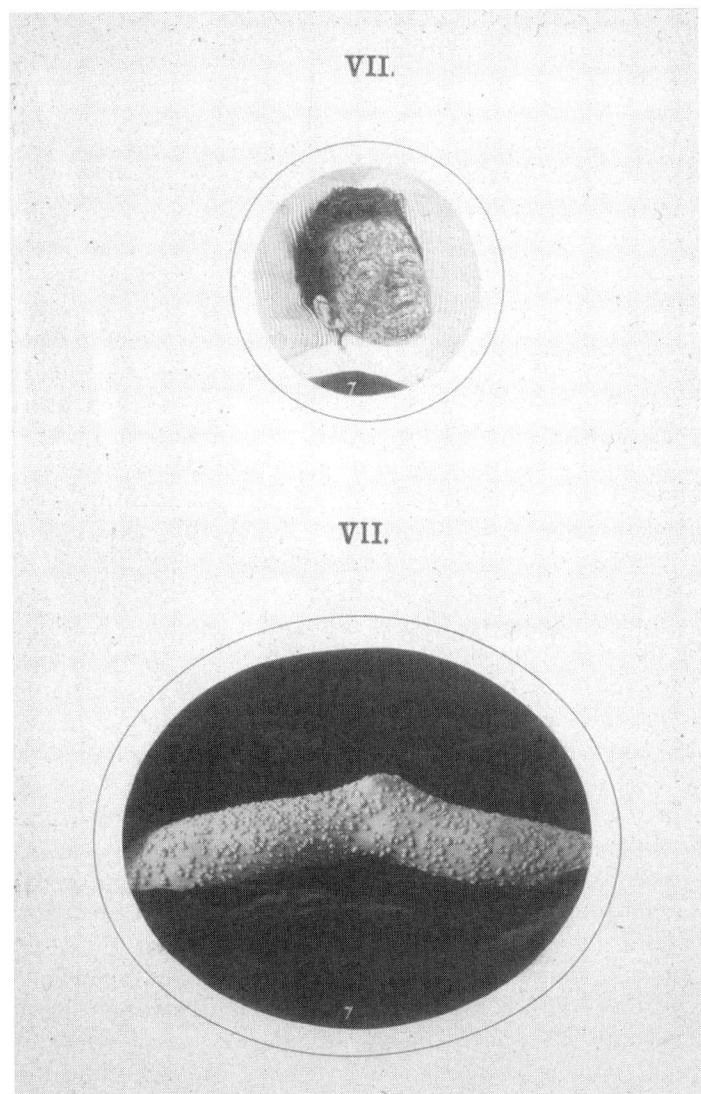

Figure 2.2 From J. Ashburton Thompson, *A Report to the President of the Board of Health: containing photographs of a person suffering from variola discreta, and accounts of the case*, Sydney, Government Printer, 1886. Copy in author's possession.

explicit ways. Despite the long-standing endemic status of smallpox in Europe, its origins are constantly sought and typically represented as 'Eastern'. This is the case both in nineteenth- and twentieth-century representations, for the *genre* of medical history as well as the deeply related discipline of epidemiology, seek origins almost pathologically. For example, the British educated physician L. H. J. Maclean told the New South Wales parliament in 1881: 'I believe it is an endemic disease of the valley of the Yang Tze and other river valleys in China . . . It never made its appearance in Europe until about 1,000 years ago. It was only about that time that communication with the extreme east of Asia became fairly common, and it was with the commencement of that communication that small-pox made its appearance and small-pox came from the East.'[37] A 1954 *Story of Medicine* states that 'smallpox was first introduced into Europe by the Crusaders who brought it home from the Holy Land where the disease was common'.[38] After ascertaining origins, most general medical histories then shift in a formulaic way to the story of inoculation versus vaccination. Inoculation, the apparently 'folk' and traditional practice of gaining immunity through infection with the actual smallpox virus is represented as rigidly and crucially distinct from vaccination, the more expert practice of infecting with the cowpox virus, innovated by Jenner in the late eighteenth century. Below I look at the distinction more closely, including a radical questioning of this distinction which in fact has gone on more or less since Jenner's time. But for now I am interested in the ways of telling the story of smallpox, inoculation and vaccination, which are organised through, and sustain, a certain orientalism.

The historian of immunology H. J. Parish used a kind of orientalist travel narrative to describe the movement from east to west not only of the smallpox virus itself but the folk practice of inoculation (sometimes called 'variolation' after the *variola* (smallpox) virus): 'After these beginnings in eastern countries various forms of variolation, like smallpox itself naturally spread westwards.'[39] Indeed in a recent edition of *Dorland's Medical Dictionary* the entry for 'variolation' informs us that as 'practised in the Orient in ancient times, the dried crusts of smallpox lesions were applied to the skin or nasal mucous membranes, or were ingested'.[40] If 'smallpox' was brought/caught from the 'East', then in an inverse move Lady Mary Wortley Montagu in her travels to the Orient 'discovered' for the West the technology of inoculation against smallpox, and brought it Home.[41] Montagu, wife of the British consul in Constantinople famously had her daughter inoculated in 1721, having noted the practice amongst Turkish women. Given the popular currency of the story of Montagu, and the Ottoman origins of the technique, both lay and expert perceptions of inoculation had the taint of the Other about it, this notwithstanding the acclaimed inoculation of various European royals. In *The Conquest of Disease* (1925) David Masters wrote scathingly of the 'ignorant' practice of deliberate infection as a preventive measure, of mothers purposefully infecting their children with measles for example. 'If any one is to be blamed in the matter, it appears to be the Turks, who were practising this method of voluntary infection long before the people in England thought of it.'[42]

After 'the story of Jenner' gained as much circulation and currency as 'the story of Lady Mary Wortley Montagu', inoculation with smallpox matter began to fall into disfavour. Via the nugatory 1840, 1853 and 1867 enactments of mass vaccination (the last two compulsory) in Britain variolation/inoculation was made illegal. The physician Alexander Collie wrote in 1887 that inoculation 'is a penal offence, and is now rarely met with'.[43] British imperial powers also declared inoculation illegal in colonies where it had been traditionally practised. For example, traditional inoculation was made illegal in India as part of the attempt to institute and render compulsory, mass vaccination.[44] David Arnold notes that for Indians under the British, '[v]accination was construed as a site of conflict between malevolent British intent and something Indian, something sacred, that was under threat of violation and destruction'.[45]

It is profitable, then, to think about the medical story of inoculation versus vaccination as being partly shaped by orientalism and colonialism. And like everything else colonial and orientalist 'inoculation versus vaccination' should also be understood as gendered. Quite clearly, inoculation appears historically as a feminine and feminised practice. This is the case through its 'eastern-ness', through the well-documented and always mentioned femaleness of the inoculators in eighteenth-century Constantinople (a 'Bedouin female servant', a 'woman from Morea' and another from Bosnia) and through its strong association with Montagu.[46] There has always been an investment in constructing it so, for this feminisation of inoculation simultaneously constructs 'vaccination' as masculine, expert and modern. For the British, vaccination as opposed to inoculation was a home-grown idea and, if originally an English folk practice, nonetheless was rendered 'expert' by a distinguished man of science – Jenner. And as for the substance itself, something that originated in English cows was better than something that originated with Turkish women and children.

Like contagious disease and like the practice of inoculation, the vaccine matter of cowpox moved around the globe, sometimes through populations, sometimes as lymph or crusts stored in a vial.[47] The vaccine would then multiply locally. There were certain global centres for source production, which sent the vaccine off to 'colonise' new regions with missionaries, traders, bureaucrats and militaries. Vaccination worked like an epidemic of contagious disease in that it was spread through the world along routes of human transport and travel, and this aspect of vaccination is perpetuated in the conventions of the historiography. For example one article is titled 'The Odyssey of Smallpox Vaccination', and is significantly organised through sections titled 'the Eastward Odyssey' (from England to the Middle East, France, Russia, the Mediterranean, North America, India and Japan) and 'the Westward Odyssey' (from Spain to Spanish America, the Philippines and China). The author concluded that 'one decade after its discovery, vaccination had girdled the world on Asian and New World voyages from Europe'.[48]

Genealogies

Typically early epidemiologists traced epidemics of infectious diseases backwards in place and time to an originary moment and person. If epidemiology was 'governing by numbers' in the phrase of Petersen and Lupton,[49] it also governed by an originary narrative which involved tracing and mapping contacts and connections to locate 'case one'. This 'natural history' of infectious disease implied control and it implied closure; a case one and a final case bounded the epidemic. Similarly, vaccination involved an imperative toward origins: the tracing of a genealogy. This was the case in two respects. First, the genealogy of the actual vaccine matter came to be understood as vitally important: vaccines had pedigrees. Second, the genealogy of the children through whom the matter had passed was investigated and monitored.

First, then, the genealogy, the 'lymphline', of the vaccine. Inoculation involved the use of smallpox matter; vaccination involved the use of cowpox matter. But the apparently new technology of vaccination was not that simple. In some cases the vaccine originated from the pustules of a cow infected with cowpox. In other cases the vaccine derived from the pustules of the cow infected with smallpox, infected deliberately from a child with the actual smallpox disease. Those who supported this practice theorised that the disease *turned into* cowpox when it was thus 'bovinised'. Sometimes doctors argued that the most effective vaccine was that which had been in circulation in the human population for the longest time – 'humanised lymph'. One doctor at the 1872 Select Committee Inquiry in New South Wales argued that 'very good authorities on the question believe that vaccine virus, which has been passing from one person to another from the time of Jenner, onwards, is as effective as that drawn direct from the cow'.[50] At other times doctors claimed that this weakened the vaccine: 'I think lymph passing through a great number of human beings ... must become to a great extent deteriorated by its frequent passage through different constitutions.' In these cases it was suggested that the vaccine matter needed to pass back through the cow periodically, in order to maintain its strength and potency – thus 'bovinised lymph' was considered the most effective. The issue of efficacy and potency was always alive as a theoretical question in the nineteenth century, and only came to be resolved strategically as governments, practitioners and parents generally came to prefer calf-lymph as a way of avoiding the transmission of other human diseases.

Whether a physician or public vaccinator considered bovinised or humanised lymph to be more potent, the specific vaccine which any one practitioner used needed to be traced and traceable in time and space – its 'line' known and verified. The question of origins involved interrogating both the source of the vaccine matter, and tracing its global travel since that origin. In the 1872 and 1881 enquiries, the 'purity' and the pedigree of vaccine matter in New South Wales came under question: could the vaccine matter be traced to Jenner's lymph? And if not Jenner's, then whose? Did the lymph originate in human or animal? And through which humans and animals had it passed on its way from England to the Australian colonies?[51] One witness at the 1872 Select Committee detailed the possible lines of origin of vaccine matter available in New South Wales:

> I have been in the habit of getting vaccine lymph from Mr Badcock, in England ... This lymph is transmitted through the cow every six or twelve months ... There are three ways in which the lymph now used in England has been obtained. 1st. The original Jenner lymph. 2nd. Lymph obtained by Mr Ceiley who variolated the cow first in 1839, and from which source Mr Badcock's supplies have been obtained; and 3rd. Vaccine brought to England by Dr Blanc from the Continent, obtained from a cow under the natural disease, and reproduced upon heifers.[52]

He said that the lymph he received from England every second mail was 'pure from Home'. It was the 'Home-ness' in this statement which advertised this vaccinator's lymph as safe and clean in a context where there was a certain competition for purity amongst practitioners. Lymph direct from 'Home' implied that it had not passed through other colonial populations – it had not passed through populations of Indian children, for example, which was another common source for vaccine matter in the British colonial world. Newspaper advertisements for vaccination during the 1881 epidemic of smallpox in Sydney invariably announced the purity of the source: 'pure lymph from heifers, 3 to 5 pm daily' or 'Pure Vaccinate from the Heifer'.[53]

But even lymph pure from 'Home' or pure from the calf was not automatically established as of clean lineage, nor were anxieties about origins thus precluded. Even the purity, or more accurately the authenticity of Jenner's vaccine was under question, both in England and in the colonies. John le Gay Brereton argued: 'the original vaccine lymph we use from the Royal Vaccine Institute has never been vaccine lymph at all, from the day it was introduced into London to the present time – it was derived from the arm of Jane King, who was inoculated from a horse with greasy heels.'[54] The 'True Pedigree of English Vaccine' as one English physician titled his chapter, was debated.[55] Charles Creighton, English author of *The Natural History of Cow-Pox and Vaccinal Syphilis* (1887) detailed the outbreak of cowpox in Gray's Inn Lane in London as 'the source of English vaccine'.

> Thus we are enabled to trace to its source Jenner's own stock of lymph ... and with which he started his own first continuous series. It was taken from Ann Bumpus, aged twenty, who was inoculated on the 6th of February from Sarah Butcher, a healthy girl, aged thirteen

[who was vaccinated from] Jane Collingridge, a healthy, active girl, aged seventeen, she herself being one of the first group inoculated with purulent matter direct from the cow's teat [in Gray's Inn Lane].[56]

Nineteenth-century concerns about the vaccine were not just medical anxieties about biological purity, but were also cultural anxieties about race, class and species mixing. Given the standard practice of arm-to-arm techniques, the purity of the vaccine drew into consideration the purity of the individual child or adult and the population through which the vaccine passed, and which necessarily became part of the vaccine matter. As I have indicated, some medical men argued for the increasing strength of vaccine the longer it stayed in the human population. But that implied contact with increasing numbers of unknown individuals, it implied connection, indeed incorporation, with wholly unknown populations. Had the vaccine matter been through a population of Indian children? Had it been through a population of children in London or inner-city Sydney? Did it have any point of connection with groups compulsorily vaccinated at one time or another, in one place or another: prisoners; Chinese in smallpox epidemics; nurses working in infectious disease hospitals? Officials, doctors, public vaccinators, governments desperately sought and not infrequently fabricated, origins and paths through populations for their particular vaccine lymph.

The possibility of the transmission of syphilis from child to child in the process of vaccination was discussed regularly and with considerable alarm. And so the genealogy of the child was also in question: the family history of the child, or more precisely the sexual history of the father, was thus raised as an issue. In one anti-vaccination pamphlet published in 1875, *Vaccination and its Evil Consequences*, the author asked: 'by taking lymph from one child and applying it to the arms of another, how do we know whether the father or mother, to say nothing of the grandfather or grandmothers, have not had Syphilis, Scrofula, Insanity ect. [*sic*].'[57] In the 1872 Select Committee on the Vaccination Bill one doctor was asked: 'How can medical men guard against the use of impure lymph?' And he responded: 'The chief protection is in a knowledge of the family history of each child which in the city is difficult to get.'[58] He suggested a protective measure which apparently was implemented in London: 'I think it would be wise to adopt a precaution they have in London, that lymph should not be taken from a first-born child in a family, because the first child would be the most likely to show a syphilitic tendency.'[59] In New South Wales, children 'of syphilitic descent' were discounted from the arm-to-arm lineage; in effect, they were considered outside the social body.[60]

Epilogue

My suggestion in this chapter is that vaccination worked in a manner contrary to the familiar quarantining logic in which the clean and the dirty were unambiguously marked and separated. Vaccination connected a contaminated body with a clean one, an immune body with a vulnerable and susceptible one. This counterintuitive logic of vaccination, and its distinction from quarantine was articulated in a 1907 parliamentary debate on the Quarantine Bill. One member supported clauses of the Bill which would require individuals to be compulsorily detained, treated and vaccinated in quarantine – the suspension of individual rights for the sake of the community, 'in just the same way that the authorities interfere when a man has a dangerously dirty back yard'. But this made no sense to another member who responded incredulously: 'But the honorable member would propose to make a man's blood dirty.'[61] Vaccinia was a contagious disease and it needed to spread on an epidemic scale in order that it effect a viable population immunity, both locally and globally. I have suggested that this 'spread' over time and space of the technologies of inoculation and vaccination, of infected/immune individuals and populations, and of the vaccinia and variola viruses themselves, has implicated smallpox and vaccination in a modern history of travel and colonisation.

A conjectural medical article about the origin of the HIV-1 virus published in 1993 brings together an almost identical cluster of concerns. It is suggested that HIV was produced from the combination of two other viruses found in cattle and sheep, the Bovine Leukaemia Virus and the Visna Virus. HIV was 'created' as a recombinant virus in the process of the production of Vaccinia, the vaccine for smallpox. This natural recombinant was 'inadvertently transferred to humans through contaminated vaccine used to inoculate millions of Africans against smallpox during the eradication program conducted in sub-Saharan Africa in the late 1960s and most of the 1970s'.[62] The author describes the process by which the vaccine was manufactured from cows and sheep, which, except for homogenisation and freeze-drying, was quite similar to the nineteenth-century procedure. One of these sheep or cows, it is hypothesised, was co-infected with the other viruses, which recombined into HIV-1 and it was the resulting contaminated batches of vaccine which made their way to parts of sub-Saharan Africa. Unknowingly rehearsing the connections between smallpox, vaccine, travel and race which shaped nineteenth-century debate, the author spends considerable time tracing human movement between Africa, Haiti and the USA, 'the Haitian connection'. Dual 'origins' are sought and speculated upon in this article. The geographical origin of HIV is sub-Saharan Africa, and the origin of the virus is animal, not human: humans have no immunity to HIV because it 'is basically an animal disease'.[63]

The fields of virology, immunology and infectious disease control have, of course, become infinitely more complicated over the twentieth century. However it is not uncommon to find, as in this article, traces of the nineteenth-century concerns in contemporary scientific, public health and epidemiological debate. In particular, the nineteenth-century contestation about the true source of vaccine matter continues in several manifestations. First, there remains an insistence on affirming or disproving Jenner's status as the originator of the technology of vaccination itself. For example a local history webpage devotes some space to 'the first recorded Smallpox vaccination' by Benjamin Jesty in Dorset in 1774.[64] Second, enquiries into the genealogy of Jenner's vaccine and the subsequent strains of the attenuated virus appear intermittently in quite the same paradigm as the nineteenth-century search for origins and authenticity, albeit overlain with twentieth-century virological and immunological insights and questions. For example, Peter Razzell's intriguing book *Edward Jenner's Cowpox Vaccine: The History of a Medical Myth* (1977) argues that the major vaccine Jenner used throughout his lifetime, and from which other vaccines were developed, derived not from the cowpox virus at all, but was an attenuated strain of the smallpox virus. Thus, he writes in a further book, this 'undermines the polarisation of vaccination and inoculation, with the one being viewed as safe and effective, the other as dangerous and demographically damaging'.[65] Razzell turns conventionally to historical documentation for evidence to support his theory. More interestingly, though, is his subsequent turn to the twentieth-century virus itself to see what traces of its own socio-biological history are readable by virological technologies available in the 1970s. In quite the same manner as any number of nineteenth-century writers, he summarises research into the relative characteristics of smallpox, cowpox and the then current strains of the vaccinia virus: 'The three viruses are very closely related . . . but differences have made it impossible to establish any clear-cut genealogical relationship between them.'[66] The riddle of origins and the imperative to trace genealogies continue. For example, this partly drives the World Health Organization's reluctance to destroy the last remaining smallpox virus, in order to apply the more recent historical and genealogical technology of DNA testing to the determination of its pedigree.

It is also possible to trace aspects of the orientalist and colonialist history of smallpox, inoculation and vaccination into the mid and late twentieth-century histories of globalisation and cold war militarisation. Over the last two centuries one can trace a nice global chase, if you like, between smallpox and its vaccine matter. As smallpox epidemics shifted from country to country, they were accompanied or followed by the vaccine in precious vials. As the vaccine matter travelled and multiplied, the smallpox matter reduced. As a result of the WHO eradication campaign, it is now the smallpox virus itself which is kept in the two 'precious vials' in the State Research Centre of Virology and Biotechnology, Russia and the Center for Disease Control and Prevention, Atlanta, Georgia, USA. If there was an obsessive concern in the nineteenth century with the lineage and location of the vaccine matter, in the late twentieth century this global obsession has been inverted: that is, there is now an imperative to know where the microbe itself is, with ensuring that it stays in those known places, that it doesn't move; an anxiety informed partly by biological warfare scares.[67] WHO's deferral of the destruction of the virus (although this has been scheduled several times) suggests that its existence in known and surveilled locations is more reassuring than the uncertainty which might accompany its destruction – that it would then be 'nowhere'.[68] In all of these sites one finds retellings of longstanding anxieties about the use of one infection to prevent another, about the production of unknown viral mutations and new diseases, about inter-species crossing, about racial/sexual transmissions and global movement in populations, now figured between the 'third' and 'first' worlds. There is still a sense, then, in which vaccination as contagion is perceived as culturally and biologically dangerous.

Notes

Sincere thanks Carolyn Strange, Claire Hooker, Roy Macleod and Glenda Sluga for their sharp readings of several versions of this chapter. Thanks also to Michelle Arrow and Maria Nugent and for quality research assistance, commentary and collegiality. Research was made possible through funding from the Australian Research Council and in collaboration with the Powerhouse Museum, Sydney.

1 F. Newman, *The Coming Revolution*, Nottingham, Bailey and Smith, 1882, p. 11, cited in D. Porter and R. Porter, 'The Politics of Prevention: Anti-Vaccinationism and Public Health in Nineteenth Century England', *Medical History*, 1988, vol. 32, p. 241; see also C. Huerkamp, 'The History of Smallpox Vaccination in Germany: A First Step in the Medicalization of the General Public', *Journal of Contemporary History*, 1985, vol. 20, p. 628; M. Clark Nelson and J. Rogers, 'The Right to Die? Anti-Vaccination Activity and the 1874 Smallpox Epidemic in Stockholm', *Social History of Medicine*, 1992, vol. 5, pp. 382–7; R. M. Macleod, 'Law, Medicine and Public Opinion: the Resistance to Compulsory Health Legislation, 1870–1907', *Public Law*, 1967, pp. 106–28, 188–211; A. Beck, 'Issues in the Anti-Vaccination Movement in England', *Medical History*, 1960, vol. 4, p. 4, 313, 317; A. Wohl, *Endangered Lives: Public Health in Victorian Britain*, London, J. M. Dent, 1983, pp. 133–4.
2 See D. Armstrong, 'Public Health Spaces and the Fabrication of Identity', *Sociology*, 1993, vol. 27, pp. 393–410; A. Petersen and D. Lupton, *The New Public Health: Health and Self in the Age of Risk*, London, Sage, 1996, p. 7; D. Lupton, *The Imperative of Health: Public Health and the Regulated Body*, London, Sage, 1995, p. 19; D. Porter, *Health, Civilization and the State*, London, Routledge, 1999, p. 38.
3 This is clearly evident in the famous anti-vaccinationist activity in Leicester where notification and isolation policies were practised in defiant and explicit opposition to compulsory vaccination laws. See Wohl, *Endangered Lives*, p. 134.
4 C. Waldby, *AIDS and the Body Politic: Biomedicine and Sexual Difference*, London, Routledge, 1996, p. 107.
5 See A. McClintock, *Imperial Leather: Race, Gender and Sexuality in the Colonial Contest*, London, Routledge, 1995.
6 E. Said, *Orientalism: Western Conceptions of the Orient*, Harmondsworth, Penguin, 1995.
7 See J. Nguyet Erni, *Unstable Frontiers: Technomedicine and the Cultural Politics of 'Curing' AIDS*, Minneapolis and London, University of Minnesota Press, 1994, pp. 69–88.

8 A. Bashford, 'Quarantine and the Imagining of the Australian Nation', *Health*, 1998, vol. 2, pp. 387–402; 'Epidemic and Governmentality: Smallpox in Sydney, 1881', *Critical Public Health*, 1999, vol. 9, pp. 301–16; ' "Is White Australia Possible?" Race, Colonialism and Tropical Medicine', *Ethnic and Racial Studies*, 2000, vol. 23, pp. 248–71.
9 The process of nineteenth-century arm-to-arm vaccination was nicely modelled by the Australian Broadcasting Commission's television news graphics team in their efforts to illustrate the famous 1999 Melissa Virus. One infected computer contaminates fifty others through direct email connections, each contaminating a further fifty. Only in the dreams of nineteenth-century vaccinationists would the process be so efficient. But the fact remains that vaccination – a process for the prevention of disease – worked through a logic of exponential infection, a logic of contagion.
10 See e.g. J. B. Buist, *Vaccinia and Variola: A Study of their Life History*, London, J. & A. Churchill, 1887, pp. 1–4.
11 W. Cleaver Woods, 'The Recent Unsatisfactory Position of Vaccination in the Commonwealth', *Australasian Medical Gazette*, 20 May 1905, p. 208.
12 D. Haraway, 'Biopolitics of Postmodern Bodies: Constitutions of Self in Immune System Discourse', in her *Simians, Cyborgs and Women*, New York, Routledge, 1991, p. 204.
13 Evidence of Alfred Roberts, Select Committee: Opinions on Compulsory Vaccination, New South Wales Legislative Assembly, *Votes and Proceedings*, 1881, vol. 4, p. 248. [Hereafter Select Committee on Vaccination, 1881]
14 A. Tauber, *The Immune Self: Theory or Metaphor*, Cambridge, Cambridge University Press, 1994, p. 6, pp. 26–7.
15 Evidence of Carl F. Fischer, Select Committee on Vaccination, 1881, p. 8.
16 J. Compton Burnett, *Vaccinosis and its Cure by Thuja: With Remarks on Homeoprophylaxis*, London, The Homoeopathic Publishing Co., 1897, pp. 128–9. Of course there was no homoeopathic consensus on vaccination. John Le Gay Brereton was also a homoeopathic practitioner, but he entirely opposed vaccination. In 1881 he said, 'I would rather be shot than have anyone of my family vaccinated.' Evidence of John le Gay Brereton, Select Committee on Vaccination, 1881, p. 25.
17 W. D. Stokes, *Truth V. Error: A Scientific Treatise Showing the Dangers of Drugs as Medicine*, Brighton, n.d., p. 452.
18 Melbourne Branch of the British Union of Vivisection, *Vaccination a Failure*, Melbourne, 1946.
19 E. Blackwell, *Scientific Method in Biology*, London, Elliot Stock, 1898, p. 65; see M. Douglas, *Purity and Danger: An Analysis of the Concepts of Pollution and Taboo*, London, Routledge, 1994; see also A. Bashford, *Purity and Pollution: Gender, Embodiment and Victorian Medicine*, Basingstoke, Macmillan, 1998, p. xi.
20 E. Robinson, 'Can Disease Protect Health? Being a Reply to Ernest Hart's Pamphlet Entitled 'The Truth about Vaccination'', London, 1880.
21 Beck, 'Issues in the Anti-Vaccination Movement', p. 315.
22 Evidence of John le Gay Brereton, Select Committee on the Vaccination Bill, *Journals of the NSW Legislative Council*, vol. 21, 1872, pp. 24, 28 [hereafter Select Committee on Vaccination, 1872].
23 J. P. Murray, *Small-pox, Chicken-pox and Vaccination*, Melbourne, George Robertson, 1869, p. 14.
24 After the 1881 epidemic of smallpox in Sydney there were calls for a vaccine calf farm to be established for those who did not want arm-to-arm vaccination. See Report on the Late Visitation of Small-pox, NSW Legislative Assembly, *Votes and Proceedings*, 1883, vol. 2, p. 10. For England, see D. Porter and R. Porter, 'The Politics of Prevention', p. 234.

25 Huerkamp, 'The History of Smallpox Vaccination in Germany', p. 630.
26 J. Beaney, *Vaccination and its Dangers*, Melbourne, RN Henningham, 1870, p. 11 [original emphasis].
27 Evidence of John T. Marx, Select Committee on Vaccination, 1872, p. 28.
28 A. Peripateticus, *Cancer: A Result of Vaccination*, Melbourne, J. C. Stephens, 1898.
29 Evidence of John le Gay Brereton, Select Committee on Vaccination, 1881, p. 28. Such theories anticipate current concerns that the sudden appearance and virulence of the Human Immuno-deficiency Virus in parts of Africa in the 1980s was a result of the intense WHO smallpox eradication campaign in the preceding decades. See R. Porter, *The Greatest Benefit to Mankind: A Medical History of Humanity from Antiquity to the Present*, London, FontanaPress, 1999, p. 491.
30 Sometimes these anxieties were well founded, sometimes they were clearly part of other mythologies. For medical histories which explore the connection between migration and infectious disease, see A. W. Crosby, *Ecological Imperialism: The Biological Expansion of Europe, 900–1900*, Cambridge, Cambridge University Press, 1986; A. Kraut, *Silent Travelers: Germs, Genes and the 'Immigrant Menace'*, Baltimore, 1991; P. D. Curtin, *Death by Migration: Europe's Encounter with the Tropical World in the Nineteenth Century*, Cambridge, Cambridge University Press, 1989; L. Manderson, 'Migration, Prostitution and Medical Surveillance in Early Twentieth Century Malaya', in L. Marks and M. Worboys (eds), *Migrants, Minorities and Health: Historical and Contemporary Studies*, London and New York, Routledge, 1997, pp. 49–69.
31 See below, Ch. 5.
32 Porter, 'The Greatest Benefit', p. 490.
33 It is no coincidence that 'immunity' has both biological and governmental/bureaucratic meanings. Its original medical usage stemmed from a Latin usage: 'exemption from military service'. See K. Walker, *The Story of Medicine*, London, Arrow, 1959, p. 230.
34 See P. H. Curson, *Times of Crisis: Epidemics in Sydney 1788–1900*, Sydney, Sydney University Press, 1985.
35 J. H. L. Cumpston and F. McCallum, *The History of Small-Pox in Australia 1909–1923*, Melbourne, Government Printer, 1925, pp. 31–2, 77.
36 Cumpston and McCallum, *The History of Small-Pox in Australia 1909–1923*, p. 15.
37 Cabinet of the NSW Legislative, *Council Opinions upon Compulsory Vaccination*, Sydney, Government Printer, 1881, p. 223.
38 Walker, *The Story of Medicine*, p. 224.
39 H. J. Parish, *Victory with Vaccines: The Story of Immunization*, Edinburgh and London, E. & S. Livingstone, 1968, p. 9.
40 *Dorland's Medical Dictionary*, Philadelphia, W. B. Saunders, 1994, p. 1796.
41 One popular medical historian depicts an orientalised, turbaned Montagu and writes that while 'inoculation was practised widely in the Near East and the Orient for centuries, it was made popular in Europe chiefly through Lady Montague's [sic] crusading'. S. R. Riedman, *The Story of Vaccination*, Folkestone, Bailey Brothers and Swinfen, 1974, p. 13. See W. Frith, 'Sex, Smallpox and Seraglios: A Monument to Lady Mary Wortley Montagu', in G. Perry and M. Rossington (eds), *Femininity and Masculinity in Eighteenth-Century Art and Culture*, Manchester and New York, Manchester University Press, 1994, pp. 99–122.
42 D. Masters, *The Conquest of Disease*, London, John Lane, 1925, p. 36.
43 A. Collie, *On Fevers, their History, Aetiology, Diagnosis, Prognosis and Treatment*, London, H. K. Lewis, 1887, p. 161. See also D. Arnold, *Colonising the Body: State Medicine and Epidemic Disease in Nineteenth-Century India*, Berkeley, Calif., University of California Press, 1993, p. 151; Beck, 'Issues in the Anti-Vaccination Movement', p. 311.
44 See Arnold, *Colonising the Body*, pp. 151–2.

45 Ibid., p. 144.
46 For careful detail of the eighteenth-century English interest in the practice of these women, see P. Razzell, *The Conquest of Smallpox: The Impact of Inoculation on Smallpox Mortality in Eighteenth Century Britain*, Firle, Caliban, 1977, pp. 2–6.
47 See J. Z. Bowers, 'The Odyssey of Smallpox Vaccination', *Bulletin of the History of Medicine*, 1981, vol. 55, pp. 17–33.
48 See Bowers, 'The Odyssey of Smallpox Vaccination', pp. 17–33. R. Porter writes of the 'spread' of variolation. See Porter, *The Greatest Benefit*, p. 276.
49 A. Petersen and D. Lupton, *The New Public Health: Health and Self in the Age of Risk*, Sydney, Allen and Unwin, 1996, pp. 27–60.
50 Evidence of Samuel Pickford Bedford, Select Committee on Vaccination, 1872, p. 790.
51 For example, this question was put to the Tasmanian Parliament in 1908. See 'Vaccination and Quality of Lymph', *Australasian Medical Gazette*, 20 Oct. 1908, p. 567.
52 Evidence of Miles Egan, Select Committee on Vaccination, 1872, p. 796.
53 *Sydney Daily Telegraph*, 14 Jul. 1881, p. 4; *Sydney Daily Telegraph*, 10 Aug. 1881, p. 4.
54 Evidence of John le Gay Brereton, Select Committee on Vaccination, 1881, p. 27.
55 C. Creighton, *The Natural History of Cow-Pox and Vaccinal Syphilis*, London, Cassell, 1887, pp. 23–8.
56 Creighton, *The Natural History of Cow-Pox*, pp. 25–6. Here inoculation means vaccination. For further nineteenth-century discussion of the origin of Jenner's lymph see E. M. Crookshank, *The History and Pathology of Vaccination*, 2 vols. London, H. K. Lewis, 1889.
57 J. Morton, *Vaccination and its Evil Consequences*, Parramatta, C. E. Fuller, 1875, p. 5.
58 Evidence of Dr Charles Taylor, Select Committee on Vaccination, 1872, p. 17.
59 Ibid., p. 18.
60 See e.g. Evidence of John le Gay Brereton, Select Committee on Vaccination, 1872, p. 27.
61 House of Representatives Debate on the Quarantine Bill, 16 Jul. 1907, *Commonwealth Parliamentary Debates*, p. 1734.
62 D. Siefkes, 'The Origin of HIV-1, The AIDS Virus', *Medical Hypotheses*, 1993, vol. 41, p. 289.
63 Ibid., p. 295.
64 'The first recorded Smallpox vaccination'. Online. Available http://home.sprynet.com/~btomp/smallpox.htm. 18 Dec. 1999.
65 P. Razzell, *Edward Jenner's Cowpox Vaccine: The History of a Medical Myth*, Firle, Caliban, 1977, p. 5; see the genealogical table on p. 23 of this book. Peter Razzell, *The Conquest of Smallpox*, p. ix. See also D. Baxby, *Jenner's Smallpox Vaccine: The Riddle of Vaccinia Virus and its Origin*, London, 1981; D. Baxby, 'The Origins of Vaccinia Virus – An Even Shorter Rejoinder', *Social History of Medicine*, 1999, vol. 12, p. 139; P. Razzell, 'The Origins of Vaccinia Virus – A Brief Comment', *Social History of Medicine*, 1999, vol. 12, p. 141.
66 Razzell, *Edward Jenner's Cowpox Vaccine*, p. 97.
67 See 'Questions and Answers on Bio-Warfare/Bio-Terrorism with Dr Ken Alibek', 17 Mar. 2000. Online. Available http://www.emergency.com/1999/alibek99.htm.
68 'Future Research on Smallpox Virus Recommended', 10 Dec. 1999. Online. Available http://www.who.int/inf-pr-1999/en/pr99-77.html.

3 Moral contagion and the will

The crisis of masculinity in fin-de-siècle France

Christopher E. Forth

Enlightenment and Romantic theories about the autonomy of the self have received their fair share of criticism in recent decades, and for some very good reasons. Many of these criticisms, whether informed by feminist, Marxist, postcolonialist, or poststructuralist theoretical frameworks, tend to agree on at least one crucial point: that the generalised concept of selfhood posited by western thinkers implicitly referred to a quite narrow group of white, bourgeois males who clothed their particularity in a rhetoric of universality. Nevertheless the overtly masculinist ideal of personal autonomy – of being 'master of oneself' or 'captain of one's destiny' – has been powerful enough to shape the contours of an entire culture, so much so that today, the very notion of a loss of control can elicit feelings of embarrassment, pity and even disgust.[1] Such responses have a long lineage, for those whose opinions and deeds deviate from mainstream prescriptions have historically been viewed as essentially weak-willed individuals slavishly beholden to the age-old power of custom, the persuasiveness of popular beliefs or the stirring of their own flesh. Since such people seemed to exempt themselves from personhood altogether, they could be scientifically categorised alongside women, children, 'primitives', criminals and the insane in the cultural imagination. Armed with the ideal of a heroically independent self, western physicians, scientists, and social critics searched for ways of understanding those 'others' who, either through congenital defects or acquired habits, seemed unable to exercise the volition considered proper to the species.

During the nineteenth century a wide range of behaviour, from fairly benign acts like yawning, facial tics, laughter and tears, to more dangerous activities like murder, rioting, madness and suicide, were typically conceived as the result of what physicians and other observers called 'moral' or 'mental' contagion. Insofar as it was said to act upon a person's unconscious and thus bypass the rational will, this form of contamination appeared to most commentators as a veritable liquidation of selfhood: 'Mental contagion ... excludes all idea of deliberation on the part of the subject who submits: it is always produced without the intervention of the "I will", of the idea of the ego as the cause that executes it.'[2] With female psychology traditionally considered to be naturally unstable and amorphous, it was thought quite natural that women would be more susceptible than men to such external influences, a view that fostered the understanding that a loss of selfhood represented a form of 'feminisation'. Putatively equipped with firm wills and a stronger sense of their own individuality, many contended that healthy men were able to resist being penetrated by external stimuli.

In order to demonstrate what can happen when the cultural ideal of subjective autonomy collides with the everyday practice of trying to live such an ideal, this chapter explores the interrelationship between theories of moral contagion and changing concepts of masculine identity in France at the end of the nineteenth century. During the turn of the century, a period recognised for a 'crisis of masculine identity',[3] fears about moral contagion often invoked contemporary anxieties about the collapse of volition in the face of the hyperstimulus of urban modernity. Conceived against the background of new developments in psychology, moral contagion served as a reminder that lapses of the will could strike any man, a realisation that prompted a widespread cultural obsession with the fortification or 'education' of the manly will during the early twentieth century. The rehabilitation of the will through physical culture and mental discipline was proposed as a means of constructing a new man capable of resisting the 'contagious' impact of unhealthy influences.[4]

Sites of contagion, crises of the will

With a history traceable to the eighteenth century, moral contagion proved a remarkably persuasive medico-social category despite widespread confusion about its actual functioning. As one physician admitted, 'Scholars have not always agreed on the causes of this contagion, but no one doubts its existence.'[5] The term 'moral contagion' was first coined in 1733 by Philippe Hecquet, a French physician who used the analogy of an epidemic to explain an incident of collective religious convulsions. As Jan Goldstein has shown, this form of contagion quickly helped expand the political role of the French medical profession against the competing interpretations of religious authorities and non-professional interlopers. Given the fact that the very notion of contagion invoked the long-standing collaboration between the medical profession and the state, the assertion that dangerous ideas could be similarly contagious conferred a significant degree of rhetorical power over medicine's expansion into matters of the mind by revealing that psychological disturbances also posed a danger to the public order.[6]

Eighteenth-century notions of moral contagion depended upon a person's susceptibility to the minute '*corpuscules*' emitted by the bodies of others, which when absorbed by one's own body facilitated the transmission of the moral qualities of the other. 'All living bodies transpire,' explained the prominent physician S. A. Tissot in 1760; 'every instant half the pores of the skin exhale a very subtle humour, that is more important than all the rest of our evacuations. At the same time another kind of pores receive [*sic*] part of the fluids which surround us, and communicate them to the vessels.' The perspiration of strong people therefore 'contains something nutritious and strengthening, which being inspired by another invigorates him', while the emanations of weaker types, being 'corrupt and putrid', threaten to enfeeble those with hardy constitutions.[7] This was the conception of the body that Philippe Hecquet had in mind: since the *corpuscules* comprising the atmosphere around bodies were imprinted with the mark of that person's temperament and physical condition, individuals in close proximity to one another transmitted psychological states through the skin, which for Hecquet explained how the ecstasies of the *convulsionnaires* could be communicated to others.[8]

Against the relatively porous body posited by Enlightenment physicians, the biomedical body of the nineteenth century was conceived in rather different terms: the skin was no longer viewed as a passively permeable boundary, but was considered more or less sealed. After the discoveries of Pasteur many physicians conceded that while microbes could penetrate the body's surfaces, these minute bodies carried diseases rather than the moral qualities of others.[9] Such conclusions, however, failed to explain how an idea could pass from person to person, animating entire groups as if their individual wills had been nullified by some external suggestion. Troubling examples of crowd behaviour during the closing decades of the century, from the violence of the Paris Commune to the antisemitic riots of the Dreyfus Affair, seemed to confirm the suspicion that dangerous ideas could 'infect' individuals and compel them to commit criminal deeds.

Despite the metaphorical nature of moral contagion, many physicians employed the language of microbiology to explain the dynamics of this special form of contamination. In his study of contagious murder, for instance, Paul Aubry described moral contagion as the *'penetration of a morbid element into a prepared soil'*.[10] That is, with healthy individuals considered to be more or less immune to contamination, the majority of those identified as having succumbed to contagious influences also suffered from hereditary degeneration, nervous disorders, or some other acquired affliction, all of which fostered a special receptivity in the person. Lodged thus in a similarly unhealthy 'soil', the morbid 'seed' would act much like a microbe: 'there the idea will germinate, grow, ripen and, at a certain moment, secrete the toxins that will transform a normal brain into a criminal brain.'[11] However, this was no simple 'penetration' at work here, for while moral contagion was in many respects 'produced from the outside in', as two other specialists noted,[12] it also acted primarily upon those whose defences had been weakened and whose capacity for self-control was compromised. In this sense moral contagion represented a double capitulation to the outer world of 'contagious' ideas and to the inner world of affects and drives: the external 'other' seemed to form an alliance with the sensual 'other' within. Not only does this suggest an *eruption* or *uprising* as well as a penetration, but it indicates that on an unconscious level the individual welcomed the collapse of the will that contagion entailed.

The suspicion that anyone could succumb to moral contagion, or, as one doctor vividly put it, that 'the most virtuous being conceals a dormant criminal',[13] necessarily invoked some of the most recent findings in psychology pertaining to hypnotic suggestion. Indeed, alongside the idea of imitation, suggestion was the most widely cited mode of transmission for morbid ideas, and medical discussions about suggestion served as a point of intersection for debates about contagion and the paralysis of the will. Although Jean-Martin Charcot's ideas about suggestion attracted great notoriety at the *fin de siècle*, largely due to the physician's dramatic public hypnotism of hysterical female patients at the Salpêtrière hospital, his theories were quite conservative when compared to those of his rival from the city of Nancy, Hippolyte Bernheim. Contra Charcot, who claimed that only hysterical patients could be hypnotised, Bernheim presented evidence that healthy individuals were also subject to visual and verbal suggestion, and that such suggestion often took place in the waking state without the use of hypnosis. 'Sensorial hallucinations' were thus not only experienced by hysterics, but were an everyday reality for all people as they lived their lives. Bernheim's findings thus blurred the distinction between the subjective interior and the outside world in a way that helped shape the manner in which moral contagion would be conceived. 'We are all suggestible,' he contended. 'No one can escape the suggestive influence of others.'[14]

The ramifications of the debate between Bernheim and Charcot during the 1880s have been addressed in a number of historical works and need not be explored further here.[15] For our purposes it is important to note how this contest illuminates the relationship between moral contagion and the will. A number of physicians and social critics agreed with Charcot that only those with pre-existing nervous disorders like hysteria were susceptible to suggestion, a position which allowed them to maintain a sharp division between 'normal' and 'pathological' (read: feminine) personality types. Bernheim's more expansive understanding of suggestion undermined any such hard and fast distinctions by tacitly calling into question the sovereignty of the will in the psychic lives of all individuals. According to him, impairment of the will remained an ever present danger for anyone who came into contact with the innumerable suggestions offered by the modern world. The psychological tendency that Charcot assigned to women emerged in Bernheim's work as something manifested by men as well.

Considered in strict medical terms, paralysis of the will (or 'abulia') was often isolated as a disorder in itself that left the patient bedridden with no desire to do anything at all. Yet more frequently the disorder appeared as the most common and troubling symptom of nearly all of the period's other afflictions, from neurasthenia and hysteria to degeneracy, agoraphobia, and sexual 'perversions'. Despite a number of cases where the problem of female volition was raised, as in kleptomania and crimes of passion, the *fin-de-siècle* obsession with willpower primarily concerned men.[16] Indeed, nineteenth-century discourses of masculinity repeatedly stressed the need for a male to *be a man*, as if manliness were the result of an act of will. As Angus McLaren observes: 'To be a man required effort and labour that was not required of women. One did not goad on a woman by force of will to "be a woman"; she was born one. Exertion and activity was required to "be a man". In effect the public accepted implicitly the notion that manliness was a constructed identity because a male had to "prove" repeatedly at work and at play that he was a "man".'[17] The overall effort required to 'be a man' was the sum of all the ways in which willpower could manifest itself, and included the ability to withstand pain, to display courage in the face of danger (especially when fighting duels), and, in short, to steel the body as a means of overcoming the sensuality of 'the flesh'. This practical logic was reinforced by medical wisdom wherein volition emerged as much more of a factor in the male psyche than it was in the female, mostly due to the assumption that women (and other countertypes like Jews, criminals and the insane) were closely tied to the flesh in ways that 'normal' men were not. Above all, as one physician noted, an inability to exert effort left one 'powerless' in the face of the 'unhealthy incitations' of the outside world.[18] In medical texts and in everyday life willpower was considered an intrinsically masculine quality and its diminishment or collapse signified a slide into effeminacy.[19]

Despite this association of manhood and willpower, in medical texts it was the collapse rather than the triumph of the will that seemed more likely. As Théodule Ribot declared in his classic study, *Les Maladies de la volonté*, the will is no natural psychological given but is rather 'the result of art, of education, of experience. It is an edifice constructed slowly, piece by piece. Observation, both objective and subjective, shows that every form of voluntary activity is the fruit of a conquest.'[20] What one 'conquered' in the act of volition was the substratum of desire, images and fantasies that constituted humanity's primitive heritage, a reservoir of irrationality threatening to engulf the person whenever the will wavered. Yet from Ribot's physicalist perspective the will was not a simple idea standing over and above the body, but was itself a reflection of material processes. Indeed, having maintained that moral precepts needed to be *felt* in order to have any sway over the individual, Ribot concluded that the 'predominance of the affective life does not necessarily exclude the will: an intense, stable, permitted passion is the very basis of all energetic wills'.[21] In light of the various diseases of the will observed at the *fin de siècle*, Ribot affirmed the rather frail nature of such a faculty and reiterated the need for constant personal vigilance: 'the will is not an entity reigning by right of birth, although sometimes disobeyed, but a resultant always unstable, always ready to decompose itself, and, to say truly, a happy accident.'[22]

In the eyes of many worried observers, the entire modern world seemed committed to toppling this already unstable faculty. Commentators from across the political spectrum bemoaned the negative effects that modern urban existence had upon the minds and bodies of both men and women, and often charted a decline of manhood that seemed to march in step with the endless parade of modern advancements. In his famous work on degeneration, the physician and social critic Max Nordau pointed to hyperstimulus as wearing away the nerves of westerners: 'Even the little shocks of railway travelling, not perceived by consciousness, the perpetual noises, and the various sights in the streets of a large town, our suspense pending the sequel of progressive events, the constant expectation of the newspaper, of the postman, of visitors, cost our brains wear and tear.'[23] Novels and the mass circulation press seemed to exacerbate the problem by serving as vehicles for 'contagious' ideas: jurists and criminal anthropologists often claimed that the newspaper coverage of sensational trials and the glorification of criminals in novels only encouraged impressionable readers to imitate the crimes described.

In his 1903 essay, 'The Metropolis and Mental Life', German sociologist Georg Simmel pointed to the expansion of mental life as a possible bulwark against the potentially debilitating effect of modernity: 'Intellectuality is thus seen to preserve subjective life against the overwhelming power of metropolitan life.'[24] Such a view would have had few champions in France, however, where since the 1880s physicians and educators alike noted with alarm the increase of *surmenage intellectuel* (intellectual exhaustion) among high school students who developed their minds while allowing their bodies to wither away. The academic reforms instituted in the wake of such findings, including the scaling back of study hours and their replacement with physical education and rest, did not cause the furore about intellectual labour to abate. Rather, as a disease associated with youth *surmenage intellectuel* found its adult complement in neurasthenia, which also traced its origins to the sedentary lives of white-collar professionals where mental activity took pride of place to manual labour. The self-help manuals of the period emphasised this point clearly: whereas the intellectual development of females was thought to produce 'mannish' women, excessive cerebrality among males threatened to generate effeminate men.[25] In short, the very faculty that Simmel believed might allow humans to thrive in modernity was viewed across the Rhine as an occasion for the victory of modernity over the will.

Crowd psychology crystallised many contemporary anxieties about the expansion of suggestion and the decline of volition in the age of the masses. In his famous study *Psychologie des foules* Gustave Le Bon developed an influential, if rather derivative, theory of the collective mind that applied the recent psychological theories of Bernheim and Charcot to social phenomena. 'In a crowd every sentiment and act is contagious,' Le Bon observed, 'and contagious to such a degree that an individual readily sacrifices his personal interest to the collective interest.'[26] Although he sometimes claimed that those who participate in mass activities often suffer from hereditary degeneration and other disorders, Le Bon also insisted that crowd formation implied a process of psychological levelling that affected all people regardless of their gender, heredity, social class or level of education. Insofar as 'suggestions are contagious in every human agglomeration', no one would be able to resist the lure of the mass: 'The conscious personality has entirely vanished; will and discernment are lost ... From the moment that they form part of a crowd the learned man and the ignoramus are equally incapable of observation.'[27] Le Bon's colleague Gabriel Tarde took this even further by arguing that a mild form of moral contagion that he called 'imitation' was the very essence of the social bond: 'A slow contagion from mind to mind, a tranquil and silent imitation, has always preceded and paved the way for these rapid contagions, these noisy and captivating imitations that characterise popular movements.'[28]

Developments such as these only exacerbated the masculinity crisis that France had experienced since the country's humiliating defeat at the hands of Prussia in 1870. The rise of the women's movement and the emergence of the career-minded New Woman at the end of the century suggested a migration of women from what many men considered their 'proper' sphere in society, an occurrence that infringed upon the traditionally male domain of public life. In addition, the growing visibility of homosexuals, usually counted among the most 'effeminate' males, seemed to testify to the replacement of 'real' men by effete copies. Finally, the *fin-de-siècle* shift in labour toward white-collar professions signalled for many the decline of physical action and courage, especially when many of these 'brain workers' ended up being diagnosed with neurasthenia. All of this flowed into the pressing issue of depopulation, what Robert Nye appropriately terms the 'master pathology' of the period. With the population of the German empire growing steadily, the decline of the French birthrate since the 1850s prompted a massive campaign to reverse this downward trend. By failing to channel their energy into marriage and family, men and women who drifted from conventional gender roles at the end of the century seemed to shirk their national duty.[29]

By the late nineteenth century French men had reason to be suspicious of traditional ideals about the autonomy of the self, for much of what they experienced in their culture seemed to mitigate such notions. Yet far from instilling a sense of fatalism in men, the gender crisis of the *fin de siècle* contributed in part to a renewed emphasis on the recuperation of manhood during the early twentieth century. There may not have been anything *naturally* autonomous about selfhood, but this did not rule out the possibility of deliberately trying to mould oneself into a cultural ideal. Physicians who insisted on innate disposition when it came to suggestibility found their claims countered by a larger group whose members cited the contagiousness of sensual distractions and the need for constant vigilance in order to sustain some semblance of masculine identity. For these authorities, whose insights had a significant impact upon the popular medicine of the day, manhood was something more or less produced by fostering willpower in men. Since manhood was indeed a construction, a veritable expression of will, doctors encouraged men to take an active role in their own fabrication.

Educating the will

In 1914, just months before the outbreak of the First World War, a new health spa opened near the French town of Chalon-sur-Saône offering treatment for nervous disorders, digestive problems and various substance addictions. In the promotional literature for the Maison de Saint-Remy, a single provocative phrase summed up the institution's overall curative project: 'Re-education of the will'. In the face of the apparent crumbling of volition and the decline of healthy manhood, the prospect that one could 'educate the will' was so attractive that it reverberated throughout French culture in the prewar years. Incorporating mental as well as physical therapy, the threefold regime practised at Saint-Remy reflected the mental and physical recommendations found in numerous self-help manuals for well over a decade: hydrotherapy, psychotherapy and rest.[30]

The apparently personal weaknesses that might lead one to a sanatorium had a distinctly national resonance that was frequently noted by critics like the social philosopher Alfred Fouillée: 'Neurosis is a danger to the individual, but it is much more a danger to the nation ... We fear a weakening of moral vigour, of courage, consistency, firmness, of all the qualities that create the life force. Intelligence is refined along with the nerves, but willpower is weakened along with the muscles.'[31] The regime at Saint-Remy was just one example of the emphasis on reversing the effeminacy of French life during the prewar years. Given the diffusion of microbiological metaphors of 'seed' and 'soil', it became imperative to transform one's inner garden into an inhospitable place for infectious thoughts. When one was not marked by hereditary taint or nervous disorder, doctors warned about the weaknesses bred through overindulgence in many modern diversions, including the reading of novels and newspapers, and the cultivation of 'filthy habits'.[32] By cultivating a strong will, a man would be in a position to protect himself from 'dangerous invasions'.[33]

The therapeutic ethos of the early twentieth century emphasised working the body as a means of overcoming crises of the will and resisting the power of moral contagion. Many health reformers approvingly cited the words of Rousseau, who in his rather austere educational philosophy expressed a similar concern for the self in an urbanised eighteenth-century world: 'The weaker the body, the more it commands; the stronger it is, the more it obeys. All the sensual passions lodge in effeminated bodies.'[34]

What some historians have seen as a virtual 'rediscovery of the body' at this time was manifested in a widespread interest in sports, gymnastics, bodybuilding and an increasing emphasis on the acquisition of 'force'. The ideal man being constructed in these medical discourses was one capable of sustaining his mental autonomy through sheer willpower. Men who succumbed to moral contagion therefore exempted themselves from the ranks of such men to take their place alongside women and children, those with weaker constitutions who by virtue of their 'impressionable' nervous systems 'receive and transform the expressive movement and consequently submit to the external influence'.[35] Even neo-Kantian philosophers, who usually contested the tendency of physicians to ground mental phenomena in the body, agreed that 'hygiene and medicine constitute the two great groups of objective means by which we indirectly submit to our personal power'.[36]

Strengthening the will and acquiring 'personal power' became so fashionable after 1900 that some men began to assert their self-mastery through the cultivation of 'magnetic' personalities. Where physicians disagreed about the many factors that contributed to moral contagion, most concurred that suggestibility was the single most important ingredient in determining one's susceptibility to outside influences. For instance, famed psychologist Alfred Binet considered congenital predisposition to play a deciding role in a person's ability to resist suggestion. Binet recognised four principal personality types that manifested different degrees of suggestibility, from those who were especially prone to suggestion to those seemingly born to exercise their powers of suggestion over others. 'We can certainly say that *les suggestionneurs* ... have a greater chance of succeeding in life than do *les suggestibles*.'[37] This belief that it was better to be a virtual hypnotist than *un suggestible* was echoed in advertisements in popular health magazines and self-help manuals that taught men how to increase their personal magnetism and secure wealth and happiness by learning how to manipulate others. Having intelligence and strong opinions are very useful for success, counselled one such author, but they are not enough: 'you must exert a sort of fascination over your peers; you must dominate them, impose your views upon them ... To have all of that, one must possess personal magnetism.'[38] Finally, this collective fantasy of achieving a sense of power through irresistible seductiveness may have had even more personal dimensions: Alain Corbin cites the rise of seduction fantasies in brothels at the end of the century, where clients began to insist on scenarios in which prostitutes played the role of helpless 'virgins' to their seductive overtures.[39]

Such flights of fantasy were often complemented by new dietary and exercise regimens as doctors virtually fell over one another in an attempt to bolster the virility of the nation. If modernity seduced men and destroyed their ability to withstand external stimuli, then the new man would have to gird himself against its sensual overtures. Leaving aside the debate about innate and acquired suggestibility, many physicians concurred that 'educating the will' was the most reliable path toward such self-mastery, either as therapy for men with weak volition or as a prophylactic measure against the ubiquitous spectre of moral contagion. As one doctor noted, 'we recommend a severe disciplining of the will; it is the will that we must fortify, that we must "train" until it is master once and for all'.[40] Whatever influences threatened to overthrow a man's inner order, the will could be trained to resist and repel them. The physician Rambosson certainly saw things in this way, and even asserted that with 'a firm will, one can cure madness just as one can prevent it'. Man differs from the animal in his ability to conquer sensual material, the doctor maintained: 'through his will, through the power he wields over his brain, man can neutralise this cerebral movement, calm it, and thus more or less resist its impulsion.'[41]

A shift in the language used to market self-help literature around 1900 attests to this emphasis on the reconstruction of virility. In earlier years writers and publishers of popular health manuals contented themselves with fairly descriptive and neutral titles, such as *L'hygiène de l'adolescence* (1887), *Hygiène: à l'usage des gens du monde* (1894), *Hygiène des fiancés* (1896), and similar works that targeted potentially vulnerable age groups and lifestyles. By 1900, however, the language acquired a new urgency, employing a rhetoric of crisis and defence that implicated all readers in an increasingly pathological world. Of course the more conventional descriptive titles remained, but they were now joined on the shelf by more urgent appeals to the imperilled customer forced into a defensive posture. In the following manuals, all published in 1900, the self was clearly under siege: *Comment on se défend contre la neurasthénie*, *Comment on se défend des maladies*, and *Comment on défend ses organes intimes*. The world had become a dangerous place, it seems, requiring one to be kept abreast, as one author suggested, of the *Amis et ennemis du corps humain* (1905). Although the preservation or recuperation of manhood may have been subtly woven into older manuals, by this time the crisis of masculinity was loudly proclaimed. Indeed, in the burgeoning field of physical culture male weakness was assumed from the start, not to mention required for book sales: *Comment devenir énergique?* (1901), *Comment devenir fort* (1902), *Comment on devient beau et fort* (1905), *Comment on devient robuste* (1909). Other books simply barked orders at the pathetic weaklings of the 1890s, such as 1902's *Portez-vous bien!* Finally, if the new emphasis on the recuperation of manhood was not apparent enough in these titles, other authors spelled it out clearly with the rhetoric of force and virility: *La santé virile par l'hygiène* (1901), *L'art de conserver la santé et de vivre longtemps. Forces viriles. Beautés féminines* (1907), and *Force et beauté pour tous* (1908).

We need not content ourselves with simply reading the titles of such books, for the message disseminated within them articulated the same contemporary concern about physical collapse and the loss of virility. In his *Hygiène de l'adolescence* (1891), for instance, a manual that promised 'to harden [*endurcir*] the body through a virile education', Pèrier recommended that young men practise cold water therapy as a means of crafting 'strong subjects who are masters of themselves and ready to conquer the life of high struggle'.[42] New trends towards physical culture, abetted largely through the efforts of Edmond Desbonnet and his chain of bodybuilding centres, placed a great emphasis on the cultivation of the will, especially when condemning those obese men who lacked the will to conquer their bodies by eating less and exercising more. Here as elsewhere in hygienic literature an economic model of the body reigned supreme, and was explicitly counterposed to the hyperstimulus of modernity: 'The intellectual and physical exhaustion of modern life ... entails immense losses for the organism that demand compensation ... The disciplining of force consists in the perfect submission of the muscles to the will.'[43]

By far the most significant and widely read manual for the cultivation of willpower was Jules Payot's *L'Éducation de la volonté* (1893), which went through thirty-seven editions in less than twenty years and was translated into most European languages.[44] A former student of Théodule Ribot, Payot addressed his work to young men between 18 and 25 years of age, most of whom he assumed would go on to some white-collar profession, or 'intellectual labour'. Admitting that emotion *per se* was not incompatible with volition, Payot identified 'sensuality' as perhaps the most significant obstacle to masculine autonomy. 'Passion, that's animality victorious,' Payot had declared, 'the blind urge of heredity which darkens intelligence, oppresses it, and, moreover, enslaves it; it is the suppression of humanity within us, the debasement of what comprises at once our honour and our raison d'être: when it growls, we assume a different rung in the zoological hierarchy.'[45] A strong will would help curb the impulses of the flesh, thus providing a foundation from which one could also resist masturbation, prostitutes, alcohol, and other tempting diversions. Unlike many anticlerical physicians who associated religious faith with a decidedly 'feminine' credulity, Payot applauded the example of the Church as an educator of masculinity: 'Virility is there, and nowhere else: it is in this mastery of oneself – and the Church is right to see in chastity the supreme guarantee of the energy of the will.'[46]

Like many other hygienic reformers who distrusted the contaminating influence of the city, Payot depicted modern urban life as fraught with seductions and excitations that could cause young men to abandon themselves to their own sensuality. The young man should keep his body scrupulously clean and exercise regularly, thus engaging in what Payot called the 'primary school of the will'. Most of Payot's prescriptions were negative, however, and generally cautioned young men about a range of dangerous influences which must be carefully avoided, including the reading of novels, oversleeping, sitting for too long, overeating, eating spiced foods or excessive meat, alcohol, coffee, and consorting with 'libidinous comrades'.[47] All of these nefarious influences tended to produce a 'scattered' or 'dispersed' personality that was ill-equipped to remain committed to a particular goal in life. Physical and mental idleness was perhaps the best way to leave oneself open to being 'invaded' by sexual suggestions, for such passionate solicitations 'only have a chance of entering when the mind is empty'. In the event that some erotic thought did arise, however, special care must be taken: 'Here courage consists in flight. To struggle, one must use cunning. To attack the enemy head on is to run into defeat ... [unlike intellectual conquests] the great conquests over sensuality are accomplished by never thinking about it.'[48]

Due to its very fragility, the will alone could not be invoked in the battle against sensuality. Scholars influenced by Bernheim's theory of hypnosis subscribed to a very controlled form of prophylactic suggestion that could be employed to build up the self's ability to cope with the menace of moral contagion, a measure that was most appropriately termed 'moral vaccination'.[49] Sometimes administered to women with hope that they might resist the 'hypnotic' temptations of would-be seducers through the implantation of virtuous ideas, something akin to moral vaccination could be prescribed to young men for very similar reasons. Indeed, in its emphasis on psychotherapy the Maison de Saint-Remy deliberately tried to counter destructive habits of both men and women through the use of suggestion. Although Payot did not use this term, his emphasis on the therapeutic and prophylactic use of suggestion subtly invoked such an idea. 'Indeed, mastering oneself implies the reconquest of the self from the thousand suggestions from the external world, but it also and above all implies the domination of intelligence over the blind powers of feeling.'[50] In order to dissipate the 'haze' of the modern world, he wrote, one must retire from external distractions into a quiet state of 'meditative reflection' and 'in this state of calm, substitute for mediocre suggestions the suggestions of a great thinker, and allow this benevolent influence to penetrate to the depths of the soul'.[51] Against the vagaries of uncontrolled contagion-through-seduction one could administer rational and measured doses of counter-suggestion to inoculate oneself against future contamination.

In conclusion, it is evident that on some level the threat of moral contagion weighed heavy on the minds of men at the dawn of the twentieth century. The boundaries that were once thought to separate self from other no longer seemed to insulate man from the sensory overload of his modern environment, and thus left him vulnerable to 'invasions' that threatened his very identity. The obsessive reiteration of willpower and the recuperation of virility articulated in self-help manuals attests to this realisation of the fragile nature of masculinity, for ultimately such frantic affirmations suggest weakness rather than strength, and tacitly concede that there is really nothing 'natural' about masculinity itself. Despite the repeated emphasis on force, willpower and muscularity, the ideal male celebrated during the early 1900s was a cultural model that was deliberately contrasted with the 'soft' man of the past decade – yet this ideal could only be approximated through constant vigilance against what was often called the 'flood' or 'contagion' of sensual stimuli. Though constructed as normative, masculine identity emerges as the unstable result of repeated effort, the 'performance', in Judith Butler's terms, of an ideal script that can never be fully mastered.[52] Erected with an eye toward his possible collapse, the new man of the twentieth century would find his will endlessly plagued by the threat of moral contagion.

Notes

Many thanks to Alison Bashford and Claire Hooker for inviting me to contribute this chapter and for their helpful comments on earlier drafts. I am also grateful to my research assistant, Francine Morgan, for tracking down some rare medical texts, and to the Centre Parisien d'Études et de Documentation pour l'Enseignement et le Rayonnement du Français (CPEDERF) for their excellent research services. Aspects of this essay were made possible through funds from the Australian Research Council's Small Grants Scheme.

1 Susan Bordo's discussion of anorexia nervosa addresses the range of this emphasis on personal mastery. See S. Bordo, *Unbearable Weight: Feminism, Western Culture, and the Body*, Berkeley, Calif., University of California Press, 1993, pp. 139–64.
2 A. Vigouroux and P. Juquelier, *La Contagion mentale*, Paris, Octave Doin, 1905, p. 19.
3 A. Maugue, *L'Identité masculine en crise au tournant du siècle, 1871–1914*, Paris, Rivages, 1987.
4 In this chapter 'masculinity' refers not to a singular gender identity accepted by all, but to ideals asserted by different groups of men, each of whom maintained the right to define what counts as legitimate 'masculine' behaviour. Men engaged in this struggle typically posited codes of manhood that were often class-specific and mutually exclusive: what counted as 'manly' among artists, for instance, often appeared rather 'effeminate' to men of the working class. I am concerned in this chapter with a particularly persuasive version of manhood articulated in medical circles and circulated in French bourgeois society through periodical and self-help literature. This medical model of manhood was an extension of the widespread medicalisation of social problems and political crises at the end of the nineteenth century, what Robert Nye describes as an 'organicist discourse of national decline' that identified the body as the topos of many contemporary anxieties and a project for overcoming them. Cf. R. A. Nye, *Crime, Madness and Politics in Modern France*, Princeton, NJ, Princeton University Press, 1984.
5 J. Rambosson, *Phénomènes nerveux, intellectuels et moraux, leur transmission par contagion*, Paris, Librairie Firmin-Didot et cie., 1883, p. 196.
6 J. Goldstein, ' "Moral Contagion": A Professional Ideology of Medicine and Psychiatry in Eighteenth- and Nineteenth-Century France', in G. L. Geison (ed.), *Professions and the French State, 1700–1900*, Philadelphia, University of Pennsylvania Press, 1984, pp. 181–222.
7 S. A. Tissot, *Onanism: or, A Treatise Upon the Disorders Produced by Masturbation*, trans. A. Hume, London, 1767 [1760]; reprint, New York, Garland, 1985, pp. 81–2.
8 Goldstein, ' "Moral Contagion" ', pp. 186–7.
9 G. Vigarello, *Concepts of Cleanliness: Changing Attitudes in France since the Middle Ages*, trans. J. Birrell, Cambridge, Cambridge University Press, 1988, p. 205. This is not to say that physical contagion was entirely divorced from morality, for many

physicians blamed the transmission of cholera and tuberculosis, for example, on the moral inability of poorer populations to make their living spaces hygienically sound. On this point see A. R. Aisenberg, *Contagion: Disease, Government, and the 'Social Question' in Nineteenth-Century France*, Stanford, Calif., Stanford University Press, 1999, pp. 25, 60.

10 P. Aubry, *La Contagion du meurtre: étude d'anthropologie criminelle*, Paris, Alcan, 1894, p. 2.

11 Ibid., p. 12. On the role of 'soil' and 'seed' in contemporary debates about tuberculosis, see D. S. Barnes, *The Making of a Social Disease: Tuberculosis in Nineteenth-Century France*, Berkeley, Calif., University of California Press, 1995.

12 Vigouroux and Juquelier, *La Contagion mentale*, p. 22.

13 A. Corre, preface to Aubry, *La Contagion du meurtre*, p. xxi.

14 As quoted in D. L. Silverman, *Art Nouveau in Fin-de-Siècle France: Politics, Psychology, and Style*, Berkeley, Calif., University of California Press, 1989, p. 87.

15 R. Harris, *Murders and Madness: Medicine, Law, and Society in the Fin de Siècle*, Oxford, Clarendon Press, 1989.

16 See A.-L. Shapiro, *Breaking the Codes: Female Criminality in Fin-de-Siècle Paris*, Stanford, Calif., Stanford University Press, 1996, and C. E. Forth, 'Educating the Will: Masculinity and Modernity in *La Grande encyclopédie* (1886–1902)', in R. G. McInnis (ed.), *Discourse Synthesis: A Volume Dedicated to the History and Theory of Knowledge Cumulation*, Westport, Conn., Praeger, 2000.

17 A. McLaren, *Trials of Masculinity: Policing Sexual Boundaries, 1870–1930*, Chicago, University of Chicago Press, 1997, pp. 33–4.

18 Corre, preface to Aubry, *La Contagion du meurtre*, p. xv.

19 J. H. Smith, 'Abulia: Sexuality and Diseases of the Will in the Late Nineteenth Century', *Genders*, 1989, vol. 6, pp. 102–24; G. L. Mosse, *The Image of Man: The Creation of Modern Masculinity*, New York, Oxford University Press, 1996, pp. 100–1. Among women diseases of the will were often cited to confirm what doctors saw as the natural feebleness of the female. Medical discussions of the female criminal corroborated such a view by debating whether or not women could be responsible for their crimes due to their naturally 'disordered' biology. The situation was considered far more dire for men, whose entire identity was predicated on a healthy dose of self-control and the possession of an iron will. Lapses of female volition were to some extent expected, and thus confirmed for many the natural weakness of the sex; lapses of the male will, on the other hand, signified unmitigated pathology.

20 T. Ribot, *Diseases of the Will*, trans. Merwin-Marie Snell, Chicago, Open Court Publishing Company, 1894 (trans. from the 8th French edn, 1888), p. 64.

21 Ibid., p. 91.

22 Ibid., p. 65.

23 M. Nordau, *Degeneration*, Lincoln, Neb., University of Nebraska Press, 1993 (trans. from the 2nd German edn, 1895), p. 39.

24 G. Simmel, 'The Metropolis and Mental Life', in *The Sociology of Georg Simmel*, trans. K. H. Wolff, New York, The Free Press, 1967.

25 A. Rabinbach, *The Human Motor: Energy, Fatigue, and the Origins of Modernity*, Berkeley, Calif., University of California Press, 1990, pp. 146–78.

26 G. Le Bon, *The Crowd*, New York, Viking, 1960 (1st edn, 1895), p. 30.

27 Ibid., pp. 31, 39, 42.

28 G. Tarde, 'Les Crimes des foules', *Archives de l'anthropologie criminelle et des sciences pénales*, 1892, vol. 7, p. 355. Tarde's theory of imitation was developed more fully in *Les Lois de l'imitation*, Paris, Alcan, 1890.

29 Nye, *Crime, Madness, and Politics*; E. Berenson, *The Trial of Madame Caillaux*, Berkeley, Calif., University of California Press, 1992, pp. 169–207.

30 Advertisements for the Maison de Saint-Remy were prominently displayed, not surprisingly, in the medical magazine it published, *L'Esprit et le corps*.
31 As quoted in Silverman, *Art Nouveau*, p. 83.
32 Aubry, *La Contagion du meurtre*, p. 11.
33 F. Paulhan, *La Volonté*, Paris, Alcan, 1903, p. 37.
34 J.-J. Rousseau, *Emile, or On Education*, trans. Allan Bloom, New York, Basic Books, 1979, p. 54.
35 Rambosson, *Phénomènes nerveux*, p. 240.
36 Paulhan, *La Volonté*, p. 240.
37 A. Binet, 'La Suggestibilité au point de vue de la psychologie individuelle', *Annales des sciences psychiques*, 1899, vol. 9, p. 75.
38 A. de Browne, *La Puissance en soi-même par le magnetisme et l'hypnotisme*, Macon, Perroux, 1903, pp. 18–19.
39 A. Corbin, *Women for Hire: Prostitution and Sexuality in France After 1850*, trans. A. Sheridan, Cambridge, Mass., Harvard University Press, 1990, pp. 118, 168, 174–5.
40 C. Mélinand, 'Peur', *La Grande encyclopédie*, Paris, Société anonyme de la Grande encyclopédie, 1889, vol. 26, p. 558.
41 Rambosson, *Phénomènes nerveux*, pp. 234, 235.
42 E. Perier, *Hygiène de l'adolescence*, Paris, Baillière, 1891, pp. vi, 78.
43 J. de Lerne, *Comment devenir fort*, Paris, Baillière, 1902, pp. 152, 196. In a recent work Peter Stearns shows how remaining slender was considered a matter of willpower in France at the *fin de siècle*, but does not explore how such associations resonated with the period's masculinity crisis. Cf. P. N. Stearns, *Fat History: Bodies and Beauty in the Modern West*, New York, New York University Press, 1997.
44 J. Payot, *L'Éducation de la volonté*, Paris, Alcan, 1912 [1893].
45 Ibid., pp. 189–90.
46 Ibid., p. 210.
47 Ibid., pp. 203, 212.
48 Ibid., pp. 212–14.
49 For more on 'moral vaccination' see Harris, *Murders and Madness*, p. 189.
50 Payot, *L'Éducation*, pp. 116–17.
51 Ibid., p. 111.
52 J. Butler, *Gender Trouble*, New York, Routledge, 1993.

4 Excremental colonialism
Public health and the poetics of pollution

Warwick Anderson

> Although they called it architecture it was in fact elaborately built toilets, decorated toilets, toilets surrounded with and by business and enterprise in order to have something to do in between defecations since waste was the order of the day and the ordering principle of the universe ... That was the sole lesson of their world: how to make waste, how to make machines that make more waste, how to make wasteful products, how to talk waste, how to study waste, how to design waste, how to cure people who were sickened by waste so they could be well enough to endure it, how to mobilize waste, legalize waste and how to despise the culture that lived in cloth houses and shit on the ground far away from where they ate.
>
> Toni Morrison, *Tar Baby*[1]

In reading the literature of American public health in the Philippines, one soon becomes immersed in a poetics of pollution.[2] Medical texts insistently contrast a closed, ascetic American body with an open, grotesque Filipino body, the former typically in charge of a sterilised laboratory or clinic, the latter squatting in an unruly, promiscuous marketplace. Reductive as it may seem, this sequence of equivalence and opposition proved remarkably pervasive and effective. American colonial health officers in the early twentieth century turned their new tropical frontier into a desolate human-waste land, imagining everything 'brownwashed' with a thin film of germs. Thus constituted, the tropical environment called for massive, ceaseless disinfection; the Filipino bodies that polluted it required control and medical reformation; and the vulnerable, formalised bodies of the American colonialists demanded a sanitary quarantine. (By definition, the American body was necessarily closed off, abstracted from its tropical dislocation.) This is an essay, then, on the medical production of colonial bodies and colonial space – in other words, an essay about faeces, orifices, and toilets.

The personal hygiene of Filipinos – never much admired by ordinary Americans in the Islands – earned more than mere aesthetic or moral disapproval in early twentieth-century medical reports. Human wastes, the Bureau of Health warned Filipinos, 'are more dangerous than arsenic or strychnine'. Recent research had proven that 'dysentery, typhoid fever, cholera, and kindred diseases are conveyed to a person, regardless of whether he be king or peasant, with minute organisms that, probably, have passed through the bowels of another person'. Accordingly, all Filipinos should learn to treat their 'evacuated intestinal contents as a poison', taking care to avoid contact with them, or spreading them about.[3] Unlike Americans, Filipinos seemed to lack control of their orifices. 'The native and Chinese population,' lamented Dr Wallace De Witt, 'tend markedly to increase the general unhygienic surroundings by reason of their uncleanly habits.'[4] Thus it was clear to Dr Thomas R. Marshall, among others, that 'the Filipino people, generally speaking, should be taught that . . . promiscuous defecation is dangerous and should be discontinued'.[5] Ideally, Americans should train Filipinos to behave as meticulously and as retentively as themselves.

The importance of excrement in the medical world should not surprise us. Of all the manifold sources of germs – whether blood, urine, pus, water, soil, mucus, or saliva – faeces appeared to public health officers the most salient and the most dangerous, just as to an earlier generation of physicians the odour of human waste had been generally the most feared of all noxious emanations.[6] Throughout much of the nineteenth century, physicians had demonstrated special sensitivity to excremental odours, and their twentieth-century successors continued to identify human waste as a rich source of pathology. But with the development of a new bacteriological frame of mind, they discounted the morbidity of stenches in favour of the dangers of germs; the dire consequences of faeces derived more from direct physical contact, than from any olfactory action at a distance. Thus prevention usually meant interment and disinfection, more than simple deodorisation and ventilation. (Human waste, as we shall see, had to be rendered invisible as well as odourless.) But despite these permutations, the crucial link between excrement and danger was remarkably resilient, apparently immune to etiological trend. Alain Corbin, echoing Freud, has called this medical preoccupation the 'implacable return of excrement'.[7]

I intend to pursue the symbolic meaning of the colonial physician's obsession with 'matter out of place'.[8] Out of place themselves, American colonial health officers used the body's orifices and its products to mark racial and social boundaries in the Philippines. Waste practices were a potent means of organising a strange, teeming, threatening environment. In this new orificial order, American bodily control legitimated and symbolised social and political control, while the 'promiscuous defecation' of Filipinos appeared to mock and to transgress the supposedly firm, closed, colonial boundaries.[9] As Americans issued formal directives, and designed toilets, they imagined Filipinos – of a lower bodily (as well as social) stratum – defiantly subverting their hygienic abstractions and shitting regardless. The worst of it was that reckless pollution behaviour in the tropics seemed to endanger the lawful and innocent (Americans) instead of the trangressors (Filipinos) – lending force to those health officers who sought to constrain such delinquency. In constructing 'symbolic inversions' of the formal body and the abstract space of American colonialism, physicians sought to extend their power to inspect and regulate the personal conduct and the social life of the errant Filipinos.[10] The colonial state – its repressions and its discontents – came to be delineated on racialised bodies (Filipino or American), intimately reduced to orifices (open or closed) and dejecta (visible or invisible).

To attempt at this distance to determine the 'true' pattern of Filipino and American excretory practices is unrewarding at best. Even if such a positivist reckoning were possible, its results would contribute little to our understanding of the contemporary meaning of an objectifying corporeal poetics. Moreover, an exonerative ethnography risks perpetuating the frames of reference that gave rise to the charges in the first place. We may assume that Filipinos frequently transmitted pathogens – but so too did Americans. No doubt Filipinos, as much as Americans, constructed boundaries and transgressions with 'matter out of place', but American assertions suffuse the historical record. Accordingly, this essay focuses on colonial strategies of self-constitution, silencing and exclusion, rather than on reinstantiating biological, epidemiological, or phenomenological foundationalisms. Instead of renaming or naturalising abjection (that is, recuperating it as another object) I want to understand what was at stake politically in performing an American sublime and a Filipino abject. In what productive forms did bodily control extend colonial modernity? How were excretory habits racialised? How was pathology embodied? What did it mean to emphasise personal hygiene more than environmental sanitation? How did the medical officer's obsession with Filipino wastes render invisible the contributions of economic exploitation and social disruption – together more effective than even the most 'promiscuous' of 'defecators' – to the spread of disease? These are some of the questions that shaped this essay.

My argument is that the production of a space for somatic disciplining of supposedly refractory Filipinos was one of the more significant aspects of the American colonial project.[11] Animated by the new focus on microscopic germs and their passage through humans, insects and the environment, bacteriology's colonial enthusiasts eagerly sought out, isolated and disinfected native reservoirs and transmitters of pathology. If the exciting cause of disease could no longer be smelled, it could certainly be rendered visible through staining and culturing specimens obtained from the body and its environment – especially, disproportionately, the Filipino body.[12] These laboratory investigations reinforced fears of bodily contact in the tropics and encouraged American and European votaries of the new tropical medicine to extend further and to harden colonial social boundaries. Evolution had apparently fashioned Filipinos as natural carriers of tropical pathogens – germs to which previously unexposed whites were peculiarly vulnerable – and promiscuous Filipino behaviour was bound to fill up these natural corporeal reservoirs to overflowing. Or so it seemed to American public health officers in the early twentieth century.[13] The only responsible course, then, was to examine systematically the whole population of the archipelago, to disinfect it, and to reform its customs and habits. The new tropical medicine thus provides an instance of a material power that operates on distinctly racial bodies to produce the sort of body that colonial society required.[14] As the Philippine archipelago was remapped, so too were the bodies of Filipinos. But this spatialising project, as we shall see, required not only a 'confession of putrescence' from Filipinos but also constant self-discipline among American residents in the tropics, a transcendence of the 'natural' body, a territorial possessing predicated on self-possession.[15] And so waste became the order of the day, the ordering principle of the colonial Philippines.

Formal bodies and grotesque bodies

Sent to Surigao in 1902, Dr Henry du Rest Phelan, a medical officer with the United States Army, found the town a 'most charming and delightful spot', on a 'picturesque' site. But its sanitary condition alarmed him. Filth abounded. The *tiendas* were 'all more or less filthy', the promenade in front of them 'a lounging place for idlers of both sexes'. The ground beneath the houses was covered with 'filth of all kinds, human excrement included'; weeds had sprouted up in the streets, and garbage accumulated in vacant lots. That the Islands had recently endured a brutal war and massive social disruption meant little to Phelan; the problem seemed one of Filipino fecklessness and lack of 'civilisation'. 'They appear to me,' he reported, 'like so many children who need a strong hand to lead them in the path they are to follow.' Filipinos were wilfully polluting the soil, even around their own houses. Accordingly, Phelan, 'necessarily somewhat autocratic', began his 'crusade against filth'. In a short time, 'the roads were clean, the marshes drained, the houses purified, and the inhabitants impressed with the necessity of adopting new rules of hygiene'. And when, despite this transition from 'squalor' to cleanliness, the mortality rate climbed, Phelan wryly speculated on whether the transition itself 'could have given the community a shock sufficient to cause such a thinning out of its ranks'.[16]

Over the next decade, disease surveys and laboratory investigations confirmed the dangers of Filipino excrement and reinforced American fears of contact with native bodies and their products. Weston P. Chamberlain reported that more than 95 per cent of lowland Filipinos showed parasites in their stools. Since most natives, unlike Americans, were inured to these organisms, disease carriage was usually asymptomatic. Therefore vulnerable foreigners would be wise to treat all Filipinos as potentially infected and dangerous. In 1908, P. E. Garrison claimed he had discovered 'one of the most striking instances in the history of medicine of a population almost universally infested with animal parasites'. Accordingly, he recognised the 'imperative need' to control 'the methods of the disposal of the excreta customary among the Filipino people'. And in the 1915 cholera outbreak, E. L. Munson, using 'laboratory facilities in the making of bacteriological diagnoses on a large scale', found that Filipino vibrio carriers 'would seem not only the most numerous but the most insidious and dangerous sources of infection'. And yet Munson conceded that:

> The work meant invasion of the accepted rights of the home and of the individual on a scale perhaps unprecedented for any community. The collection of the fecal specimens necessarily might fairly be regarded as repulsive to modesty. Add to this the facts that the search was made among persons apparently healthy to themselves and others who could scarcely fall even within the class of suspects, and that those found positive were subjected to all the inconveniences of isolation, separation from family, loss of earning capacity, etc.[17]

In 1909 alone, the hard-pressed staff of the Manila Bureau of Science examined over 7,000 faecal specimens, almost all from Filipinos; and then in 1914, at the beginning of the cholera epidemic, they were overwhelmed by more than 126,000 jars of faeces.[18]

If the supply of water in the cities and villages was 'generally contaminated and noxious',[19] this was now seen to derive from poor Filipino hygiene rather than from peculiar emanations from the tropical environment. An American physician declared that 'the cleaning of the Augean stables was a slight undertaking in comparison with purifying the Philippines ... No imagination can make the Filipino customs with respect to [defecation] worse than actuality.'[20] Indeed, the model disease survey of the town of Taytay pointed to many dangerous waste disposal 'customs'. The investigators reported, for instance, that most residents in the mornings would empty, in any convenient place, vessels containing their excreta, or else they defecated in the bushes at the edge of town. Only a quarter of the dwellings had separate outhouses, and even these were generally holes in the floor, through which human waste dropped onto the ground, where the pigs scavenged it.[21]

Thus a grotesque, defecating Filipino body regularly irrupted into medical reports and scientific papers. Like the grotesque body that Bakhtin has found in the work of Rabelais, this medically produced Filipino body appears unfinished, outgrowing itself, transgressing its own limits. This open body, all apertures, 'is not separated from the world by clearly defined boundaries; it is blended with the world, with animals, with objects', with other reservoirs of pathology.[22] Especially in times of cholera and typhoid, physicians overwhelmed with faecal specimens were inclined to reduce the Filipino body – in practice – to little more than a gaping anus, and two soiled hands. But unlike the Rabelaisian grotesque, this medical homunculus offered no celebration of the lower bodily stratum; the abundance of the medical grotesque is more destructive than regenerating, more debasing than liberating. Physicians thus construed the Filipino body as an essential negation: of health, of discipline, of civilisation.

The colonising process must therefore be a 'civilising' process. Americans at all levels of colonial society (but especially women and public health officers) set out to train childlike Filipinos in the correct techniques of the body, 'under the watchword of civilité', rationalised as hygiene.[23] The medical reformulation, and reinforcement, of the conventional sense of disgust permeated American social life in the Philippines. Since bodily contact now implied particular medical risk, servants warranted relentless scrutiny and regulation. At times, the 'half-naked, dark-skinned creatures' employed by Mrs Edith Moses gave her the impression of 'trained baboons', especially a 'monkey-like coolie' who polished the narra floors; but on other occasions her servants were simply 'like children', fun-loving and filthy. Accordingly, when cholera struck in 1902 'we hosed off the "China" boys and Filipinos with disinfectants', for 'in spite of all my lectures and my practice, our Chinese do not understand the first principles of sanitary cleanliness'.[24] Nevertheless, Moses persisted in her efforts to teach her servants to avoid handling food, to set tables decorously, to dispose of their wastes fastidiously, and to wash their hands regularly. She housetrained them. And when Emily Bronson Conger stormed into the archipelago, she too experienced 'a wild desire to take those dirty, almost nude creatures in hand and, holding them at arm's length, dip them into some cleansing caldron'. For 'it never occurs to them to wash their hands', and they never used soap or towels. 'They rub their bodies sometimes with a stone,' she noted. 'It does not matter which way you turn you see hundreds of natives at their toilet. One does not mind them more than the caribou [*sic*] in some muddy pond, and one is about as cleanly as the other.'[25]

But if Mrs Conger claimed indifference to these infractions, her peers did not; most were convinced that such uncivilised, indeed dangerous, behaviour required reformation. Thus, in Lilian Hathaway Mearns's *Philippine Romance*, the heroine, Patricia, expresses the nobility of her character when she assures her suitor that 'everyday I have made a visit to the *barrio*, and have preached soap and water without ceasing'.[26] In the interests of hygiene and the American way of life, Patricia was teaching 'barbarous' Filipinos to contain their bodily wastes and not spread them around. Less noble, perhaps, were the methods of Mr and Mrs Campbell Dauncey. When they moved to Iloilo, Mrs Dauncey was appalled to find that her new house was next to 'a rabbit warren of low-class Filipinos, who keep all sorts of animals in the rooms, and throw all their refuse out into the narrow alley between this and the next house'. She put out bowls of disinfectant to ward off her new neighbours, but to no avail. Far more effective was her husband's response to these 'transgressions of the laws of cleanliness and decency'. He followed the simple plan of 'leaning out of the window when the people below do anything he does not like, and calling them "*Babuis*" (pigs), or "*sin verguenza*" (without shame) in a very loud voice, which they don't like at all'.[27]

If the anus was a synecdoche for the medicalised Filipino body, the mouth just as surely symbolised American presence. In this sense, American physicians were doubly spokesmen for the body. Unlike Filipinos, they produced abstractions, by mouth and by hand, not shit – or, at least, not dangerous and visible shit. The American colonialists imagined themselves inhabiting the 'classical body': a completed body, isolated and closed off from other bodies, something individual and expressive.[28] Americans talk, write, report, police, supervise servants, hunt, fish and fight; but after reading the medical documents produced in the Philippines in the first decade of the century, one suspects that they rarely, if ever, went to the toilet. Whatever happened to *their* lower bodily functions? These retentive colonialists imagine themselves to have achieved the transcendence of the 'natural' body that modern industry demanded.[29] An American sublime that demanded such relentless self-discipline made the labour of Filipino suppression as much a labour of American repression.[30] American bodies became the idealised, enclosed bodies of automata in the new machine culture, abstracted from the filthy exuberance of the tropics and represented as truly 'civilised' models for Filipinos.[31]

The outbreak of typhoid at Ludlow Barracks during November 1909 provides us with an example of the unfortunate materiality of the medical grotesque. The post surgeon reported that 'my first effort was to discover a possible carrier. The natives and kitchen force around Co. "I" were tested for "Widal" reaction and later the cooks of other companies were examined.'[32] No asymptomatic carriers were detected. Yet the surgeon decided – regardless of the bacteriological result – to issue orders 'forbidding natives, laundrymen, etc, to sleep under barracks ... Natives were prohibited from touching or eating from any dish used by soldiers.'[33] Although it was later determined that the typhoid outbreak arose from drinking contaminated water, and no native disease carriers had ever been identified, his report concluded, in part, that: 'Natives are uncontrolled as to their personal hygiene and are undoubtedly a source of disease. Malaria, filarial diseases, cholera, dysentry [*sic*] and hookworm diseases as well as typhoid must be distributed by these natives who as laundrymen, kitchen and dining room servants, woodchoppers and private servants swarm around every barracks.'[34] Americans on these occasions are reduced to consumers of food and writers of reports (and all of course transcend their excreta), while Filipinos, even when 'proven' otherwise, are open, threatening, excreting animals.

The laboratory and the market

The 'civilising process' in the Philippines depended on the medical production and filling of a closed, colonial space – the reproduction of 'abstract space'.[35] Each society produces its own space. Abstract space, according to Henri Lefebvre, is above all formal and quantitative, dominated by the rationality of exchange and calculation. In such bourgeois spaces 'history is experienced as nostalgia, and nature as regret – as a horizon fast disappearing behind us'.[36] This is the reductionist space of the grid and the map, hierarchical and segregated. It emphasises the primacy of the visual such that 'space has no social existence independently of an intense, aggressive and repressive visualization'.[37] Coercion is intrinsic to this modernising abstraction: thus 'operating procedures attributable to the action of a power which has its own location in space appear to result from a *simple logic of space*'.[38] In this sense, then, the spatial practices of the laboratory (and the toilet) work in the Philippines to produce a formal body, a body abstracted, fragmented. Indeed, only such relentlessly poeticised spaces render possible the transcendent body, and condition its misrecognition as aspatial and ahistorical.

Where better to produce this abstract space of colonialism than a medical laboratory, as much sign as signifier of difference.[39] In focusing on the laboratory as a representational space, we are inclined to forget that this modern workplace had its own distinctively 'abstract' spatial texture. It was (and is) a delibidinised place of white coats, hand washing, strict hierarchy, correct training, isolation, inscription – in short, a place of somatic control and closure, organised around the avoidance of contamination. Just as the laboratory's spatial representations – its reports and scientific papers – reduced the tropics (the lower regional stratum) to a series of controllable, visualised, abstracted specimens, so too did the spatial practices producing these inscriptions depend on its workforce of mostly young, single males transcending the lower bodily stratum and setting themselves apart from the filth outside. Even more than the factory or the school, the laboratory thus becomes the exemplary locus of colonial modernity.

As early as July 1901 the Philippines Commission had established a Bureau of Government Laboratories, which consisted, initially, of a biological and a chemical section.[40] The biological laboratory was expected to provide 'adequate facilities for investigation into, and scientific report upon, the causes, pathology and methods of diagnosing and combating the diseases of man and of domesticated animals', as well as to perform any 'routine' biological work required by other government departments.[41] The chemistry laboratory investigated food, drug and plant composition, and mineral resources. Paul C. Freer, the first director of the bureau, declared that the new Manila laboratories provided 'a position for the higher type of educated American investigator, not only for the actual material results which he may obtain, but also for the benefit which will accrue by his very presence in the community'.[42] Indeed, Freer never tired of extolling the value of scientific work in the Philippines. Nor did he hesitate to point out that 'the work is of so difficult a nature, so important, and, if imperfect methods are used, so subject to error, that a poor equipment both in the literature of medical biology and in apparatus would be the precursor of failure'. He thus presented his demands for 'the highest type of trained investigators, a complete library, and exceptional facilities'.[43] In 1904 he got his 'properly equipped biological laboratory', with large rooms ('well lighted without direct sunlight') and a supply of microscopes, incubators, sterilisers, microtomes, glassware, stains, chemicals, and small animals.[44] The new laboratory buildings, decorated externally in a modified Spanish style, occupied a fine site near the heart of the city on the old Exposition Grounds.

Laboratory design was predicated on a transcendence of the tropical environment. A modern power plant provided the rooms with vacuum, air pressure, and steam and supplied light to all the laboratory buildings. To ensure good ventilation and coolness in the two-storey building, on each floor the rooms were grouped on either side of a large, main corridor, ten feet wide and running the entire length of the building. When the hallway was open, Freer noticed that 'a breeze is almost continually passing through it, generally supplying a suction as it passes the doors of the individual laboratories so that a constant circulation of air is produced'.[45] The largest part of the building was the main laboratory structure, facing toward the south and divided into two symmetrical portions, one for the biological laboratory, and the other for the chemical laboratory. In the rooms of the biological wing, a microscope table ran along the entire window front. So that 'the strange breezes which prevail in this country' should not play havoc with materials on this work table, the windows were placed well above the desks.[46] In the centre of the room, two tables provided ample space for the general work of the laboratory, particularly for any heating, filtering, or distilling. Along another wall of each biological room, was a chemical worktable furnished with gas, water, and vacuum. A hood occupied the opposite wall; its flue extended up into the attic and connected with the main exhaust tanks, producing a strong draft. On the ground floor a special room was given over to the preparation of culture media; here, steam was provided for sterilisers and the main autoclaves of the building. Each floor of the biological wing included a room for the refrigerating boxes, and for the incubators, each heated by Bunsen burners. A separate house, behind the biological wing, held the cages of the experimental animals.

To assay accurately the tropical environment, and to gauge the character of its inhabitants, the investigators – all correctly trained 'higher types' – needed to compare new specimens with standard reference material. The museum was therefore one of the more important sections of the laboratories. Typical examples of anatomical and histological pathology were carefully preserved, along with a collection of local parasites and insects.[47] But the scientific library was perhaps of even more use to investigators trying to formalise and abstract the apparent chaos of the tropics. The scope of the library meant that 'no one need fear a lack of literature' in Manila.[48] The library, the 'central depository of scientific books for the entire Government', boasted an extensive holding of monographs and periodicals.[49] An assiduous researcher could find there all the major British, German, and French publications dealing with tropical science. But constant vigilance was required to protect this defining resource from tropical depredation. The environment it codified threatened constantly to consume it. 'Books must be inspected daily,' Freer lamented, 'and wiped off very frequently during the rainy season, on account of the mold.' Unruly insects, particularly cockroaches, could destroy overnight the texts that stigmatised them. To protect the books, the covers were varnished, and the legs of the bookcases rested in cans of petroleum. Freer took comfort in the fact that 'white ants have never attacked the library', although they had come close.[50]

For American optimists, the whole of the Philippine archipelago was an incipient colonial laboratory. With much time and effort the chaos and promiscuity of the Islands might be subdued, and the colonial space might then replicate the controlled conditions of the Bureau of Science. 'The Philippines may be considered today as a laboratory,' declared James A. LeRoy, 'where an experiment with important bearings on the "race problem" is being conducted.'[51] Joseph Ralston Hayden, a vice-governor of the Islands, claimed that 'one of the great achievements of the period [was] that within the Philippines government an essentially scientific attitude should have been substituted for the unscientific ways of Spanish days'.[52] This was more than an effort to make laboratory work possible; it was the attempt to render the tropics laboratory-like. Bruno Latour has described how the followers of Pasteur a few decades earlier had worked to 'enrol' outsiders in their laboratory science and to capture others' interests, thereby connecting everyday activities with the proceedings of the laboratory. Society, Latour argues, was made to conform to laboratory requirements. 'In this succession of displacements,' Latour declares, 'no one can say *where the laboratory is* and *where the society is*.'[53]

But initially the demarcation in the Philippines was for many all too clear. That most of the laboratory workers – all college graduates – lived in small rooms and ate out at the local restaurants appalled Freer. (After all, this risked exposing the Americans as bonded to intimate activities involving excretion and contamination.) Outside the abstract space of his idealised laboratory even 'higher types' might become obviously degraded. 'In a country like this where hygienic surroundings are of the highest importance and where sickness causes such a large decrease in the normal efficiency of a working force, it is highly desirable that members of a staff should be able to find suitable and healthful accommodations upon their arrival.'[54] Above all, it was imperative that young American scientists avoid the filth of Philippine markets. Imagined as a centre of pollution and disorder, the market was evidently the chief impediment to rendering the Philippines laboratory-like. Regarded as a negation of American formality, the open market, like the grotesque Filipino body, came to appear a 'deathly obstacle to ideal aspirations', ever in need of scientific reformation.[55]

For many American colonialists, the Philippine marketplace provided a fascinating combination of sensuality and danger, however bland the social life of these public spaces may in fact have been. Although such places do not seem to have retained the 'utopian folk element' – the revelling, games, clowning, and so on – that Bakhtin found in an earlier European carnivalesque, entering the market undoubtedly continued to produce a discomforting sense of a suspension of hierarchy, of freedom and familiarity.[56] The marketplace was readily represented as a locus of promiscuous contact and contamination, a space quite unlike the ideal laboratory that was formally documenting its dangers. If Americans were scorned and ridiculed, surely they were most exposed to such inversions of colonial relations in the marketplace. This necessarily perverted place was (and still is) imagined as a place of risk, both symbolically and materially. James LeRoy found that 'unless there be rigid and efficient supervision', the markets were 'foci of infection'.[57] Whenever he wandered through these places, Nicholas Roosevelt assumed that 'many varieties of intestinal germs and parasites may lurk in most foods'.[58] For Daniel R. Williams, the markets were simply 'unwholesome and death-dealing plazas'.[59] 'No one who has not travelled in the Orient can conceive of the noise and confusion,' William Freer wrote of Manila's street life. 'Words fail utterly to describe it.'[60]

But how to render this teeming, promiscuous environment more laboratory-like? Just as the laboratory had constructed – or, rather, informed and rationalised – the problem of contact, so too did it offer solutions. When Katherine Mayo visited the 'Isles of Fear' in the early 1920s she was pleased to note the strict control of potential 'disease carriers' in hotels or restaurants. No servant could handle food 'without a health certificate showing he was free from germs likely to convey disease'.[61] Washing and disinfecting hands were constantly emphasised. Governor James F. Smith was himself convinced that cholera attacked only those 'people drinking from *esteros*, eating with fingers and refusing to recognise the importance of sanitary laws'.[62] In order to protect consumers in the public sphere, new *sanitary* markets were constructed in Manila. The buildings, all of supposedly hygienic reinforced concrete, were 'supplied with ample water facilities, enabling them to be kept scrupulously clean'.[63] Sanitary inspectors patrolled the aisles, checking regularly to ensure that the stallholders wore clean clothes, kept their hands spotless and their nails trimmed, and used only clean white wrapping paper.[64] To prevent shoppers engaging in 'the old custom of handling one piece of meat after another with the fingers', forks were provided. In case this was not enough, meat was placed in 'substantial screen cages made of copper wire with sliding doors', in this way protecting it further, not only from 'promiscuous handling but also from contamination by flies'. Such modern markets, constructed throughout the archipelago, became 'educational features . . . doing much to spread the doctrine of cleanliness throughout the Islands'.[65]

Despite improvements to the water supply, sanitary inspectors still detected 'bacilli of the colon type' in samples of drinking water dispensed in the stores or *tiendas*. The director of health therefore stipulated that in order to obtain a licence each *tienda* must provide a teakettle 'for rendering water sterile'. Instructions – printed in Spanish, Tagalog and Chinese – required the kettle, filled from the city pipes, to 'boil violently' for at least fifteen minutes, before it was poured.[66] The Bureau of Health also recognised that the common drinking cup served to transmit several kinds of infectious diseases. In institutions and churches the 'necessity' of the individual cup appeared particularly urgent. A disposable cup was the only practical and progressive solution. The bureau suggested a method of making an individual drinking cup from a square sheet of tough paper. 'Inmates of institutions soon learn to make their own cups,' Dr Victor G. Heiser reported, 'and take great delight in the thought of protective cleanliness which is afforded by their use.'[67]

When the author of *Interesting Manila* first visited the city in 1900 he observed that the *tiendas* were 'so open to the street as to be practically in the highway', and those of the Chinese were 'always repulsive and dirty'. But after ten years they were far cleaner, better enclosed – 'interesting' even. As for the markets, 'before the days of American sanitation', he recalled, 'the condition of these places was always indescribably bad, but modern regulations and efficient inspectors have changed all this to comparative cleanliness and good order'.[68] Similarly, Frank G. Carpenter remembered that in 1900 the largest marketplace in Tondo 'consisted of ten acres of rude sheds, roofed with straw matting or galvanized iron laid upon a framework of bamboo poles'. But by 1920 it was a building of concrete and steel, hosed down every night.[69]

Dipesh Chakrabarty has argued that in colonial India the discourse on filth in public spaces was a 'language of modernity, of civic consciousness and public health, of even certain ideas of beauty related to the management of public space and interests, an order of aesthetics from which the ideals of public health and hygiene cannot be separated'.[70] More than anything else – more, even, than the rebuilding of the markets – it was the American toilet that would, in the Philippines, permit an extension of the boundaries of modern hygienic space.

The toilet in the tropics

Observing the early failures to inculcate American excretory habits in Filipinos, Allan McLaughlin lamented that 'it requires a long time completely to change the habits of a people and it will probably require another generation to complete the work'.[71] When the 'native custom' of eating with one's fingers was not easily suppressed, Heiser saw 'years of discouraging struggle ahead of us before they can be broken of so fixed a habit, the menace of which as yet is entirely beyond their comprehension'.[72] Dr Thomas W. Jackson, having lived 'surrounded by Filipino neighbors' in a provincial town, where it had been 'impossible to avoid an intimate knowledge of their manner of life', endorsed the general pessimism.[73] The first seven years of American control had seen only minimal improvement in the condition of the market, the disposal of garbage, and in 'such personal habits as defecation, urination, expectoration, and eating with the fingers'.[74] Jackson concluded that the teachings of sanitary principles might be the 'necessary and preliminary foundation' for disease prevention, but the introduction of such sanitary teachings 'into the home by schoolchildren must be a slow and tedious process, unlikely to produce results within a generation'.[75] The unsanitary local customs and habits were thus regarded almost as racial characteristics, subject to change only over decades. Until then, close supervision and regulation would be warranted. In the opinion of an editor of the influential *Cablenews-American*, for the moment 'only by force can the lower classes of natives' be made to abstain from food and drink 'laden with germs'. Despite noble educational efforts, 'the densely ignorant adult native persists in compassing his own death', and the deaths of innocent Americans – although 'with the coming generation this fatal ignorance will largely pass'.[76]

To combat the apparent racial obstacles, health experts vigorously promoted educational and publicity projects in the second decade of the century. The health service began issuing a semi-weekly bulletin, never more than a page in length, dealing with some topical public health question. This was published in all the daily papers (in English, Spanish and Tagalog) and mailed to medical officers and other government officials throughout the Islands. From 1915, women's clubs conducted discussions on maternal and infant welfare, and issued their own bulletins. Sanitary commissions visited selected towns, surveying health conditions in the community, giving practical demonstrations of how to prepare balanced diets from the local food supply, and instructing the local inhabitants in personal hygiene, home cleanliness and the care of the sick. The health service also maintained permanent exhibits of model sanitary houses, methods of sewerage disposal, and sanitary and unsanitary *barrios*. Photographs, 'moving pictures', parade floats, and (in 1921) a 'healthmobile' sent out to fairs and fiestas illustrated modern methods of hygiene.[77] Cartoons in English and Tagalog also showed promise as effective means of persuading infantilised Filipinos to change their unhygienic habits. Warnings abound about the 'poisonous' nature of faecal matter, the evils of handling food, and the dangers of 'the promiscuous spitting habit'. No wonder, then, that when exercise was advised it was 'for the purposes of enabling the body to eliminate its waste products and become clean'.[78] The general message was that Filipino bodies were filthy – had not the microscope shown it to be so? – and personal contact or loose behaviour would only distribute the filth.

The public schools became a major sanitary venue. Teachers would compile a 'health index' for every child in their class. The Bureau of Education's idealised 'healthy child' had a 'well-formed body', 'clean and shining hair', 'a clear skin of good color', 'ears free from discharge', 'a voice of pleasing quality', 'an amiable disposition', and so on.[79] A premium was thus placed on the Filipino child's formal, expressive qualities. Furthermore, every child was to be weighed once a month and the height measured at least twice a year. If anything was amiss, the teacher reported it to the local health officer. But this was not enough. It was also the duty of a teacher to 'instruct pupils to care for themselves and to put into practice both in the school and at home miscellaneous health principles'.[80] The transcendence of the lower bodily stratum was also to animate everyday life; in this reculturation, the body was treated (in Bourdieu's formulation) as a memory.[81] Through training, children learned of the dangers of raw vegetables, impure water, poorly ventilated houses, a sedentary way of life, and deformed posture. Every child had to carry a clean handkerchief, drink at least a cup of milk each day, sleep from ten to twelve hours a night (under a mosquito net), bathe daily, wear shoes, wash the hands before eating – and never touch the food. So that the non-contaminating abstract space of the classroom should be faultlessly extended – to retrace domestically the body-as-memory – health experts urged that 'the construction of a toilet, either in his own home or in that of a neighbor, be a project for each seventh-grade boy'.[82]

In this very material sense, the production of colonial space required that Filipinos confess repeatedly their filthiness. In submitting to the Americans' craze for building toilets, Filipinos voiced their own impurity. Untreated, their excrement could have no regenerating power in the fields; rather, it had become a source of shame, to be admitted, then sealed off and enclosed. Americans, though they doubtlessly suspected that they too were rotten, would not avow it; they could transcend all that. And yet Filipinos, whatever their misgivings, were compelled from infancy to confess this 'putrescence' in order that the formalising American colonial institutions may recognise them – if only to retrain them. Not altogether unlike the 'torture victims' Certeau describes, a Filipino becoming 'civilized' is abandoned to equipment that 'unrelentingly works to prove to him that he is a betrayer, a coward, a pile of shit'.[83] Only with the confession of this rottenness could Filipinos be admitted to an American modernity; once fallen, they could then help raise themselves up. As de Certeau claims, 'what goes on in the kitchen is quite different from what happens in the parlor'; however, it is only through assenting to the toilet, and to disinfection, that Filipinos ever gain entry even to the American colonial kitchen.

Toilets soon were cropping up everywhere. The Bureau of Health from the beginning had urged all Filipinos to treat their 'evacuated intestinal contents as a poison', taking care to avoid contact with them. 'Let those who are able to put in septic tanks and flush closets do so' – all others should install a pail closet, at a cost.[84] In the smaller communities where cholera had prevailed in the early 1900s, sanitary officers had found the pail system – the digging of pits and covering of excreta with lime or clean earth at regular intervals – to be effective, although it seemed initially that 'the cost of maintenance and inspections as a regular measure is prohibitive and only warranted by emergency conditions'.[85] But public health officials hoped that widespread use of the pail could yet be made feasible and affordable. Heiser suggested that a pail system might even be profitable in routine conditions if it was installed along 'with an after-treatment of the night soil which would render it suitable for fertilizing mulberry trees, thus promoting the silk industry'.[86] (He was, however, vehemently opposed to the plan 'followed in many oriental countries' of letting out private contracts for the collection of night soil from private residences, for it was 'established custom' to use this untreated waste to fertilise vegetables – often with mixed cultures of amoebae, cholera bacilli, and other pathogens.)[87] And if the profit motive was insufficient, then taxation might make the pail system commonplace. Householders soon had to choose between paying quarterly charges of seven and a half pesos for individual pails kept on the premises or one peso to use the public pail system.

Much attention also had been given to the design of a cheaper and more efficient 'sanitary pail'. The bureau recommended a raised frame of four posts set at a height that allowed an 'ordinary five-gallon kerosene can' to be slipped under the bottom of the seat. By covering the hole with a self-closing, hinged seat, the designers had carefully ensured that no flies or other insects could gain access to the contents. But the 'container for the can has the advantage of being entirely open, which fact secures good ventilation and leaves no opportunity for the collection and retention of disagreeable odors', which had been an unfortunate consequence of the superseded boxlike designs.[88] The ordinary carabao cart could haul far more of the light cans than it could the old-fashioned wooden pails, so the costs of collection were also much reduced. With the savings, an attendant could be hired to supervise 'a suitably located central pit' where the contents of the cans were dumped.[89]

Even after such improvements in efficiency and reductions in cost, many years passed before the pail system was widely used. The poorer sections of Manila continued to depend on a few scattered public collections of 'insanitary closets', or none at all. Until the 1920s, approved systems of waste disposal remained a rare sight in the provinces. When David Willets visited the Batanes Islands in 1913 he reported bluntly that 'a suitable method for disposing of human excrement is lacking'. Water closets were very rare, 'and furthermore the people have not learned to use

Public health and the poetics of pollution 91

them'.⁹⁰ But if the local inhabitants continued to disregard sanitary advice and regulation, when emergencies arose sanitary officers could still forcibly disinfect them and their surroundings. When McLaughlin took charge of the sanitary response to the 1908 Manila cholera outbreak, he organised more than 600 men into disinfecting squads that went about spraying carbolic over dwellings and 'liming all closets and places where fecal matter existed or was likely to be deposited'. Each day in the 'strong material districts', squads disinfected the closets, while 'in the light material districts, the effort to disinfect the dejecta of the entire population necessitated the disinfection of entire districts. It was necessary to disinfect practically the whole ground area.'⁹¹ Anyone who tried to obstruct the disinfecting squads was arrested and fined. The amount of disinfectant dispersed was enormous: more than 150,000 pounds of lime and 700 gallons of carbolic acid were used. When the entire stock of disinfectant in the Islands had gone, supplies had to be ordered from Hong Kong. When they ran out of lime, squads took to digging ditches and cleaning up the yards until new stocks came in.

But by 1920 such forcible disinfection was no longer a major part of the sanitary response to enteric diseases. Filipinos were generally obeying the provisions of sanitary code that required 'any building of whatever character' to include 'adequate privies or toilet accommodations, constructed according to plans approved by the Director of Health'. A sanitary inspector could now demand to see, at the very least, 'a pit not less than one and a half meters in depth, securely covered by a slab of stone or concrete ... a seat, provided with a cover, so devised to close automatically when not in use; a vertical conducting pipe ... leading from the seat to within the pit; and a vent pipe not less than ten centimeters in diameter leading from the pit to one meter above the eaves of the building'. The capacity of the pit was set liberally at one cubic metre for each resident. Though 'adequate facilities for ventilation' were crucial, this 'Antipolo toilet' was not permitted to 'communicate' with any other room, and had to have 'a tight-fitting door'.⁹²

From fiesta to Clean-Up Week

José Rizal has provided us with an almost rhapsodic account of a Filipino fiesta in the 1890s. On the eve of the fiesta it seemed to the community that 'the air is laden and saturated with gladness'. And on the day, while 'everything is confusion, noise, uproar', it was an amiable confusion, not at all contaminating or threatening. Banners waved in the streets as processions passed by; the community gathered to watch, join in the parades, sing, dance, and attend the cockfights and games of chance. People sauntered about at will. In the plaza, on a bamboo stage, the comedy from Tondo began its songs, dance, and mimicry. All members of the audience were dressed in their best clothes and, according to Rizal, a scent 'of powder, of flowers, of incense, of perfume' permeated the town. If, in the pushing and the crush of the crowd, one caught a whiff of 'human animal', this contact with one's fellows was more to be cherished than feared. And so the romance of the fiesta continued, until at the end of the day 'lights and variegated colors distracted the eyes, melodies and explosions, the ears'.[93]

But Mrs Dauncey had quite another impression of the 1904 fiesta that commemorated the death of Rizal. The crowds 'swarmed out' into the town of Iloilo in the evening. 'They hang out flags and lanterns,' she reported, 'and every Filipino knocks off what little work he ever does, and crawls about on the streets and spits … while the women slouch along in gangs with myriads of children.'[94] To her eyes it was a time of promiscuous, animalistic contact. In June 1900, Edith Moses, newly settled in Manila, heard of the dangers of such gatherings. 'Many officers seem to think that the fiesta is a mask for an uprising on a large scale,' she wrote, 'and all American women and children have been warned not to go into the streets.'[95] Clearly the fiesta represented a challenge to the American control of colonial public space, if not to the actual institutions of government. And though sceptical of the 'dangerous fiesta', Mrs Moses later heard 'insurrectos whispering under my bed and coming up the ladder', invading even her domestic refuge, her personal enclosure.[96] Thus the communal fiesta comes to appear an earthy, open site for the subversion of American modernity.

To the materialists in the Bureau of Health the uncontrolled fiesta meant principally a concentration of 'an extraordinary amount of foodstuffs, most of which are improperly prepared and handled, and exposed to contamination'.[97] It sometimes involved the congregation of sick, often infected, people at some religious shrine. The 'lack of sanitary preparation to accommodate the crowds' thus dispersed diseases across the archipelago. In order 'to meet this menace', the Bureau of Health demanded that local authorities provide 'clean, disinfected, and otherwise supervised' convenience stations where people concentrated, a clean water supply, and food prepared and served 'in a cleanly manner'.[98] To ensure this occurred at Antipolo during the 1915 pilgrimage to the shrine of 'Nuestra Señora de la Paz y Buen Viaje', the Bureau of Health had dispatched an auxiliary corps of sanitary inspectors. Thus, 'instead of proving a menace to the people of the town', the event became 'a means for educating and improving them'.[99] But the bureau did not have the resources to supervise all the local fiestas.

In the first decade of the twentieth century, the colonial government decided to establish an 'institutional Carnival' in Manila as an alternative to these dangerous fiestas. By February 1918, the 'big fiesta' was a lavish occasion, a 'Red Cross Carnival' resembling a small city. Designed to 'combine pleasure with the noble spirit of business and democratic understanding between all who live and trade in the Orient', the carnival now consisted of a patriotically decorated piazza, commercial establishments (including a few 'curious Chinese concessions'), a motor industry display (housed in 'buildings constructed in Roman style'), a merry-go-round, some instructive government exhibitions, and an auditorium 'where the Queen of the Great Festival is crowned'.[100] Not surprisingly, the 'atmosphere of patriotic solemnity' was supposed to 'convinc[e] the people that the Red Cross Carnival was not merely an occasion for mirth and frivolity'. One imagines that after watching the parade of Red Cross Women who reflected on their faces 'the beautiful rays of Christian charity and unbounded patriotism', the 'martial columns' of school cadets, and 'the allegorical floats of the different establishments, institutions of learning and bureaus of Insular Government', that the attentive crowd found its sense of frivolity was suitably muted. But just in case, any eager revellers had been told to wait until the end, 'when they could throw confetti right and left without offence or undue familiarity and when they could feel to have come in tacit understanding to enjoy themselves without encroaching the unwritten code of good manners'.[101] This was not, one suspects, a carnival that Rizal – or Rabelais – would recognise. Indeed, one irreverent reporter observed that the conspicuous presence of recruiting stations 'gave the general atmosphere of merriment an aspect of the grim reality of life in army camps'.[102]

Of all the exhibitions, perhaps the most elaborate, and the most telling, was the Philippine Health Service's display of a Sanitary Model House, complete 'to the minutest detail' with an exemplary water closet. 'Beautifully surrounded by a flower and vegetable garden, [the model] made a lasting impression on thousands of home lovers.'[103] Perhaps more reliable is the description of the carnival as 'one big gambol' – even if such unadulterated pleasure was illicit – followed by a dutiful admonition to 'those of us who have spent the last eight evenings dancing, throwing confetti and visiting side-shows' to take a little time to view the government exhibitions. These were as 'instructive' as ever, the breezy report noted, which 'leaves very little to be said'.[104] More prudish commentators lamented the behaviour of dedicated revellers. While many of the subversives who took part in 'the hubbub, the jollities, the fooleries, and the emptying-purses', were students, it seems they had little time for the edifying structures of the Red Cross Carnival. Rather, students went straight for the 'hurly-burly dancing, pitching handfuls of confetti at some giggling lasses', or they strolled 'around the city of mirth throwing a few centavos here and there ... to the fake freaks of nature exhibited in the side-shows'. Evidently this institutional carnival could scarcely contain the carnivalesque, let alone reform it. As a result of such 'unbridled pleasure', the students awoke the next morning 'haggard-looking', with 'a dull head, unable to concentrate their minds on their lessons'.[105] If only – one hears the reproach – they had lingered longer at the Sanitary Model House.

While the Manila Carnival occurred in February each year, Clean-Up Week – the other alternative to the traditional fiesta – usually took place the week before Christmas. Promising 'the sanitation and the beautification of the Philippine towns', it was chiefly a time for 'the cleaning of private and public premises, the gathering and burning of rubbish ... the construction of drains, the repair of fences, the trimming of hedges, the construction of toilets ...',[106] all done with appropriate mirth and ardour, of course. In the past, it had been 'the custom to have a municipal clean-up before town fiestas', but what used to be merely preparation for a festival had become the *raison d'être* of community activity.[107] In this sense, it was promoted as a 'nation-wide' revival of a 'good custom of our grandfathers, only to be done in a more systematic way'.[108] The first such celebration of Hygeia took place in 1914 – to a 'distinct lack of cooperation and interest on the part of everybody'.[109] But eagerness picked up after 1920, when the government began offering 100 pesos to any 'charitable or social institution in a town in each province, which will make the best effort to have the greatest number of houses and lots cleaned and improved'.[110] By 1922, Clean-Up Week was well observed. It had been divided into special days, including weed-rubbish day, draining day, privy day, repairing day, scrubbing day, and house-furnishings day. On privy day, of course, all were expected to build or repair their toilets. The week opened with decorous parades and band music and closed with speeches and prizes. A policeman, often assisted by a teacher or councillor, went about with standardised forms scoring all dwellings and shops in the district. 'Line up folks,' the Filipino townspeople were exhorted. 'Roll up your sleeves. Get ready for the great national event.'[111]

Conclusion: replacing matter

American physicians in the early twentieth century sought to ensure that the colonial Philippines were inhabited with propriety. The new tropical medicine, informing an expanded apparatus of surveillance and regulation in the archipelago, worked to reproduce in parallel the formalised body and the abstract space of colonial modernity. By enforcing this sealed orificial order, the public health officials would ideally bring about a seamless reformation of supposedly grotesque, open Filipino bodies and would, furthermore, re-territorialise the marketplace and the fiesta, both of which had figured in the American imagination as places of promiscuous, threatening contact.[112] For as American corporeality was erased, Filipinos became the chief, and most generous, sources of contaminating matter. Uncivilised, even bestial, Filipinos were seen as 'promiscuous defecators', transgressing colonial safe havens, imperilling the innocent Americans who had managed to transcend nature.

But how convincing was this assumption of 'transcendence'? Americans clearly were still fascinated by defilement and the boundaries – both social and spatial – it marked in a manner so excitingly assailable. Much as they denied it, Americans were themselves victims of the abject, for even as

Filipinos were isolated and disinfected, the rejected Other could never be radically excluded from the colonialists' own embodiment. This secret rottenness remained a non-assimilable alien, an abiding structure within even the most apparently abstracted of bodies, always there to disturb as much as constitute American identity. And so it was that the effort to suppress this abject Other, this alter ego, required relentless self-control and sublimated productivity – the development and further expansion, that is, of a conflicted colonial modernity.[113]

And yet American scientists, as we have seen, obsessively collected any specimens of Filipino faeces they could lay their gloved hands on. To what can we attribute their surprising immunity from the 'dangers that would kill uninitiated men'?[114] For scientists in the Philippines human excrement was as practically creative as it was potentially destructive. If Filipinos were not allowed to spread their faeces on their fields, and ordinary Americans were not allowed to touch the stuff, the 'ritual frame' of the laboratory permitted accredited scientists to smear the pulverised, reduced material on their microscope slides and agar plates with abandon.[115] Thus when Ernest L. Walker and Andrew W. Sellards conducted their investigations into the etiology of dysentery, they did not hesitate to feed their Filipino 'clinical material' with organisms cultured from the stools of acute cases and carriers of the disease, and to analyse their subjects' faeces for the answer to the problem.[116] The decent, delibidinised, closed space of the modern laboratory had conferred on shit the 'epistemological clarity' of just one more specimen among many.[117] On the resulting abstractions and inscriptions did the colonial scientists' reputations and career prospects depend. 'Within the ritual frame,' Douglas reminds us, 'the abomination is ... handled as a source of great power.'[118] The abomination propelled Richard P. Strong, for instance, from Manila – where he helped identify the dysentery bacillus – to the first chair of Tropical Medicine at Harvard.

Shit, as Barthes points out, has no odour when written.[119]

Notes

I am grateful to the University of Chicago Press and the editors of *Critical Inquiry* for permission to reprint this essay with minor revisions. For their comments on earlier versions of the essay I would like to thank Vince Rafael, Mary Steedly, Dipesh Chakrabarty, Caroline Jones, Charles Rosenberg, Anna Tsing, Vernon Rosario, Jill Carrick and Mari Schindele.

1 T. Morrison, *Tar Baby*, New York, New American Library, 1981, pp. 203–4.
2 I call this a 'poetics' in order to emphasise the effort of public health officials to close the structure of medical metaphor and to erase any relations of these texts to a history of political practice. In effect, the expression of a figure outside of time works as a modernising strategy. The medical symbolic is thus fixed in a system especially discomposed by recognition of its historical and geographical specificity. Accordingly, this essay can be read as a critique or re-encoding of a certain poetics of space (and bodies and culture) which claims 'no past,

at least no recent past, in which preparation and appearance could be followed', G. Bachelard, *The Poetics of Space*, trans. M. Jolas, Boston, Mass., Beacon Press, 1994 [1958], p. i. 'Poetics' here means rather more than James Clifford's 'constant reconstitution of selves and others through specific exclusions, conventions, and discursive practices' ('Introduction: Partial Truths', in J. Clifford *et al.* (eds), *Writing Culture: The Poetics and Politics of Ethnography*, Berkeley, Calif., University of California Press, 1986, p. 24); and yet rather less than R. Jakobson's well-known formalist definition ('Closing Statement: Linguistics and Poetics', in T. Sebeok (ed.), *Style In Language*, Cambridge, Mass., MIT Press, 1960, pp. 357–68).
3 Bureau of Health, *The Disposal of Human Wastes in the Provinces*, Health Bulletin no. 13, Manila, Bureau of Printing, c.1912, US National Archives, Washington, DC (USNA), Record Group (RG) 350, File 3465–184, pp. 4–5.
4 W. De Witt, 'A Few Remarks Concerning the Health Conditions of Americans in the Philippines', *Yale Medical Journal*, 1904–5, vol. 11, pp. 56–63, at 56.
5 T. R. Marshall, *Asiatic Cholera in the Philippine Islands*, Manila, Bureau of Public Printing, 1904, p. 9.
6 See esp. A. Corbin, *The Foul and the Fragrant: Odor and the French Social Imagination*, trans. M. L. Kochan, R. Porter and C. Prendergast, Cambridge, Mass., Harvard University Press, 1986. D. Laporte, in C. Bourgois (ed.), *Histoire de la merde*, Paris, 1979, has suggested that 'apprenticeship in smelling [was] directed entirely toward excrement', p. 60, and that the rise of a strong state led to the privatising, and constrained circulation, of smell-producing excrement.
7 Corbin, *The Foul and the Fragrant*, p. 231. Georges Vigarello argues that the microbe 'materialised' the risk previously associated with odour, in *Concepts of Cleanliness: Changing Attitudes in France since the Middle Ages*, trans. J. Birrell, Cambridge and Paris, Cambridge University Press, and *Éditions de la maison des sciences de l'homme*, 1988 [1985], p. 203. On 'excremental vision' see N. O. Brown, 'The Excremental Vision', in *Life Against Death: The Psychoanalytic Meaning of History*, 2nd edn, Middletown, Wesleyan University Press, 1985 [1959], pp. 179–201. ('Excremental Vision' was also the title of a chapter in J. Middleton Murry, *Jonathan Swift, A Critical Biography*, London, Jonathan Cape, 1954, pp. 432–48.) See also K. Burke, 'The Thinking of the Body: Comments on the Imagery of Catharsis in Literature', in *Language as Symbolic Action: Essays on Life, Literature and Method*, Berkeley, Calif., University of California Press, 1966, pp. 308–43; and A. H. A. Rushdy, 'A New Emetics of Interpretation: Swift, his Critics and the Alimentary Canal', *Mosaic*, 1991, vol. 24, pp. 1–32. While the literary excrementalism of Swift and Rabelais is well known, the symbolism of medical excrementalism has been relatively neglected, with the notable exceptions of Corbin, *The Foul and Fragrant*, Laporte, *Histoire de la merde*, and P. Stallybrass and A. White, 'The City: The Sewer, the Gaze and the Contaminating Touch', in *The Politics and Poetics of Transgression*, Ithaca, NY, Cornell University Press, 1986, pp. 125–48.

More could be made – but in another essay – of Freud's writing on anal character during this period. See 'Character and Anal Eroticism', in J. Strachey (ed.), *Pelican Freud Library*, 15 vols, Harmondsworth, Penguin, 1973–86, vol. 7, pp. 209–25; and 'On the Transformations of Instinct as Exemplified in Anal Eroticism', ibid., pp. 39–169. A corollary of this paper's argument is the correspondence of Freudian categories with a modernist colonial discourse. On Freud the Orientalist, see C. E. Schorske, 'Freud's Egyptian Dig', *New York Review of Books*, 27 May 1993, pp. 35–40.
8 M. Douglas, *Purity and Danger: An Analysis of Concepts of Pollution and Taboo*, London, Routledge & Kegan Paul, 1976 [1966], p. 35. W. James, in his lecture on 'The Sick Soul' (*The Varieties of Religious Experience*, Cambridge, Mass., Harvard

University Press, 1985 [1901–2], p. 114), also refers to the challenge that 'matter out of place' presents to any system – 'evil' can thus be represented as 'an alien unreality, a waste element, to be sloughed off and negated', and the 'ideal' is 'marked by its deliverance from all contact with this diseased, inferior, and excrementitious stuff', p. 113. Of course James warns us against 'medical materialism', that is, reducing symbolic systems to a medical explanation. (James was a friend and correspondent of some of the senior colonial administrators in the Philippines, in particular of W. Cameron Forbes, a governor-general of the Islands.)

9   On the body as a medium of social expression, see M. Mauss, 'Techniques of the Body', *Economy and Society*, 1973, vol. 2, pp. 70–88. According to M. Douglas: 'Interest in [the body's] apertures depends on the preoccupation with social exits and entrances, escape routes and invasions' (*Natural Symbols: Explorations in Cosmology*, Harmondsworth, Penguin, 1978 [1970], p. 98).

10 Barbara Babcock has described 'symbolic inversion' as 'any act of expressive behavior which inverts, contradicts, abrogates or in some fashion presents an alternative to commonly held cultural codes, values and norms' (*The Reversible World: Symbolic Inversion in Art and Society*, Ithaca, NY, Cornell University Press, 1978, p. 14). Of course I am not arguing that Filipinos were, in fact, 'promiscuous defecators', just that it was necessary for colonial physicians to represent them as such. As Stallybrass and White point out: 'the classificatory body of a culture is always double, always structured in relation to its negation, its inverse', *Transgression*, p. 20.

11 I develop this argument further in 'Leprosy and Citizenship', *Positions*, 1998, vol. 6, pp. 707–30.

12 This is a model for the more general *fin-de-siècle* realist project of making visible. As Mark Seltzer points out: 'Relations of power in the realist text are insistently articulated along lines of sight', *Bodies and Machines*, New York and London, Routledge, 1992, p. 96.

13 W. Anderson, 'Immunities of Empire: Race, Disease and the New Tropical Medicine', *Bulletin of the History of Medicine*, 1996, vol. 70, pp. 94–118.

14 M. Foucault, 'Body/power', in C. Gordon (ed.), *Power/Knowledge: Selected Interviews and Other Writings, 1972–77*, trans. C. Gordon, L. Marshall, J. Mephan and K. Soper, Brighton, Harvester Press, 1980; and *Discipline and Punish: The Birth of the Prison*, New York, Pantheon, 1977. See esp. J. and J. Comaroff, 'Body Reform as Historical Practice', in *Ethnography and the Historical Imagination*, Boulder, Colo., Westview Press, 1992, pp. 69–91.

15 On the 'positioning of the subject under the sign of refuse', see M. de Certeau, 'The Institution of Rot', in *Heterologies: Discourse on the Other*, trans. B. Massumi, History and Theory of Literature series, vol. 17, Minneapolis, University of Minnesota Press, 1986, p. 40. On the late nineteenth-century American 'invention of bodies in the abstract', see Seltser, *Bodies and Machines*, p. 64. The relation I am sketching here between the 'technologies of domination of others' and the 'technologies of the self', Foucault, in his later work, has called 'governmentality'. See 'On Governmentality', *Ideology and Consciousness*, 1981, vol. 8, pp. 3–14; and 'The Political Technology of Individuals', in L. H. Martin, H. Gutman and P. H. Hutton (eds), *Technologies of the Self: A Seminar with Michel Foucault*, Amherst, Mass., University of Massachusetts Press, 1988.

16 H. du Rest Phelan, 'Sanitary Service in Surigao, a Filipino Town on the Island of Mindanao', *Journal of the Association of Military Surgeons*, 1904, vol.14, pp. 1–18.

17 W. P. Chamberlain *et al.*, 'Examinations of Stools and Blood among the Igorots at Baguio, Philippine Islands', *The Philippine Journal of Science*, 1910, vol. 5B, pp. 505–14. P. E. Garrison, 'The Prevalence and Distribution of Animal Parasites of Man in the Philippine Islands, with a Consideration of their Possible

Influence upon Public Health', *The Philippine Journal of Science*, 1908, vol. 3B, pp. 191–210, p. 205. E. L. Munson, 'Cholera Carriers in Relation to Cholera Control', *The Philippine Journal of Science*, 1915, vol. 10B, pp. 1–9, pp. 5, 9. See also O. Shöbl, 'Observations concerning Cholera Carriers', *The Philippine Journal of Science*, 1915, vol. 10B, pp. 11–17. On the discovery of carrier status in the 1890s and its political uses in the US, see J. Walzer Leavitt, ' "Typhoid Mary" Strikes Back: Bacteriological Theory and Practice in Early Twentieth-Century Public Health', *Isis*, 1992, vol. 83, pp. 608–29. On the new public health, see B. Gutmann Rosenkrantz, *Public Health and the State: Changing Views in Massachusetts, 1842–1936*, Cambridge, Mass., Harvard University Press, 1972, and A. Brandt, *No Magic Bullet: A Social History of Venereal Disease in the United States Since 1880*, New York, Oxford University Press, 1985.

18 P. C. Freer, *Eighth Annual Report of the Director of the Bureau of Science, for the Year Ending August 1, 1909*, Manila, Bureau of Printing, 1910, RG 350/3466–21, USNA, p. 16. A. J. Cox, *13th Annual Report of the Director of the Bureau of Science, for the year ending December 31, 1914*, Manila, Bureau of Printing, 1915, RG 350/3466–30, USNA, pp. 11–12.

19 W. H. Taft, 'Report of the Secretary of War on the Philippines', in *Report of the Philippines Commission to the President*, 1907, 3 vols, Washington, DC Government Printing Office, 1908, vol. 3, pp. 284–5.

20 F. Chamberlin, *The Philippine Problem*, Boston, Mass., Little, Brown, 1913, pp. 113–14.

21 R. P. Strong *et al.*, 'Medical Survey of the Town of Taytay', *The Philippine Journal of Science*, 1909, vol. 4B, pp. 247–52.

22 M. M. Bakhtin, *Rabelais and his World*, trans. H. Iswolsky, Bloomington, Ind., Indiana University Press, 1984 [1964], pp. 26–7. Unlike Bakhtin I do not argue for the *authenticity* of a grotesque folkloric; and the communal bodies that I describe are isolated by fracture lines of race rather than class.

23 N. Elias, *The Civilising Process*, vol. 1: *The History of Manners*, trans. E. Jephcott, New York, Pantheon, 1978, p. xiv. Stephen Greenblatt also points out that control of the body's products 'marks the entrance into civility' ('Filthy Rites', *Daedalus*, 1982, vol. 3, pp. 1–16, p. 2). Pierre Bourdieu has argued more generally that the reformation of manners 'extorts the essential while seeming to demand the insignificant', ensuring that 'the concessions of *politeness* always contain *political* concessions' (*Outline of a Theory of Practice*, trans. R. Nice, Cambridge, Cambridge University Press, 1977, p. 90. It is surely worth exploring how this sense of disgust had to be suppressed in 'scientific' ethnography – for it to conform to a positivist 'value-free' representation – just as it was being licensed in tropical medicine.

24 E. Moses, *Unofficial Letters of an Official's Wife*, New York, D. Appleton, 1908, pp. 14, 16, 221, 226. Her husband was secretary of public instruction.

25 E. Bronson Conger, *An Ohio Woman in the Philippines*, Cleveland, Oh., Arthur H. Clark, 1904, pp. 51, 70.

26 L. Hathaway Mearns, *A Philippine Romance*, New York, Aberdeen Publishing, 1910, p. 77. Patricia felt out of place among these 'barbarous people just emerging from centuries of superstition, fear and medievalism', p. 36.

27 Mrs C. Dauncey, *An Englishwoman in the Philippines*, New York, E. P. Dutton, 1906, p. 242.

28 Bakhtin, *Rabelais*, p. 321. On the labour of bourgeois culture to produce a 'sublimated body', paralleling the classical body, see Stallybrass and White, *Transgression*, p. 93.

29 T. Veblen, *The Theory of the Leisure Class: An Economic Study of Institutions*, New York, New American Library, 1953 [1899], pp. 26–9. And yet the implacable Mrs Campbell Dauncey, an Englishwoman, found the Americans still

frightfully common, their manners those 'of ordinary European peasants'. She thought it 'a pity that such rough diamonds should represent to these natives the manners and intellect of a great and ruling white nation', and she despised 'the half-finished, skin-deep, hustling modernity of Americanised Manila'. *An Englishwoman*, pp. 12, 13, 133.

30 The 'American sublime' is a rhetorical sublime, not a metaphysics of the unpresentable. It is a colonial displacement of the 'sublimated spectacle of national empowerment' that R. Wilson has described in *American Sublime: The Genealogy of a Poetic Genre*, Madison, Wis., University of Wisconsin Press, 1991, and 'Techno-Euphoria and the Discourse of the American Sublime', *Boundary 2*, 1992, vol. 19, pp. 205–29, p. 208.

31 On the character of American machine culture, see Seltzer, *Bodies and Machines*. Seltzer suggests that such a 'materialist *reduction* of the life process to matter and mechanics is also the systematic *abstraction* of the life process', p. 225. This is, in a sense, the operationalising of the 'ascetic body' of Alfred Thayer Mahan's victorious 'new navy'. For, according to Ronald T. Takaki, 'republican "iron cages"' demanded 'the rational domination of the instinctual life ... [E]xpansionists imputed to "primitive" Filipinos and "savage" Chinese the emotional self republicans sought to deny, and sublimated republican repression to the violent domination of the "undeveloped races"' ('The New Empire: American Asceticism and the "New Navy"', in *Iron Cages: Race and Culture in 19th-Century America*, Seattle, University of Washington Press, 1979, pp. 226–79, p. 277). Donna Haraway describes this masculine American relation to the natural world in 'Teddy Bear Patriarchy: Taxidermy in the Garden of Eden, New York City, 1908–1936', in *Primate Visions: Gender, Race and Nature in the World of Modern Science*, New York and London, Routledge, 1989, pp. 26–58. On Teddy Roosevelt and the disciplined, strenuous life, see T. Lutz, *American Nervousness, 1903: An Anecdotal History*, Ithaca, NY, and London, Cornell University Press, 1991, pp. 77–84. More generally, on the development of bourgeois values of discipline and productivity, and the rise of the martial spirit, see J. Higham, 'The Reorientation of American Culture in the 1890s', in *Writing American History: Essays on Modern Scholarship*, Bloomington, Ind., Indiana University Press, 1973; and T. J. Jackson Lears, *No Place of Grace: Antimodernism and the Transformation of American Culture, 1880–1920*, New York, Pantheon Books, 1981. I discuss the medical construction of colonial masculinities in 'The Trespass Speaks: White Masculinity and Colonial Breakdown', *American Historical Review*, 1997, vol. 102, pp. 1343–70.

32 Quoted in Chief Surgeon, Philippines Division, to Surgeon-General, Washington, DC, 31 Dec. 1909, RG 112–E26/24508–120, USNA, p. 21. On the use of the Widal test to diagnose typhoid, see V. G. Heiser, 'Typhoid Fever in the Philippine Islands from the Sanitary Standpoint', *The Philippine Journal of Science*, 1912, vol. 7B, pp. 115–18.

33 Quoted in Chief Surgeon, Philippines Division, p. 17.

34 Ibid., p. 23.

35 H. Lefebvre, *The Production of Space*, trans. D. Nicholson-Smith, Oxford, Blackwell, 1991 [1971], esp. pp. 285–91. Lefebvre describes the production of abstract space from the sixteenth century, as it in part supplanted the 'space of accumulation', typically the marketplace. Similarly, Seltzer in *Bodies and Machines*, pp. 143–4, contrasts the space of the market (where movement confers agency) with the space of the factory (which implies automatism). Michel Foucault writes more generally that 'extension was substituted for localisation' ('Of Other Spaces', *Diacritics*, 1986, vol. 16, pp. 22–7, p. 23). On the understanding of a history of space, see E. W. Soja, *Postmodern Geographies: The Reassertion of Space in Critical Social Theory*, London and New York, Verso, 1989.

36 Lefebvre, *The Production of Space*, p. 51.
37 Ibid., p. 286.
38 Ibid., p. 289 (my italics). Mary Louise Pratt has commented on colonial visualisation in *Imperial Eyes: Travel Writing and Transculturation*, London and New York, Routledge, 1992. On the imposition of the square and grid in colonial Africa, see Comaroff and Comaroff, *Ethnography*, pp. 279–84; on French colonial urbanism, see Paul Rabinow, *French Modern: Norms and Forms of the Social Environment*, Cambridge, Mass., MIT Press, 1989. Although I do not explicitly deal with resistance here, I do not mean to imply that these spaces ensure submission; see Lefebvre on 'differential space', *The Production of Space*, pp. 352–400.
39 H. Bhabha, 'Signs Taken for Wonders: Questions of Ambivalence and Authority Under a Tree outside Delhi, May 1817', *Critical Inquiry*, 1985, vol. 12, pp. 144–65. On the space of the early laboratory, see O. Hannaway, 'Laboratory Design and the Aim of Science: Andreas Libavius versus Tycho Brahe', *Isis*, 1986, vol. 77, pp. 585–610; and S. Shapin, 'The House of Experiment in Seventeenth-Century England', *Isis*, 1988, vol. 79, pp. 373–404. In Bachelard's terms the colonial laboratory was a 'felicitous space ... that may be defended against adverse forces, the space we love', *The Poetics of Space*, p. xxxv.
40 See RG 350/3466–0, USNA. Act no. 607 (30 June 1903) transferred the serum laboratory of the Board of Health to the Bureau of Government Laboratories. Act no. 1407 (26 Oct. 1905) reorganised the laboratories into the Bureau of Science. See J. R. Velasco and L. Baens-Arcega, *The National Institute of Science and Technology, 1901–1982: A Facet of Science Development in the Philippines*, Manila, 1984; and E. Quisumbing, 'Development of Science in the Philippines', *Journal of East Asiatic Studies*, 1957, vol. 6, no. 2, pp. 127–53.
41 See RG 350/3466–0, USNA. Act no. 156, section 2.
42 Ibid., p. 10.
43 P. C. Freer, *Description of the New Buildings of the Bureau of Government Laboratories*, Manila, Bureau of Printing, 1904, RG 350/3466–17, USNA, p. 8.
44 Freer, *Description*, p. 8.
45 Ibid., p. 13. This is the original building, still standing on the campus of the Philippines Medical School. In 1912, a new wing was opened to contain a division of mines, the section of fisheries and fish products, the entomological collections and laboratories, and a new herbarium and library. See P. C. Freer, *Tenth Annual Report of the Director of the Bureau of Science, for the Year Ending August 1, 1911*, Manila, Bureau of Printing, 1912, RG 350/3466–25, USNA, pp. 3–5. More generally on the siting, design and equipping of tropical laboratories, see W. Byam and R. G. Archibald (eds), *The Practice of Medicine in the Tropics*, 2 vols, London, Hodder & Stoughton, 1921, vol. 1, ch. 24.
46 Freer, *Description*, p. 21.
47 P. C. Freer, *Third Annual Report of the Director of the Bureau of Science, 1903–4*, Manila, Bureau of Printing, 1905, pp. 16–18.
48 Freer, *Description*, p. 29. Freer described the herbarium as 'a card catalogue of the economic and scientific aspects of Philippine botany', *Fourth Annual Report of the Director of the Bureau of Science, 1904–5*, Manila, Bureau of Printing, 1906, p. 4. He further emphasises the importance of reinscribing the environment: 'To determine the identity of a Philippine plant with the same individual of a surrounding country, it is essential to ascertain the correct scientific name of the species, because the native name is of no value in this respect', p. 5.
49 Freer, *Third Annual Report*, p. 11. For a complete list of the library's holdings, see pp. 27–48.
50 Ibid., p. 26.

51 J. A. LeRoy, *Philippine Life in Town and Country*, New York and London, G. P. Putnam's Sons, 1906, p. 54. The experiment was to decide whether 'the Oriental' was capable of hygiene and development.
52 J. R. Hayden, *The Philippines: A Study in National Development*, New York, Macmillan, 1942, p. 644.
53 B. Latour, 'Give me a laboratory and I will raise the world', in K. Knorr-Cetina and M. Mulkay (eds), *Science Observed: Perspectives on the Social Study of Science*, London, Sage, 1983, p. 154 (Latour's italics). On the efforts of French bacteriologists to reorder colonial societies through the laboratories of the Pasteur Institute, see Latour, *The Pasteurisation of France*, Cambridge, Mass., Harvard University Press, 1988, esp. pp. 140–5.
54 Freer, *Third Annual Report*, p. 24.
55 Bakhtin, *Rabelais*, p. 23. I use the term 'market' rather loosely (as it was used by Americans) to exemplify the Philippines public sphere. See also Seltzer, *Bodies and Machines*, on the differences between market culture and machine culture. (Following Seltzer one might argue that movement in the market confers agency, while movement in the laboratory implies automatism, p. 144.) Lefebvre describes the 'space of accumulation', the marketplace, in *Production of Space*, pp. 264–8. In a more general sense, I am describing here a materialisation of Foucault's 'heterotopia of the colony', in 'Of Other Spaces', p. 27.
56 Bakhtin, *Rabelais*, pp. 217–76. See Stallybrass and White, *Transgression*, on the carnivalesque as a mode of understanding, pp. 6–19. They suggest that 'repugnance and fascination are the twin poles of the process in which a *political* imperative to reject and eliminate the debasing "low" conflicts powerfully and unpredictably with a desire for this Other', pp. 4–5. This vulnerable assumption of superiority actually depends on the construction of the low-Other. (I am implying that this holds also for the spatial practices producing these bodies.) On colonial ambivalence, see H. Bhabha 'Difference, Discrimination and the Discourse of Colonialism', in F. Barker *et al.* (eds), *The Politics of Theory*, Colchester, UK, University of Essex, 1983. Remarkably little is known about the character of the Philippines public sphere in the early twentieth century, so I make no claims about the *accuracy* of American representations of Filipino public life. For a suggestive account, see W. G. Davis, *Social Relations in a Philippine Market: Self-Interest and Subjectivity*, Berkeley, Calif., University of California Press, 1973.
57 LeRoy, *Philippine Life*, p. 54.
58 N. Roosevelt, *The Philippines: A Treasure and a Problem*, New York, J. H. Sears, 1926, p. 233.
59 D. R. Williams, *The United States and the Philippines*, New York, Doubleday, 1924, p. 125.
60 W. B. Freer, *The Philippine Experiences of an American Teacher*, New York, Charles Scribner's Sons, 1906, pp. 7–8. For a similar account of the 'filth' and the 'swarming masses of people' in primitive markets, see C. Lévi-Strauss, *Tristes tropiques*, New York, Athenaeum, 1975 [1955], pp. 143–5.
61 K. Mayo, *The Isles of Fear: The Truth about the Philippines*, New York, Harcourt Brace, 1924, p. 174. According to the *Proposed Sanitary Code*, 1920, sect. 49: 'Every person engaging in the despatching, transportation, handling or manipulation of food products . . . shall be provided with a certificate from the district health officer . . . [to] show that he is in good health and he is not a carrier of pathogenic germs', p. 22.
62 J. F. Smith to Secretary of War, 22 Nov. 1908, RG 350/3465-91, USNA. In the early 1900s, when Ralph Kent Buckland visited a *barrio* in the Visayas, he found 'not a knife, fork, nor spoon, nor a tumbler in the whole *barrio*. I had to eat with a piece of bamboo cut in the form of a paddle.' *In the Land of the Filipino*, New York, Every-Where Publishing Co., 1912, p. 184.

63 V. G. Heiser, *Annual Report of the Bureau of Health of the Philippine Islands, July 1, 1912– June 30, 1913*, Manila, Bureau of Printing, 1914, RG 350/3465–59, USNA, p. 29.
64 C. Fox, *Handbook for Sanitary Inspectors*, Manila, Bureau of Printing, 1914.
65 Heiser, *Annual Report of the Bureau of Health of the Philippine Islands*, pp. 29–30. Heiser argued that the 'habit of eating with the fingers' was the 'largest factor in the transmission of cholera and intestinal diseases', V. G. Heiser, 'Unsolved Health Problems Peculiar to the Philippines', *The Philippine Journal of Science*, 1910, vol. 5B, p. 176.
66 Heiser, *Annual Report of the Bureau of Health of the Philippine Islands*, p. 28. The *tienda* proprietors generally were a cause of considerable concern: 'The *tienda* owner . . . shall wear clean clothes with or without an apron. The hands must be kept clean and the finger nails short and well trimmed.' So too were street peddlers: 'The peddler must be neatly dressed. His hands should be clean and the nails short.' In J. P. Bantug, P. Gabriel and M. Aguelles, *A Simple Manual for Sanitary Inspectors*, Manila, Bureau of Printing, 1923, pp. 12, 14.
67 Heiser, *Annual Report of the Bureau of Health of the Philippine Islands*, pp. 67–8.
68 [G. A. Miller], *Interesting Manila*, Manila, E. C. McCullough, 1912, p. 191. In more ways than the metaphysical, then, 'The Anglo-Saxon lives in the concrete, the Oriental in the shadows', p. 17.
69 F. G. Carpenter, *Through the Philippines and Hawaii*, Garden City, NY, Doubleday, Page, 1925, p. 24.
70 D. Chakrabarty, 'Open Space/Public Space: Garbage, Modernity and India', *South Asia*, 1991, vol. 14, pp. 15–31. Chakrabarty is concerned mostly with filth rather than germs, and (accordingly) with spaces more than bodies. See also the other essays in vol. 14 of *South Asia*, a special issue entitled 'Aspects of "the public" in colonial South Asia', ed. S. B. Freitag.
71 A. MacLaughlin, 'The Suppression of a Cholera Epidemic in Manila', *The Philippine Journal of Science*, 1909, vol. 4B, p. 55.
72 Heiser, 'Unsolved Health Problems', p. 176.
73 T. W. Jackson, 'Sanitary Conditions and Needs in Provincial Towns', *The Philippine Journal of Science*, 1908, vol. 3B, p. 432.
74 Jackson, 'Sanitary Conditions', p. 432.
75 Ibid., pp. 435–6.
76 *Cablenews-American*, Manila, 30 May 1909.
77 J. D. Long, Director of Health, to W. H. Greenleaf, 7 Jan. 1918, RG 350/3465–97, USNA, provides a detailed account of these activities. See also V. de Jesús, 'Circular W-82', Philippine Health Service, Manila, 20 Nov. 1924, RG 350/3465–132, USNA; and Heiser to Commissioner of Education, Dept of the Interior, Washington, DC, Sept. 27, 1913, RG 350/3465–55, USNA.
78 Jesús, 'Circular W-82'. In this regime, the increasing emphasis on diet and food consumption generally can be read as transformative.
79 Bureau of Education and Philippine Health Service, *Health: A Manual for Teachers*, Manila, Bureau of Printing, 1928, consolidates instructions to teachers from the previous decade.
80 Ibid., p. 33.
81 Bourdieu, *Outline of a Theory*, p. 94.
82 *Health: A Manual for Teachers*, p. 49.
83 De Certeau, 'The Institution of Rot', p. 42. De Certeau argues that despite these confessions, a withholding of true affirmation occurs, since there is always 'that which exceeds', p. 44.
84 *Health: A Manual for Teachers*, p. 5. On the development of the water closet in the late nineteenth century, see L. Wright, *Clean and Decent: The Fascinating History of the Bathroom and the Water Closet*, London, Routledge & Kegan Paul,

1960; and J. Goubert, *The Conquest of Water: The Advent of Health in the Industrial Age*, trans. A. Wilson, Cambridge, Polity Press, 1989 [1986], pp. 91–7. The water closet is an invention of the last decades of the nineteenth century; Wright goes so far as to call 1870 the 'annus mirabilis of the water closet', p. 201. On the enclosure of the bathroom as a private space from 1880 onwards, see Vigarello, *Concepts of Cleanliness*, pp. 215–25.
85 Heiser, 'Unsolved Health Problems', p. 173.
86 Ibid.
87 Ibid., pp. 173, 174.
88 *The Disposal of Human Wastes in the Provinces*, pp. 5–7.
89 Ibid., pp. 7–9.
90 David G. Willets, 'General Conditions Affecting the Public Health and Diseases Prevalent in the Batanes Islands', *The Philippine Journal of Science*, 1913, vol. 8B, p. 51. Still, one was less likely to be as embarrassed on the boat to Capiz as Buckland was in 1903: 'A walk around the deck failed to disclose any of the conveniences that Americans have come to regard as absolute necessities. There was not a sign of a bathroom nor even of a lavatory any place on the main deck.' *In the Land of the Filipino*, p. 62.
91 MacLaughlin, 'The Suppression of a Cholera Epidemic in Manila', pp. 43–58, pp. 49, 50.
92 Bureau of Health, *Proposed Sanitary Code*, Health Bulletin no. 22, Manila, Bureau of Printing, 1920, pp. 15–17. This describes the Antipolo type of toilet. The director of health in his report for the fiscal year 1919 had urged 'preferential attention [be] given to the disposal of human wastes', RG 350/3465–108, USNA, p. 15. A description of the 'Antipolo system of toilet' is provided in M. Tianco (under the direction of J. D. Long, director of health), *Philippine Health Service Sanitary Almanac for 1919 and Calendars for 1920 and 1921*, Health Bulletin no. 19, Manila, Bureau of Printing, 1918, RG 350/2394–63, USNA, pp. 13, 16–19.
93 J. Rizal, *Noli Me Tangere*, trans. P.G. Valencia, Manila, National Book Store, 1967, pp. 166–92.
94 Dauncey, *An Englishwoman in the Philippines*, p. 52.
95 Moses, *Unofficial Letters of an Official's Wife*, pp. 45–6.
96 Ibid., pp. 47, 67. On public gatherings as sites of resistance, see R. C. Ileto, *Pasyon and Revolution: Popular Movements in the Philippines, 1840–1910*, Quezon City, Ateneo de Manila University Press, 1979; and A. S. Riggs, *The Filipino Drama*, Manila, Intramuros Administration, 1981 [1905].
97 Bureau of Health, 'Sanitary Measures in Connection with Local Fiestas', Provincial Circular no. 124, 6 Oct. 1915, RG 350/3465–86, USNA. On the dangers of fiestas, see also Marshall, 'Asiatic Cholera', p. 8.
98 'Sanitary Measures in Connection with Local Fiestas'.
99 Ibid. See also *Annual Report of the Bureau of Health of the Philippine Islands, July 1, 1912– June 30, 1913*, p. 33.
100 Anon., 'A Highly Artistic Red Cross Carnival', *Philippine Review*, 1918, vol. 3, Jan., p. 95.
101 Anon., 'The 1918 Philippine Red Cross Carnival', *Philippine Review*, 1918, vol. 3, Mar., p. 196.
102 Ibid., p. 197.
103 Ibid., p. 198.
104 Anon., 'Commercial Exhibits', *Philippines National Weekly*, 9 Feb. 1918, p. 3.
105 Anon., 'The Carnival and the Student', *Philippines National Weekly*, 9 Feb. 1918, p. 6. For a report emphasising sanitation in the 1922 Carnival (and describing the first 'Health Parade') see Anon., 'Manila Carnival and Commercial-Industrial Fair', *The American Chamber of Commerce Journal*, 1922, vol. 2, pp. 9–12.

106 'Clean-Up Week', Provincial Circular (unnumbered), 21 Oct. 1914, RG 350/3465–80, USNA. Clean-Up Week was also observed in many US towns. Frank Crone instructed teachers in the Philippines to explain to their students the meaning of Clean-Up Week. 'If 'Clean-Up Week' is carried out successfully the Philippines will be cleaner than ever before in their history,' he declared. 'Public health will be improved accordingly.' 'Clean-Up Week', Board of Education Circular no. 142, 3 Nov. 1914, RG 350/3465–80, USNA.

107 'Clean-Up Week', Provincial Circular (unnumbered), 2 Nov. 1915, RG 350/3465–80, USNA.

108 *Clean-Up Week: A Patriotic Message to all Patriotic Citizens*, Manila, Bureau of Printing, 1922, RG 350/3465–80, USNA. This pamphlet also suggests that 'unsanitary condition is not compatible with our national pride and aspiration'.

109 'Clean-Up Week', Public Welfare Board Circular, 30 Oct. 1920, RG 350/3465–80, USNA.

110 Ibid.

111 *Clean-Up Week: A Patriotic Message*, p. 8. Clean-Up Week was still popular in the 1930s; see D. D. Davis, 'Significance of Clean-Up Week', *Monthly Bulletin of the Philippine Health Service*, Jan. 1930, RG 350/3465–80, USNA. Davis, Governor General of the Islands, pointed out that: 'The formation of health habits is an important factor in the prevention of diseases. Health habits include sanitation, personal cleanliness, plenty of fresh air, good nourishing food, sleep, sunshine, and exercise', p. 7. See also the delightfully specific *Organization and Activities of Clean-Up Week for 1924*, Manila, Bureau of Printing, 1924, RG 350/3465–80, USNA. This is prefaced with a 'proclamation' from Leonard Wood, then Governor General, who insists that 'unattractive unsanitary surroundings are inconsistent with the best traditions and ideals of a progressive people', p. 5. B. Anderson's *Imagined Communities: Reflections on the Origins and Spread of Nationalism*, 2nd edn, London, Verso, 1991, is relevant to an understanding of these rituals of citizenship.

112 There is an obvious genetic link to the disparagement of the personal hygiene of foreigners and African-Americans in the United States itself that occurred during this period. The public health discourse was certainly similar, though perhaps enforced more rigorously and anxiously in the colonial tropics. For many immigrant groups in America – for generations of 'aliens' – 'civics' courses reproduced the colonial experience. The exploration of these parallels would require another essay. See A. M. Kraut, *Silent Travelers: Germs, Genes and the 'Immigrant Menace'*, New York, Basic Books, 1994.

113 On abjection 'which modernity has learned to repress, dodge or fake', see J. Kristeva, *Powers of Horror: An Essay in Abjection*, trans. L. S. Roudies, New York, Columbia University Press, 1982 [1980], p. 26. She describes the abject as 'something rejected from which one does not part, from which one does not protect oneself as from an object', p. 4. Accordingly, it is 'not lack of cleanliness or health that causes abjection, but what disturbs identity, system, order. What does not respect bodies, positions, rules. The in-between, the ambiguous, the composite.' At the same time as one condemns the abject, one also, paradoxically, yearns for it. (But while Kristeva – like so many colonial health officials – appears interested in naturalising the abject, admittedly with the uncolonial intention of privileging it, my goal has been to uncover a pragmatics of abjection related to identity politics.) See also G. Bataille, 'L'Abjection et les formes misérables', in *Essais de sociologie: Oeuvres complètes*, vol. 2, Paris, Gallimard, 1970. Despite the derivation of Kristeva's notion of abjection from the work of Bataille, it would seem that the colonial naming and enactment of the abject is designed (unsuccessfully) to control or evade Bataille's more

corroding *informe*. Homi Bhabha has written persuasively on colonial desire and psychic projections, and at one point he expresses this politics of identity in a form that is in this context particularly apposite: 'The white man does not merely deny what he fears and desires by projecting it on "them": Fanon sometimes forgets that paranoia never preserves its position of power, for the compulsive identification with a persecutory "they" is always an *evacuation and emptying* of the "I"' (my italics), in H. Bhabha, 'Remembering Fanon: Self, Psyche and the Colonial Condition', in B. Kruger and P. Mariani (eds), *Remaking History*, Discussions in Contemporary Culture Series, no. 4, Seattle, Bay Press, 1989, pp. 131–50, at 142.
114 Douglas, *Purity and Danger*, p. 170.
115 Ibid., p. 165.
116 See E. L. Walker and Andrew W. Sellards, 'Experimental Entamoebic Dysentery', *The Philippine Journal of Science*, 1913, vol. 8B, pp. 253–329.
117 Douglas, *Purity and Danger*, p. 108.
118 Ibid., p. 165. 'Epistemological clarity' is from Stallybrass and White, *Transgression*, p. 108.
119 R. Barthes, *Sade/Fourier/Loyola*, trans. R. Miller, Berkeley, Calif., University of California Press, 1976, p. 137. More particularly, in this case shit becomes 'cultured' and so reduced, abstracted and named, though in the process it is evidently rendered more powerful as a discursive resource.

5 Leprosy and the management of race, sexuality and nation in tropical Australia

Alison Bashford and Maria Nugent

A history of the control and prevention of leprosy – that culturally loaded infectious disease which always seems to stand for so much more than itself – exposes the powerful and complicated interplay between the management of 'race' and the management of 'health' in early to mid-twentieth-century Australia. Leprosy came quite suddenly into renewed European prominence in the late nineteenth century. Across the western and into the colonial worlds, including the Australian colonies, leprosy funds were established, international leprosy conferences organised, new legislation passed which permitted compulsory segregation, leper colonies or 'lazarets' created where there had been none. No remarkable increase in the disease itself prompted this action. Rather, leprosy became freshly significant for European cultures grappling with the implications of colonialism and changing economies of race.[1] The modern study of leprosy took place largely within new theories about racial differences and acclimatisation arising out of the deeply colonial discipline of tropical medicine.[2] Although leprosy was not exclusively a colonial issue in this period,[3] for most governments, scientists, epidemiologists and public health officers, leprosy was thoroughly organised through, situated in, and productive of, questions and imperatives of race relations and colonialism. For people who suffered from leprosy, their identity as Indian or British, Chinese, Aboriginal or European, Filipino or American, African or French, directly affected their experience of medical and governmental powers battling over the cause of leprosy and the modes for its prevention, in particular the justifications for compulsory and often lifelong isolation.

Although there was disagreement over the aetiology of leprosy well into the twentieth century, it was known that it was not spread between people with anything like the virulence of other diseases – plague, cholera, tuberculosis, or smallpox, for example. This was part of the reason for the currency and longevity of the ideas that leprosy was not contagious or that it was hereditary.[4] Even for those who did subscribe to theories about its contagiousness through the action of a bacillus (first identified in 1874) it was understood that it took prolonged contact, often measured in years, for the disease to spread from person to person. Nonetheless it was with respect to leprosy specifically – not those other virulent diseases – that extremely coercive and rigid systems of isolation arose (or more correctly re-emerged) in the nineteenth century. Of course, this was not incidentally, but rather intimately (one might even argue causally) related to the colonial context of much leprosy management; the non-whiteness of so many people with the disease. The spatial techniques through which 'race' was managed in colonial situations were often similar to the techniques through which 'health' was managed – separation, isolation and containment, sometimes culturally encouraged, sometimes legally enforced. In attempts to prevent, treat and manage leprosy these spatial techniques of health and race management were intertwined with particular intensity and poignancy.

The clustering of issues of contact and contagion, race and health around leprosy was especially notable in Australia. The disease of leprosy, though never numerically significant, had become profoundly symbolic during the late nineteenth century, a period of intense race-based Australian nationalism; it stood for a threatened contamination of the mythically 'white' nation-in-the-making by Chinese men.[5] In the 1880s and 1890s, a system of compulsory isolation on island lazarets had been put in place to control the spread of leprosy, a development that was intimately tied to the problem of foreigners in, and the introduction of foreign diseases to, Australia. By the early twentieth century and the interwar period preventive policy had come to be partly structured around a peculiar theory that leprosy was a sexually transmitted disease: moreover, that it became a public health problem for 'white' Australia specifically because of sex between races, between Chinese, South Pacific Islanders, Aborigines, Torres Strait Islanders and Europeans or whites. Thus leprosy management became entangled with anxieties about miscegenation, with the complicated and paradoxical policies of assimilation of so-called half-castes, and with nationalist politics of immigration restriction and racial purity.

In this chapter we explore the ways in which the management of leprosy and the management of race (and by implication nation) became mutually constitutive in Australia, with a particular focus on Queensland in the interwar period. And we ask: how did the interconnecting questions of race, sexuality, leprosy and power play out in the early and mid-twentieth century?

The banished leper in early modern Europe is one of the figures through which Michel Foucault illustrated crudely coercive or 'sovereign' power. In *Discipline and Punish* he wrote that this practice of 'exile-enclosure' did not really 'produce' anything except separated clean and unclean communities: 'The leper was caught up in a practice of rejection, of exile-enclosure; he was left to his doom in a mass among which it was useless to differentiate.' By contrast, Foucault's 'plague town' was managed, monitored and internally differentiated. It was 'traversed throughout with hierarchy, surveillance, observation, writing ... this is the utopia of the perfectly governed city ... the exercise of disciplinary power'.[6] Much critical medical history and sociology has taken up this model of shifting modes of power, tracing changes from crude quarantining measures to more sophisticated internalised hygienic practices and the production of healthy subjectivities often associated with modern understandings of responsible citizenship.[7] Warwick Anderson has recently done so with respect to leprosy, arguing that the history of isolation should not be seen as a rigid and non-productive exclusion.[8] Rather, isolation was precisely about the productive training of lepers into civic subjectivity, at least in his early twentieth-century example, Culion, in the Philippines. What he calls 'the usual sad tale of stigmatization and segregation' did not apply at Culion, rather, 'the leper colony became a laboratory of modern citizenship'.[9]

We suggest that leprosy management involved both repressive practices of 'exile-enclosure' *and* the creation of raced civic and national subjectivities of the type Anderson identifies at Culion. In the problematic zone of tropical Australia these two modes of power were broadly racialised, though not in clear-cut ways. While not all incarcerated lepers were indigenous people in Australia, there is a clear sense in which the whole system of island isolation continued to be implemented and justified in the first half of the twentieth century because *most* lepers were Aboriginal or Torres Strait Islanders. Further, as the rest of the world gradually abandoned compulsory isolation, powerful Australian public health policy-makers argued for its continued use into the 1950s and 1960s explicitly on the grounds of Aboriginal people's *non* citizenship, or more precisely, the perception of their *incapacity* for modern citizenship. Yet, although Aboriginal people were always treated more coercively by the public health system than whites, to view Aboriginal lepers as simply 'banished' to the lazarets is to ignore evidence of limited civic subjectivities exercised within those sites of isolation, although this was never the intention of authorities in the way that Anderson suggests of Culion.

We also argue that capturing the complicated play of race and power requires analysis of the social spaces either side of the cordon sanitaire. That is, leprosy management went on not only within the confines of the lazaret, as the international historiography would imply, but also without, in the social domain.[10] The historiographical focus on leprosy management inside the lazarets has masked the range of formal and informal segregating practices which were considered or established in the social arena. Cordons sanitaire were not limited to the shores of the island lazarets, but were pursued in such conflated racial/hygienic measures as the 'leper line' in Western Australia and the system of reserves for the containment of Aboriginal people. Moreover, the cultivation of white conduct in the tropics was aimed toward a social and sexual separateness. It is possible to argue that leprosy management outside the lazaret was a productive process where racial/sexual separation and what we identify as 'interior frontiers' of whiteness were cultivated rather than enforced.

This chapter, then, is an initial presentation of the complex interplay between race and health, contagion and separation, with respect to leprosy, complexities which will be fully detailed in forthcoming work.[11] In the first section we outline the development of the island-isolation system and the race-based justifications for it. We then consider the peculiar situation of the Peel Island lazaret in Queensland, the only lazaret in Australia in which sometimes equal numbers of Aboriginal and non-Aboriginal lepers shared the place and the experience of segregation and exile.[12] Aiming to look beyond official meanings,[13] we examine the modes of protest and resistance employed by the inmates of Peel Island. As historian Suzanne Saunders has suggested, for many Aboriginal inmates the coercion and forced containment in lazarets was an extension of the reserve systems whereby movement of Aboriginal people was limited, and in which people and families were forcibly removed from one another.[14] Yet the avenues of complaint, of written protest, the sense of right of access to the highest judicial bodies, seems to have been rather more possible from the subject position of 'leper' than from the subject position of 'Aboriginal' or 'half-caste' regulated by the 'normal' systems of race management in interwar Australia, partly because the space and experience of isolation-as-leper was shared with whites. The archival fragments of inmates' lives suggest the complicated significance of race and disease in the making of individual and collective subjectivities, and in the contestation over the meanings of 'exile-enclosure'.

Leprosy management had social effects well beyond the shores of the island-lazarets, in large part because leprosy was such a deeply inscribed way of thinking about race, both internal relations between Europeans and indigenous people and external relations between Europeans and Asians. In the final section of this chapter we focus on just one of the ways in which leprosy was managed outside the lazarets, which derived from the linking of the disease with interracial sex: the health policy whereby white women were encouraged to settle in the tropical north of Australia in order to stabilise 'proper' sexual relations between the races, thus preventing the spread of leprosy. We are interested in the ways in which white women came to be thought about quite literally as public health solutions or even therapies which helped keep society in tropical Australia racially and sexually separated; that is, to stop white men having sex with Aboriginal women. We argue, then, that while race and disease was managed through crude measures of isolation and the imposition of rigid borders, this was not the only mode of power and governance at work. Racial and sexual identity and difference was also produced by a cultivation of 'settled', healthy and sexually separated white society in the precarious tropical north; a cultivation of the white self in which the influence and work of women was understood to be central.[15]

Leprosy, race and enforced isolation

Australian epidemiologists and public health administrators became suddenly interested in leprosy from the very late 1880s and 1890s, and this interest escalated with the funding and support which tropical medicine received from the new Commonwealth government after the British colonies were federated in 1901. The disease was initially associated with the Chinese population, as well as with South Pacific Islanders in northern New South Wales and Queensland, many of whom had come to Australia as indentured labourers.[16] A small number of Aboriginal people were also reported with leprosy in this late nineteenth-century period. In the late 1880s in northern and tropical Australia, where most leprosy first appeared, a system of island-isolation for people diagnosed with, or suspected as having, leprosy was instituted and legislated.[17] While the majority of people diagnosed with leprosy, and compulsorily confined, were 'coloureds', a small but growing number of 'white lepers' were identified, in Queensland especially.[18] There, a dual system of island lazarets emerged in the early 1890s – one for coloureds, one for whites. But by 1907 this had been replaced by Peel Island lazaret in Moreton Bay off Brisbane, where all lepers in Queensland (both white and coloured) were confined.[19]

By the interwar years, a changing demographic was noted. If in the 1890s lepers were mainly Chinese and Pacific Islander men, by the 1920s they were mainly Aboriginal men and women, and in the case of Queensland, white men. While 'coloured' immigrants, particularly the Chinese, were held primarily responsible for its introduction to 'leprosy-free' Australia, it was Aboriginal people, considered especially vulnerable to the disease, who came to be understood as the cause for its spread to the European, or white, population. The number of people with leprosy in Australia was not large, compared with other infectious diseases. Table 5.1 from J. H. L. Cumpston's 'Health and Disease in Australia' shows the proportionately increasing number of 'Australians' and Aborigines, and is typical of the national and racial categorisation which shaped nearly all early epidemiology on leprosy.

The relatively small numbers of people with leprosy did not preclude extensive (excessive) medical, epidemiological, legislative and popular concern. In part, the interesting problem for epidemiologists was that white people acquired leprosy in Australia, but not in England. This presented a curious problematic for those interested in contemporary theories of racial immunity and susceptibility. It was central to an Australia-wide survey of the epidemiology of leprosy conducted by Dr Cecil Cook between 1923 and 1925, a study funded by the London School of Tropical Medicine. His conclusions about the contagiousness of leprosy, and particularly his explanation about the process of its transmission, were to have long-standing ramifications. In his subsequent dual role as the Chief Medical Officer and Protector of Aborigines in the Northern Territory,[20]

Table 5.1 Nationality of recorded cases of leprosy in Australia

	Chinese	Kanakas	Aborigines	Other coloured aliens	Americans or other whites	Australians	Total
1850–60	unknown	—	—	1	—	—	1
1860–70	30+	—	—	—	4	1	35
1870–75	15	—	—	—	—	3	18
1875–80	11	—	—	—	3	2	16
1880–85	18	—	—	—	2	2	22
1885–90	31	1	—	2	4	5	43
1890–95	27	10	7	3	5	19	71
1895–1900	27	41	13	1	18	8	108
1900–05	15	43	7	5	14	19	103
1905–10	14	39	35	5	8	21	122
1910–15	6	14	22	4	10	17	73
1915–20	4	5	31	1	7	27	75
1920–25	3	5	54	—	9	22	93
Total	201	158	169	22	84	146	780

Source: J. H. L. Cumpston, 'Health and Disease in Australia: A History', unpublished typescript, vol. 1, 1928, p. 318. Courtesy, Burkitt–Ford Library, University of Sydney.

Cook consistently advocated isolation as the main measure for the prevention of leprosy in Australia, and this in the face of considerable local and international disagreement.[21] He opened his monumental study by framing leprosy squarely as a question of racial immunities and susceptibilities:

> With the exception of Northern and North-Western Australia, the country to be considered is occupied solely by a European race of whom 98 percent are British. Leprosy, virtually unknown in the Mother Country except as an importation, is found, nevertheless, spreading amongst these Australian whites. What was the origin of the disease and why should a race, so rarely affected in its own country, become more subject to infection in Australia?[22]

The ongoing international discussion in the 1920s and 1930s about the aetiology of leprosy, its contagious capacities, and the possibility of inheritance, was also always a debate about its treatment and prevention, in particular the perennially contentious question of compulsory isolation. The medical and legal justifications for isolation were strongly debated and heavily resisted, not only by people in lazarets whose liberties were suspended, but also by many doctors and epidemiologists who specialised as leprologists.

Notwithstanding the presence of white people, we suggest, like Suzanne Saunders, that it was the linking of leprosy with Aboriginality, which underpinned the continued use of islands for isolation well into the twentieth century in Australia.[23] Public health experts' opinions on the sociality of Aboriginal people were informed by, as well as themselves shaped, the prejudicial dominant culture which specifically excluded Aborigines from citizenship in Australia.[24] If, as medical sociologists Petersen and Lupton have argued, the 'good' citizen in the modern world is the 'healthy' citizen,[25] there were ways in which perceptions about Aboriginal people's inability to perform 'health and hygiene' appropriately placed them outside the citizenry. Conversely, in that Aboriginal people were already outside the citizenry, questions about the legality and liberality of their compulsory isolation were deflected.[26]

Repeatedly, Cook and Dr Raphael Cilento, the other prominent figure in interwar tropical medicine and Aboriginal health, marked Aboriginal people as incapable of responsible citizenship and self-management when it came to the prevention of leprosy.[27] In terms that reflected popular representations of Aboriginality, the threat of Aborigines in relation to leprosy was due in part to their perceived 'careless and irresponsible habits' that 'render it impossible to keep him under observation, or to submit himself to a course of treatment unless he is under restraint'.[28] In answering international criticism about the continued enforced isolation of suspected leprosy cases in Australia, Cook typically justified the practice in terms of the special problems posed by the presence of the disease among the

Aboriginal population, arguing that since Aboriginal people could not be trusted to seek treatment, 'all lepers should be isolated in a lazaret without recourse to a bacteriological examination'.[29] In 1934, it was explicitly stated that 'the effective control of leprosy and its eventual eradication are closely bound up with the supervision of the health of the Aboriginal population and other coloured peoples'.[30]

Underpinning Cilento's commitment to the practice of isolation of people believed to be infected with leprosy was his perception about the particular vulnerability of Australia to introduced infectious diseases. For Cilento, it was the combination of tropical conditions and the presence of leprosy among Aboriginal people with their unpredictable patterns of sociality, that justified island isolation. For example in Cilento's review of leprosy policy in Australia, prepared for the Federal Health Council in 1934, he argued:

> When the case of the aboriginal was investigated, the problem was seen to be infinitely complicated. The native habits of changing the name repeatedly further disguises relationships already masked by the haphazard use of the terms 'brother', 'father', 'cousin', 'uncle', etc. His complete dread of the white man's medicines, surgical possibilities, and hospitals (obvious in all areas, including those where leprosy is found most frequently) renders it utterly impossible to contemplate any system other than segregation for him.[31]

In 1950 the National Health and Medical Research Council (NH&MRC) presented a 'Standard Procedure in Respect of the Control of Leprosy'. The procedures again dealt with the isolation of Aboriginal people specifically:

> full-blooded natives who fall into one of four categories should be isolated. The categories are: i. all those with active leprosy whether bacteriological examination gives positive results or not; ii. all those with clinically suggestive conditions, whether bacteriological examination gives positive results or not; iii. those patients liable to relapse who cannot be kept under satisfactory supervision outside an institution; iv. crippled or other subjects who cannot, outside an institution, maintain a comfortable standard of living or be calculated to maintain an adequate resistance to the advance of the disease.[32]

In 1956 a special conference reviewed the NH&MRC's 1950 procedures. Yet on the question of isolation the conference reiterated the opinions expressed in the 1950 report that it was necessary for Aboriginal people. Indeed, despite a worldwide move away from compulsory segregation as the main treatment and prevention strategy for dealing with leprosy, Australian health authorities argued that '[t]he time is not ripe in

Australia for abandoning the present prophylactic system. It is in the interest alike of the patient and the general public that all cases of leprosy should be isolated and placed under treatment if necessary in special hospitals.'[33] There is a clear sense, then, in which the shift to a liberal and voluntary model of public health in which self-governance in hygienic matters was the primary mode of action, was explicitly considered not applicable to indigenous people. Aboriginal people were considered outside the supposedly responsible white citizenry who would take on health and hygiene as part of their civic duties.

Peel Island lazaret – a shared site of exile

It is very clear that compulsory segregation of lepers was justified on the grounds of the perceived threat of the Aboriginal-other to the white population, and especially the pathologising of Aboriginal patterns of sociality as constituting a risk to public health. However, focusing only on this official and expert literature would mask the ways in which the inmates of lazarets, Aboriginal, white and especially those who were identified and identified themselves as 'half-caste', exercised a certain agency despite, or perhaps because of, their exile.

Perhaps more than any other institution charged with the management of leprosy in Australia, Peel Island lazaret in Queensland, especially in the 1920s and 1930s, exposes the complex interplay between race, leprosy and power. A complicated and often ambiguous picture of the island institution emerges from the considerable archive pertaining to Peel Island, an archive that includes correspondence produced by both government and inmates. While there is not sufficient space here to fully explore it, the extant correspondence between inmates and various officials suggests a struggle of meaning between the island as a place of coercion, of 'exile enclosure', and a place where new kinds of civic subjectivities were unwittingly produced.[34]

From an official point of view, the Peel Island institution was clearly constructed as a site of enforced isolation, in which little or no attempt was made by health officers to train inmates in modern citizenship, in the ways that Anderson describes at Culion. Cilento, the government public health official in Queensland almost solely responsible for the retention of compulsory isolation in the management of leprosy, understood Peel Island predominantly as a place of confinement aimed at protecting the general population from possible infection, rather than necessarily about treatment. In 1939, he informed the Under Secretary that 'we have to consider not the 26 white lepers who are confined at Peel Island, but the one million people of Queensland many of them children of the most susceptible ages'.[35] Yet, if Cilento was not overly concerned about the treatment of inmates on the island, there were many others who were. Throughout its history, Peel Island lazaret constantly drew the attention of politicians, lay people and the judiciary. Official and semi-official visits to the island were intermittently made to investigate conditions.[36]

Some external and independent reviews of Peel Island emerged from concerns about, and questioned the rightfulness of, the enforced banishment of leprosy patients. The question of race appears equivocally in these reviews and in this public protest. On the one hand, implicit and sometimes explicit in the public protest was the fact that whites were compulsorily confined on the island, moreover that they were confined *with* Aborigines. But while the confinement of all lepers was the effect of the racial reasoning of Cilento, Cook and others, that prejudicial reasoning was not itself subject to protest. In this way, the public outcry about whites on Peel Island did not explicitly address race, but rather was directed at the matter of enforced isolation *per se*.

One of the effects of public concern about Peel Island lazaret was that inmates were provided with access to various forms of complaint and protest, particularly since, as part of the review process, patients were encouraged to make their own concerns known and to report incidents of maltreatment to public health and other government officials. Inmates wrote letters to governors, prepared petitions and appeals to politicians, and organised citizen support groups both within the confines of the island and outside it. They appealed to the officials of the Queensland Department of Health and Home Affairs which had responsibility for the management of the lazaret as well as to a level of government beyond that.[37] The appeals of inmates of the island were publicised in metropolitan newspapers, and some independent medical practitioners with an interest in leprosy advocated publicly on their behalf. Their concerns were often internal to the institution – about their treatment by resident staff, living conditions on the island and their rights as inmates. Aboriginal inmates especially made appeals for better living conditions, which by all reports were substantially worse than those provided to whites.[38] For example, in 1925, an Aboriginal woman wrote directly to the Home Secretary asking 'why cant [sic] they give me dicent [sic] beds like the other wimmen [sic] here'.[39] Another man officially classified as 'coloured' asked the Home Secretary

> if you are going to give me one [of the new huts] as you know they have gave G.W., the jarvanese and Italians and the half-caste Chinese proper places to live in so I consider myself as good as any of them in fact just as good as any of the white inmates, so I ask you if you would grant me the same.[40]

For those responsible for the day-to-day running of the lazaret, the repeated demands and protests of inmates, which were sometimes expressed in more immediate and direct ways than written complaints to the metropolitan bureaucracy, were interpreted as a kind of lawlessness. The overseers found this particularly offensive in relation to the 'coloured' inmates, whom it was claimed 'have an idea that being leper patients the law cannot touch them, in consequence of which they are impertinent and defy everyone on the island'.[41] Thus, rather than considering themselves simply outcasts, there is a sense in which inmates of the lazaret had a sense of exceptional (or special) rights produced by their very exile.

Arguably the Aboriginal lepers confined on Peel Island had a greater sense of a capacity to complain to officials and to expect redress on the leper colony than on any of the government reserves or stations, the other sites where the movement and liberties of Aboriginal people were contained.[42] Within the lazaret, their modes of exercising civic capacities mirrored those used by non-Aboriginal lepers with whom they shared the space of exile. Indeed, despite their sometimes semi-literacy, the surviving letters of Aboriginal inmates of the Peel Island lazaret indicate explicit recourse to a discourse of civic rights, and to a system of authority that existed beyond, over and above the onsite, micro-governance of the lazaret.[43]

During the 1930s, inmates of Peel Island became increasingly vocal in their criticism about compulsory isolation as a prophylactic measure in the control of leprosy. They repeatedly criticised Cilento's position, providing evidence of international opinion that leprosy was not highly contagious and did not warrant enforced isolation.[44] Armed with this evidence the inmates established their own welfare association through which they appealed to government authorities. In a petition to the governor of Queensland, the inmates asked him

> to intercede on our prolonged and wrongful detention on the grounds appearing henceforth that worlds [*sic*] recognised authorities and scientists have arrived at the conclusion that the condition commonly known as Leprosy is not transmitted by 'bacteria' of any kind from person to person.[45]

The consistent point of inmates' appeals was that isolation was unnecessary for the control of leprosy, particularly as it became increasingly evident that the disease was not highly contagious. Inmates, some of whom believed that they were being treated for leprosy while only displaying symptoms that resembled leprosy, petitioned parliament about problems associated with the efficacy of examination procedures.[46] In 1939 the Peel Island Welfare Association secretly sent an inmate to Canberra to lobby federal parliamentarians for a royal commission into Peel Island.[47] Yet, despite the protests of inmates and their supporters, Cilento continued to argue that the compulsory isolation of lepers was critical to the management and control of leprosy in tropical Queensland. With the endorsement of the Commonwealth government, the practice continued until the 1960s.[48]

Interior frontiers: sexuality and contagion

The prevention of leprosy in Australia was not only enacted by the exclusion of lepers from the social body – Peel Island being just one lazaret among many – but also by a range of measures in the racially contested zone of 'tropical' Australia. The practice of compulsory isolation was only one component of a broader campaign. According to Maguire, 'the need for the rapid colonisation of northern Australia added urgency to the search for medical and social means to contain the diseases inhibiting white adaptation to the tropics'.[49] It was leprosy conceived as a public health problem intimately tied to the 'successful colonisation of tropical Australia' that gave rise to the engineering and production of internal frontiers beyond the shores of island lazarets in the interwar period.

Two contextualising points need to be made here: first, the northern boundaries of Australia, the tropics, were especially significant in early twentieth-century race-based Australian nationalism; second, the discipline of tropical medicine (within which leprosy was studied) was put to explicit use in the production of this nationalism, that is, in the pursuit of 'white Australia'. The north of Australia, and in particular the edges of the north – the boundaries of the new island-nation – became significant for a racist nationalist culture which needed to differentiate itself from those 'others' over the northern border – Asian cultures persistently constructed as contaminating. 'Australia' was now the whole island and 'white Australians' had to fill it, or at least fill its edges. The discipline of tropical medicine was implicated closely in this national political and racial aspiration. Securing the white population of the north fell very much within the domain of public health generally and tropical medicine particularly. Thus, the burgeoning field of tropical medicine in Australia was driven by the question 'Is White Australia Possible?' – that is, can 'white man' live viably and reproduce in the tropics of Australia? From the point of view of government, it was economically and politically essential to overturn the long-standing assumption of British and some American literature that whites could not permanently settle the tropics.[50]

The tropics needed securing as white, and this process of 'settling' in the north involved not only being there, as it were, but feeling settled: the white self needed cultivating. This process might be thought of as the development of 'interior frontiers', borrowing from the theorist of nationalism Etienne Balibar.[51] Analysing the early nineteenth-century political philosopher Fichte's work, Balibar writes that an internal border or interior frontier is that which constitutes a community through internalised individual identity; for Fichte the borders of a 'spontaneous linguistic community', for Balibar 'the inner nation, the invisible nation of minds'.[52] Or, as Ann Laura Stoler writes: internal borders mark 'the moral predicates by which a subject retains his or her national identity despite location outside the national frontier and despite heterogeneity within it'.[53] Purity and integrity of an imagined national community can be threatened externally or internally.

Within the racially loaded context of northern and tropical Australia, both Cecil Cook and Raphael Cilento developed and researched the idea that leprosy was sexually transmitted, and that this transmission involved sex between racially differentiated people. Once figured as a sexually transmitted disease, and as a contagion produced and spread through miscegenation, leprosy became even more disproportionately socially and culturally invested – disproportionate, that is, to the number of people with the disease. Stoler has written of shifts in the meaning of indigenous women's sexual relations with colonising European men in other contexts. At one time considered protectors of colonial men's well-being, in the early twentieth century, they became 'bearers of ill-health and sinister influences ... now sources of contagion and loss of the (white) self'.[54] In early to mid-twentieth-century Australia, experts like Cilento and Cook perceived that whiteness was under threat from the contact with Chinese men and Aboriginal women which leprosy implied. Both Cilento and Cook were crucial policy-makers because they were deeply involved not only in health management but in the implementation of policies pertaining to Aboriginal people in Queensland and the Northern Territory.[55] Significantly, Cook was a central figure in the new policies of assimilation of 'half-castes' into white culture and white populations. Cilento wrote voluminously on the viability of the tropics for whites, as well as on Aboriginal health.[56]

The theory that leprosy was sexually transmitted existed as a minor strand in international medical literature, often working in an inferential way through a linking with syphilis.[57] In Australia, there was a larger interest in the sexual transmission of leprosy than seems to have been the case in other colonial and national contexts. The very strong connection in white Australian popular and political culture between Chineseness, leprosy and national invasion, which was not uncommonly represented as sexual invasion of virginal white womanhood, may well have been the fertile cultural ground from which these medical/epidemiological links were made.[58] At an 1884 Sanitary Conference the delegate from Western Australia confidently stated that leprosy was spread by 'the prevalence of prostitution of white women to Chinese'. And a Queensland delegate argued that '[w]e have never had the disease amongst the aboriginals in Queensland ... Simply because the black women will not cohabit with the Chinese'.[59] By the mid-1920s Cook had developed his theory thus: Chinese and Pacific Islander men, infected elsewhere, entered the Australian colonies as immigrants, or as indentured labourers during the nineteenth century. The problem, argued Cook, was that there were no women of the same race, and so, they had sex with Aboriginal women who later had sex with Aboriginal men and with white men. For Cook, the only possible conduit for the spread of leprosy was Aboriginal women. He discounted not only the possibility of sex between men, but the possibility of sexual connection between 'coloured aliens' and white women:

> White prostitutes would be unlikely to risk the stigma of association with a leper, such cases usually being regarded by the people as syphilitic. Should she do so openly, the likelihood of whites consorting with her would be small ... White women consorting with Kanakas were rare, and lost caste. They were usually faithful to their dark consorts or confined the distribution of their favours (of necessity) to coloured men. They did not, therefore, constitute a serious menace to the white male population.[60]

In an epidemiology which, in its own terms, subjected every inference to rigorous tests of logic, the assumptions about sexual behaviour here are stunning. Without any effort to verify his claims, Cook then proceeded to describe what he thought was the key to the whole question of leprosy in Australia:

> The matter of aboriginal gins is much more important, since the alien, deprived of the society of women of their own kind, and unable, except in very rare instances, to overcome the racial prejudices of the white women, fell back for conjugal relationship upon the salacious aboriginal. In this way the races came into the most intimate contact ... Herein lay the danger to the white ... Although the whites did not become directly associated with the Chinese and kanakas, there was ... a definite link between the two races by means of which the diseases of the latter could be transmitted to the former.[61]

In the logic of this epidemiology the cause and therefore the main mode of preventing leprosy hinged on sex and race demographics, and on the sexual practices and prejudices which existed between races. The situation which most threatened public health, argued Cook, was when Chinese, Pacific Islander or European men were located in a population of considerable numbers of Aboriginal people and few white women.[62] The causative demographic condition was the 'lack of an adequate white female population' and the presence of Aboriginal women.[63] According to this rationale, Cook concluded: 'A Chinese or South Sea Islander leper is, generally speaking, only to be considered as constituting a menace to the white population where there is (i) a considerable Aboriginal population, and (ii) a scarcity of white women.'[64] Thus it was surmised that the infection of the white population could only happen 'per medium of the aboriginal'.[65]

For race and health managers like Cilento and Cook, public health could be secured by stabilising boundaries between racial groups, by creating a newly permanent and stable social system in 'frontier' and tropical Australia, in which contact between races was prevented or discouraged. One manifestation of this social plan was the encouragement of 'healthy' numbers of white women to the tropics; women who were influential in normalising and settling the tropics as racially and sexually stable. This interest in the numbers of white women in the north worked at several material and symbolic levels. Their sexual availability to white men supposedly resulted in a reduction in interracial sex. The familial and domestic cultures which they were meant to introduce represented 'settlement' and permanence in the tropics. And, as Anne McClintock has argued of women in South Africa and elsewhere, white women were markers of the nation at its precarious borders. In many national cultures, white women often symbolised the purity of an imagined community.[66]

Cook wrote about the town of Derby in Western Australia as the type of healthy community to be developed in the tropical north: 'In Derby, being a permanent European settlement, the sexes amongst Europeans are comparably represented, and apart from that degree of association contingent upon domestic service, there is no intimacy or fraternization between the races.'[67] This public policy of encouraging white women to the north involved a range of 'civilising' and 'domesticating' meanings and processes. White tropical conduct was to be effected by women, and to be produced in and symbolised by, domestic arrangements. An industry in instruction in Australian tropical domesticity flourished between the wars. This included the minutiae of daily conduct; diet, exercise, clothing, literature to be read, leisure activities to be pursued, timetables for daily routine, as well as 'Attitude towards Native Assistants'.[68] While apparently effecting a reduction in sexual contact between the races, white women were perceived to be able to properly manage domestic and social contacts between Aboriginal people and the white world in their supervision of domestic help. All this was part of the cultivation of conduct specifically as white; the development of interior frontiers through an understanding of conduct which began with the domestic and the familial. It can be thought about as the introduction of a 'proper' private sphere to the north, intended to displace the illegitimate private, sexual conduct of white men and Aboriginal women which had ostensibly resulted in contagion and ill-health. This was a private conduct which was performed in, and symbolised by, domesticity and family. In Stoler's words this linking of 'domestic arrangements to the public order, family to the state' was imperial/national biopolitics at work.[69] The domesticity which white women symbolised marked the tropical north as settled, as opposed to being in a process of colonisation.

White women were understood, indeed simply assumed, to effect a reduction in sexual contact between white men and Aboriginal women. Cook based all kinds of conclusions on this assumption. For example, studying leprosy in the Queensland town of Bundaberg he concluded that the considerable numbers of European women indicated 'a degree of civilization and refinement in the community rendering combo-ism (cohabitation between white males and aboriginal females) highly improbable, even where there was a sufficiently numerous aboriginal population to encourage it'.[70] He suggested that a 'natural antipathy' between European and Aboriginal needed 'fostering' and that this would result from the presence of white women:

> As to the prevention of association between European and aboriginal, it is to be feared legislative enactments will be unavailing. On the other hand there exists in the white a natural aversion to these practices, which is only overcome after prolonged familiarity with degrading conditions and suppression of the sexual instinct. The fostering of the natural antipathy and the encouragement of female immigration such as will inevitably follow the development of the primitive regions where these conditions at present prevail, will do far more to segregate the races than a tome of prohibitive Statutes.[71]

In this report, although the radical and forced limitation of movement of Aboriginal people is suggested as possible and desirable, the forced limitation of the sexual practices of white men is understood to be impossible. Rather, their desires needed to be manufactured. This report announced a separation of races secured not coercively or through regulatory bodies, but rather through internalised lines of hygiene and as modes of gendered conduct. The presence of white women was perceived to separate the white social body, first from the Aboriginal community, and second from past invasion by Chinese men.

While the development of these kinds of interior frontiers aimed to bring about a healthy, clean and viable (separate) white identity, this did not mean that more coercive segregating measures of leprosy prevention were not employed in the 'general community' beyond the leper colonies. For Cook and Cilento, infectious disease and other forms of ill-health were often produced by what they saw as illegitimate movement, sexual contact and intermingling of racial groups: the migration of people from their proper place to an improper place. Cook, for example, argued that leprosy was most prevalent in India where tribes had left 'their native seclusion, but have not yet adopted modern sanitary measures'.[72] He suggested the containment of 'pure' Aboriginal groups as permanently separate: 'In the virgin country of North Kimberley where the natives continue in their pristine state, the disease [of leprosy] is quite unknown.'[73] Conversely, the health of a community could be achieved by preventing such 'illegitimate' movement in the first place, by putting people back where they 'belonged'. This had been partially achieved by Queensland and Commonwealth Immigration Restriction Acts which controlled the entry of non-whites into Australia, not infrequently on the grounds of infectious disease control.[74] In his major work *The White Man in the Tropics* Cilento warned readers about 'the repeated emphasis history places on purity of race' as a way of maintaining the health of a community.[75] Rather than addressing leprosy isolation as an exceptional policy, this interest in purity and segregation as a way of pursuing public health should be seen both as characteristic of the period, and as taking place outside the lazarets, in the Australian case, on the mainland.

The system of reserves to contain Aboriginal people in this period should also be taken into account in arguing for the continuity of practices either side of the cordon sanitaire of the lazarets. In some ways, the reserves also functioned as policed quarantined spaces. Cilento certainly approached them thus, and in the 1930s and 1940s researched the transmission of leprosy in several largely closed Aboriginal communities, part of a general increase in research interest in health and Aboriginal communities funded by the Commonwealth's NH&MRC.[76] Leprosy-specific segregating practices were considered and, in some cases, implemented on the mainland. Indeed Cook went so far as to consider a blanket racial segregation:

> Segregation of the race, it would appear, would be an efficient prophylactic measure ... Nor is it entirely impracticable. The enforcement of the existing prohibition against aborigines entering certain areas occupied by coloured aliens in Western Australia and the Northern Territory has not been seriously attempted. Even an abortive effort would not be without its advantages where a disease like leprosy is concerned.[77]

In 1941 the Western Australian government, through a recommendation of its Health Department, drew a 'leper line' across the State. Aborigines – not people with leprosy – who lived north of the twentieth parallel were forbidden to travel south, a restriction in place, if not enforced, until 1963.[78] Even for those epidemiologists who argued against compulsory isolation – against the system of island-lazarets – racial segregation in the general community was nonetheless to be pursued as a public health measure. For example, E. H. Molesworth was a leprologist keenly active in the movement to abandon isolation. Yet in a heated debate with Cook in 1927 he argued for the importance of 'prevention of contact on the part of whites ... with aboriginals and Asiatics'.[79] Moreover, Molesworth conceptualised the advancing European frontier as a macabre, indeed deadly, public health solution. He thought that the colonisation of the north in the form of a 'settled' white community would eventually bring about the disappearance of Aborigines altogether. So, while Aborigines were indeed considered the 'cause' of leprosy, 'with the rapid dying out of the aboriginals as a result of infection with tuberculosis, syphilis and other diseases and as the line of settlement advances', Molesworth argued, 'this problem will probably resolve itself'.[80] Just who was infecting whom in this strangely twisted logic?

Conclusion

The management of leprosy, both within and without the lazaret, was also always about the management of race. Lines of hygiene were racial lines. They took the form of the prison wall shores of the island-lazarets, the limitation of Aboriginal people's movement through reserve systems, the policing of borders like the 'leper line', and the interior frontiers by which whites separated themselves from other groups in the social domain. The island-lazarets themselves have become so compelling for historians, not without good reason, that the range of measures implemented in the social domain are either often ignored or not linked to the practice of isolation. Yet, as we have argued throughout, historians need to look both inside and outside the lazaret for the effects and imperatives of leprosy prevention in the modern and colonial period.

Because of this focus on the lazarets, the compulsory isolation of lepers is usually understood as an extraordinary measure of coercion in the pursuit of public health; leper colonies are typically thought through in terms of the denial of liberties and the forced limitation of movement. Yet once they are contextualised within other practices of racial management, they become somewhat less exceptional. As an Aboriginal person in Queensland, for example, being confined on a leper colony was possibly more similar to than different from other forms of confinement: unfreedom characterised life not only on Peel Island or any of the other lazarets, but also on government reserves like Cherbourg or Palm Island. In part this is what distinguished the experience of white lepers from Aboriginal lepers.

In Australia, preventing sexual contact between races was a twin preventive strategy to the 'exile-enclosure' on island-lazarets. Not only understanding sexual practices, but understanding sexual practices between races came to be one way to conceptualise leprosy as manageable and preventable in the community. This involved not only forced separation and containment, but also the cultivation of 'interior frontiers' of racial identity and difference. Public health, race, sexual practices and a racialised nationalism were all domains shaped by the regulation of contact and separation, contagion and quarantine. The problem of leprosy was one in which all these fields overlapped. The integral connection between public health and racial management, admittedly most clearly apparent in the case of leprosy, needs to be seen as general and problematically normative for the period and the place, rather than specific and exceptional.

Notes

Research for this chapter was funded by the Australian Research Council, in a collaborative project with the Powerhouse Museum, Sydney, and by a Wellcome Trust Travel Grant in the History of Medicine.

1 The most extensive study of race and leprosy in this period is Z. Gussow, *Leprosy, Racism and Public Health: Social Policy in Chronic Disease Control*, Boulder, Colo., Westview Press, 1989.
2 For colonialism, race and tropical medicine, see W. Anderson, 'Immunities of Empire: Race, Disease and the New Tropical Medicine 1900–1920', *Bulletin of the History of Medicine*, 1996, vol. 70, pp. 94–118; D. N. Livingstone, 'Human Acclimatization: Perspectives on a Contested Field of Inquiry in Science, Medicine and Geography', *History of Science*, 1987, vol. 25, pp. 359–94.
3 Norway, for example, was one remaining pocket of leprosy in Europe, and the preventive and treatment policies implemented there were globally influential. See Gussow, *Leprosy, Racism and Public Health*.
4 The 1865 Royal College of Physicians' survey of colonial responses to leprosy concluded that the disease was not contagious. Royal College of Physicians, *Report on Leprosy*, London, Eyre & Spottiswoode, 1867. See also J. M. Creed, 'Leprosy in its Relation to the European Population of Australia', *Transactions of the Intercolonial Medical Congress of Australasia*, 1889, pp. 501–3.
5 See e.g. R. Evans, K. Saunders and K. Cronin, *Exclusion, Exploitation and Extermination: Race Relations in Colonial Queensland*, Sydney, Australia and New Zealand Book Company, 1975, pp. 302–8. For a more general discussion of Australian nationalism and attitudes towards Chinese see: H. McQueen, *A New Britannia: An Argument Concerning the Social Origins of Australian Radicalism and Nationalism*, Ringwood, Penguin, 1986, pp. 32–40; B. Scates, *A New Australia: Citizenship, Radicalism and the First Republic*, Melbourne, Cambridge University Press, 1997, pp. 160–2.
6 M. Foucault, *Discipline and Punish*, Harmondsworth, Penguin, 1991, p. 198.
7 See e.g. A. Bashford, 'Epidemic and Governmentality: Smallpox in Sydney, 1881', *Critical Public Health*, vol. 9, no. 4, 1999, pp. 301–16. See also, D. Armstrong, 'Public Health Spaces and the Fabrication of Identity', *Sociology*, vol. 27, pp. 393–410; A. Petersen and D. Lupton, *The New Public Health: Health and Self in the Age of Risk*, London, Sage, 1996.
8 W. Anderson, 'Leprosy and Citizenship', *Positions*, 1998, vol. 6, pp. 707–30.
9 Ibid., p. 708.
10 For other studies of lazarets in the context of colonialism, see M. Vaughan, 'Without the Camp: Institutions and Identities in the Colonial History of Leprosy', in *Curing their Ills: Colonial Power and African Illness*, Stanford, Calif., Stanford University Press, 1991; S. Kakar, 'Leprosy in British India, 1860–1940', *Medical History*, 1996, vol. 40, pp. 215–30; R. Smith Kipp, 'The Evangelical Uses of Leprosy', *Social Science and Medicine*, vol. 39, 1994, pp. 165–78; Anderson, 'Leprosy and Citizenship'.
11 Further work is in progress: M. Nugent, 'Places of Isolation: Revisiting Histories of Exclusion and Exile'; A. Bashford, *Public Health and the Imagining of Australia* (forthcoming).
12 The situation is peculiar to Queensland because in the first half of the twentieth century it was the only state in Australia in which there was a considerable number of 'white lepers'. See S. Saunders, *A Suitable Island Site: Leprosy in the Northern Territory and the Channel Island Leprosarium*, Darwin, Northern Territory Historical Society, 1989, p. 8.
13 Many histories of leprosy are limited to and by the existence of records produced by government or medical/administrative authorities. See Anderson, 'Leprosy and Citizenship'; Vaughan, 'Without the Camp'. But for the leper's perspective see S. Kakar, 'Leprosy in India: The Intervention of Oral History', *Oral History*, 1995, vol. 23, pp. 37–45; Gussow, *Leprosy, Racism and Public Health*. The move in mainstream medical history to write from the viewpoint of the patient is rendered far more complex when thought through in terms of colonial relations

and the postcolonial theoretical concern for the voice of the 'subaltern'. Doubly 'subaltern', non-white lepers offer one point of departure for the writing of a postcolonial history of medicine. See also W. Anderson, 'Where is the Postcolonial History of Medicine', *Bulletin of the History of Medicine*, 1998, vol. 72, pp. 522–30.

14 S. Saunders, 'Isolation: The Development of Leprosy Prophylaxis in Australia', *Aboriginal History*, 1990, vol. 14, pp. 168–81.

15 There is a substantial literature which analyses the effects of European women, and the domesticity they ostensibly represented, on colonial societies and sexual cultures. See e.g. J. N. Brownfoot, 'Memsahibs in Colonial Malaya: A Study of European Wives in a British Colony and Protectorate 1900–1940', in H. Callan and S. Ardener (eds), *The Incorporated Wife*, London, Croom Helm, 1984; C. Knapman, *White Women in Fiji 1835–1930: The Ruin of Empire?*, Sydney, Allen & Unwin, 1986; H. Callaway, *Gender, Culture and Empire: European Women in Colonial Nigeria*, London, Macmillan, 1987; A. L. Stoler, 'Making Empire Respectable: The Politics of Race and Sexual Morality in Twentieth-Century Colonial Cultures', in A. McClintock, A. Mufti and E. Shohat (eds), *Dangerous Liaisons: Gender, Nation and Postcolonial Perspectives*, Minneapolis, University of Minnesota Press, 1997, pp. 344–73.

16 See e.g. J. Ashburton Thompson, *A Contribution to the History of Leprosy in Australia*, London, The New Sydenham Society, 1897, pp. 221–3; Cook, *Epidemiology*, pp. 14–15, p. 262; Saunders, *A Suitable Island Site*, p. 7; T. Blake, *Peel Island Lazaret Conservation Plan: A Report for the Department of Environment and Heritage*, Brisbane, Robert Riddel Architect, 1993.

17 See Saunders, *A Suitable Island Site*, for a history of the Mud Island lazaret near Palmerston (now Darwin), p. 21, pp. 24–8.

18 'Report on the Lazaret at Dunwich, February 1892–1895', Queensland Home Secretary's Office (QHSO), Queensland State Archive (QSA), COL 322. By 1906, there were reportedly twenty-one white inmates at the Dunwich lazaret on Stradbroke Island, near Brisbane. See P. Ludlow, *The Exiles of Peel Island*, Queensland, Stones Corner, 1991, p. 9.

19 From 1907 until 1940, the Peel Island lazaret was the only lazaret in Queensland, after which time an Aboriginal-only lazaret was established on Fantome Island off Townsville. See Blake, *Peel Island Lazaret*, pp. 3, 11; J. Maguire, 'The Fantome Island Leprosarium', in R. Macleod and D. Denoon (eds), *Health and Healing in Tropical Australia and Papua New Guinea*, Townsville, James Cook University, 1991, pp. 142–8.

20 See E. Kettle, *Health Services in the Northern Territory – a History 1824–1970*, vols 1 and 2, Darwin, Australian National University North Australia Research Unit, 1991.

21 See for example, C. E. Cook, 'Leprosy in Australia', *Medical Journal of Australia* (*MJA*), 27 Sept. 1924, pp. 336–7; C. E. Cook, 'Leprosy Problems', *MJA*, 11 Dec. 1926, pp. 801–3; C. E. Cook, 'Correspondence–Leprosy', *MJA*, 7 Feb. 1931, p. 183. For those opposing compulsory isolation see: L. Rogers, 'When will Australia Adopt Modern Prophylactic Measures against Leprosy?', *MJA*, 18 Oct. 1930, pp. 525–7; E. H. Molesworth, 'The Leprosy Problem', *MJA*, 18 Sept. 1926, pp. 365–81.

22 Cook, *Epidemiology*, p. 9. See also L. Rogers and E. Muir, *Leprosy*, Bristol, John Wright, 1925, p. 52.

23 Saunders, *A Suitable Island Site*, pp. 4–6.

24 For recent studies on Aborigines and citizenship, see N. Peterson and W. Sanders (eds), *Citizenship and Indigenous Australians: Changing Conceptions and Possibilities*, Melbourne, Cambridge University Press, 1998; J. Chesterman and B. Galligan, *Citizens Without Rights: Aborigines and Australian Citizenship*, Melbourne, Cambridge University Press, 1997, esp. ch. 2 on Queensland.

25 Petersen and Lupton, *The New Public Health*, pp. 61–88.
26 See e.g. Chesterman and Galligan, *Citizens Without Rights*, pp. 31–57, in which they outline the legislative control over the lives of Aborigines beginning in the late nineteenth-century period, a central component of which was the restriction of Aboriginal people's movement and their confinement on reserves. Chesterman and Galligan argue that through legislation and other means, the Queensland government 'ensured that Aboriginal Queenslanders were denied basic citizenship rights' and that 'one of the key limitations imposed upon Aborigines in Queensland was the restriction of their movement. Next to their exclusion from the franchise, this was the most clear statement of their citizenship status.'
27 See esp. Cook, 'Leprosy in Australia', *MJA*, 27 Sept. 1924, pp. 326–7; Cook, 'Leprosy Problems'; Cook, *Epidemiology*; R. Cilento, 'Brief Review of Leprosy in Australia and its Dependencies', Appendix 3, Report of Seventh Session, Federal Health Council, 1934; R. Cilento, 'Leprosy in Australia as a Problem of Preventive Medicine', Appendix 1, Report of the Second Session, National Health and Medical Research Council, 1937.
28 Cook, *Epidemiology*, p. 298.
29 Ibid.
30 'Leprosy in Australia', Newsclipping, 12 Apr. 1934, QHSO, QSA, COL 324.
31 Cilento, 'Brief Review of Leprosy in Australia and its Dependencies'.
32 A. H. Humphry, 'Leprosy among Full-Blooded Aborigines of the Northern Territory', *MJA*, 26 Apr. 1952, p. 571.
33 'Leprosy and its Management', *Health: Journal of the Commonwealth Department of Health*, 1958, vol. 8, p. 21.
34 A series of letters from Aboriginal inmates of Peel Island are contained within the files relating to the lazaret held by QSA. To protect the privacy of individuals and their families, in referencing the archives correspondents are referred to by their initials. See e.g. I.B. to the Home Secretary, 8 June 1925; C.F. to Commissioner of Public Health, 4 May 1925, 11 May 1925, 9 May 1925; G.W. to Hon. George Farrell, 6 Oct. 1924, Queensland Department of Health and Home Affairs Records (QDHHAR), QSA TR115815/F5; Statement of T.M. on behalf of coloured inmates before the Visiting Justice, 16 Jul. 1909, QDHHAR, QSR, COL 322.
35 Cilento to the Under Secretary, 13 Oct. 1939, QHSO, QSA, COL 323.
36 A series of inquiries were held into conditions on the island. See e.g. Ludlow, *Peel Island*, p. 23; Blake, *Peel Island Lazaret*, p. 17; Correspondence, 1924, QPWD, QSA, TR1158/5–F5.
37 See e.g. Correspondence and petitions, 1937–1940, QHSO, QSA, COL 323 in particular Dr Molesworth to Mrs Brown, Peel Island, 9 Nov. 1937, QHSO, QSA, COL 323; Report, Office of the Visiting Justice, Brisbane, 15 Oct. 1924, QPWD, QSA, TR1158/5–F5; Correspondence, 1924–5, Queensland Public Works Department (QPWD), QSA, TR1158/5–F5.
38 See e.g. Blake, *Peel Island Lazaret*, p. 7, p. 9, pp. 15–16.
39 I.B. to the Home Secretary, 8 Jun. 1925, QPWD, QSA, TR1158/5–F5.
40 G.W. to Hon. George Farrell, 6 Oct. 1924, QPWD, QSA, TR1158/5–F5
41 Government Health Officer to Home Secretary's Office, 18 Nov. 1921, QHSO, QSA, COL 322.
42 See e.g. C. D. Rowley, *Outcasts in White Australia: Aboriginal Policy and Practice*, Canberra, Australian National University Press, 1971, pp. 109–12, where he details the oppressively strict regulations and forms of control practised on government reserves in Queensland. In this period, Aboriginal people considered 'trouble-makers' were sent to Palm Island – a place known among Aborigines as the 'punishment place'. See Dawn May, 'A Punishment Place', in B. Gammage

and P. Spearritt, *Australians 1938*, Sydney, Fairfax Syme and Weldon Associates, 1987. Presumably for Aboriginal inmates of Peel Island, there was no other island-exile to which they could be sent.
43 For examples of Peel Island inmates' protests, see P. Ludlow, *Peel Island, Paradise or Prison?*, Stones Corner, Queensland, 1987, pp. 23–5 and pp. 41–8.
44 Petition from inmates of Peel Island to the Governor of Queensland, 27 Sept. 1939, QHSO, QSA, COS 323.
45 Petition from inmates of Peel Island to the Governor of Queensland, 27 Sept. 1939, QHSO, QSA, COS 323.
46 Peel Island Welfare Association to Premier of Queensland, 29 Feb. 1940, QHSO, QSA, COL 323.
47 See Ludlow, *Peel Island*, p. 45.
48 Maguire, 'The Fantome Island Leprosarium', p. 147.
49 Ibid., p. 145.
50 See A. Bashford, ' "Is White Australia Possible?" Race, Colonialism and Tropical Medicine', *Ethnic and Racial Studies*, 2000, vol. 23, pp. 248–71; W. Anderson, 'Geography, Race and Nation: Re-mapping "Tropical" Australia', *Historical Records of Australian Science*, 1997, vol. 11, pp. 457–68; D. Walker, 'Climate Civilization and Character in Australia, 1880–1940', *Australian Cultural History*, 1997/98, no. 16, pp. 77–95.
51 E. Balibar, 'Fichte and the Internal Border', in *Masses, Classes, Ideas: Studies on Politics and Philosophy Before and After Marx*, trans. James Swenson, New York, Routledge New York and London, 1994, p. 63.
52 Ibid., p. 76, p. 84
53 A. L. Stoler, 'Sexual Affronts and Racial Frontiers: European Identities and the Cultural Politics of Exclusion in Colonial Southeast Asia', in F. Cooper and A. L. Stoler (eds), *Tensions of Empire: Colonial Cultures in a Bourgeois World*, Berkeley, Calif., University of California Press, 1997, p. 199.
54 Stoler, 'Making Empire Respectable', p. 360.
55 Cook, for example, was both Chief Protector of the Aborigines and Chief Medical Officer in the Northern Territory for many years
56 For Cook and assimilation, see P. Jacobs, 'Science and Veiled Assumptions: Miscegenation in Western Australia, 1930–1937', *Australian Aboriginal Studies*, 1986, vol. 2, pp. 15–23. For the complicated connections between assimilation policies and anxieties about leprosy as a contagion of miscegenation, see Bashford, *Public Health and the Imagining of Australia* (forthcoming). For Cilento and tropical medicine, see Bashford, ' "Is White Australia Possible?" ', pp. 248–71.
57 For an instance of the connection between syphilis and leprosy see 'Leprosy', *Australian Medical Journal*, 1889, vol. 11, pp. 383–6; Vaughan, 'Without the Camp', p. 82. But see also the discussion of sexual relations between indigenous women and white men in Jamaica and Hawaii in Rogers and Muir, *Leprosy*, pp. 84–5.
58 See Evans, Saunders and Cronin, *Exclusion, Exploitation and Extermination*, pp. 302–7.
59 Minutes, The Australasian Sanitary Conference of Sydney, 1884, pp. 17–25.
60 Cook, *Epidemiology*, p. 20.
61 Ibid.
62 Ibid., p. 21.
63 C. E. Cook, Report upon the Activities of the Commonwealth Department of Health from 1909 to 1930, Appendix F 'Leprosy in Australia', p. 1. When Cook embarked on his leprosy study he had just completed a study of Aboriginal people and venereal disease. See C. E. Cook, 'Report', Health Department of Western Australia, File 888/1923 cited in E. Hunter, *Aboriginal Health and History: Power and Prejudice in Remote Australia*, Melbourne, Cambridge University Press, 1993, p. 61. Cilento was also very interested in the control of venereal diseases

in the indigenous population. See R. Kidd, *The Way We Civilise*, St Lucia, University of Queensland Press, 1997, pp. 80–115.
64 Cook, *Epidemiology*, p. 20.
65 Cook, 'Leprosy in Australia'.
66 See A. McClintock, *Imperial Leather: Race, Gender and Sexuality in the Imperial Contest*, New York and London, Routledge, 1995, pp. 352–89.
67 Cook, *Epidemiology*, p. 62.
68 See e.g. Cilento, *The White Man in the Tropics*, pp. 75–92; P. Cilento and R. Cilento, 'The Mother and the Child in the Tropics of the Austra-Pacific Zone', n.d., Cilento Papers, Fryer Library, Queensland, Mss 44/137.
69 Stoler, 'Sexual Affronts and Racial Frontiers', p. 199.
70 Cook, *Epidemiology*, p. 93.
71 Cook, 'Leprosy in Australia' in 'Report', p. 1.
72 *MJA*, 29 Apr. 1933.
73 Cook, *Epidemiology*, p. 63. See also Vaughan, 'Without the Camp', p. 81.
74 Australian historians often overlook the infectious disease clause in the infamous 1901 *Immigration Restriction Act* (Commonwealth) which was the basis for what popularly became known as the 'white Australia policy'. See Bashford, 'Quarantine', pp. 397–400.
75 R. Cilento, *The White Man in the Tropics*, Melbourne, Government Printer, 1925, p. 57.
76 For Cilento, this research demonstrated the infectiousness of leprosy and thus supported his commitment to compulsory isolation. See Minister for Health and Home Affairs to Mr Bedford MLA, 8 Dec. 1938, QHSO, QSA, COL 323.
77 Cook, 'Leprosy in Australia' in 'Report', p. 1.
78 See Hunter, *Aboriginal Health and History*, p. 39, p. 67.
79 E. H. Molesworth, *MJA*, 12 Mar. 1927, p. 389.
80 Ibid.

6 Sanitary failure and risk
Pasteurisation, immunisation and the logics of prevention

Claire Hooker

Pasteurisation and immunisation are two public health practices, not usually considered together, which have become normalised during the last seventy years. I examine the nature of these instruments and ask how they came to be near-universal practices. Pasteurisation refers to the heat treatment of milk to kill harmful bacteria. Immunisation refers to the introduction of disease material into the body in order to stimulate the body's internal production of antibodies to the disease.[1] The first would therefore seem to operate through a logic of sterilisation, and the second, as Bashford argues in this volume, through a logic of contagion.[2] Entirely different as procedures, I argue that the two were historically related and that their commonalities illuminate important shifts in the logics of prevention structuring modern Australian public health. Adopted more or less contemporaneously, they signified a new form of public health which both incorporated, and superseded, the strategies that preceded their introduction. Pasteurisation and mass immunisation were primarily constructed through a logic of risk reduction and population protection, different to other infectious disease control policies. Above all, they were signs of the perceived failure of sanitary strategies which were focused on locating and controlling dangerous individuals, and a sometimes reluctant shift to population-level preventive policies based in social protection and risk minimisation. Described in their own terms, they shifted public health policy from practices that aimed at cleanliness to those ensuring safety.

Pasteurisation and immunisation were designed to be the new primary instruments in the hierarchy of infectious disease prevention practices, superseding but not banishing other techniques. I argue that these other techniques, including notification, isolation, disinfection and the location and control of healthy 'carriers' of illness, were bound together by a similar sanitary logic, grounded in Australia in public health characterised by localism and voluntary action. In using the word 'sanitary' to describe this logic I refer to a common commitment to ideas of cleanliness and 'freedom from deleterious influences'.[3] A moral aspect was intrinsic to this logic, an aspect that altered, but was never lost, throughout the transformations wrought by bacteriology and bureaucracy in public health. The language of cleanliness – the sanitary control of milk, water and households, the constant references to personal, mental, physical, racial and moral hygiene – especially dominated public health literature between 1850 and 1950. 'Sanitation' connotes cleanliness and purity in the pursuit of health; 'hygiene' connotes health and the practices through which it is produced. Though 'sanitation' referred more to inanimate objects and 'hygiene' more to humans and their activities, the terms were often used interchangeably throughout this period.

The word 'sanitary' was prominent in the language of public health between 1920 and 1950, the period in question here. Sometimes it was a derogatory term, as when 'modern', bacteriological public health was favourably contrasted by its proponents with 'older', 'sanitarian' cleansing practices and mistaken miasmatic theories. Historians and sociologists have tended to follow this lead. David Armstrong, for example, defined 'sanitary science' as those mid-nineteenth-century practices which distinguished the space of bodies from their environment. He argued that the beginning of the twentieth century saw a shift to an era of 'personal hygiene', characterised by practices that focused on the space *between* bodies.[4] For Deborah Lupton and Alan Petersen, 'sanitation' refers to the broad environmental and social policies eclipsed by the advent of bacteriology, which they (among many others) argue refocused public health ideology and practice around narrow, individuated, 'microbe-hunting' policies.[5] Nancy Tomes, examining personal practices rather than policies, agrees with the argument but significantly alters the periodisation by showing that germ theory was at first merely incorporated into existing frameworks of 'sanitation'; her history found that the 'gospel of germs' only waned in favour of individuated, microbe-hunting public health in the 1920s.[6] 'Sanitation' has thus come to refer above all to the classic practices of mid-nineteenth-century British public health (sewerage and water purification systems, garbage removal and Nuisance Acts, Poor Law reforms),[7] to a public health characterised by broad environmental and social reforms as opposed to the control of individuals. Saturated in moral implications, it preceded and was differentiated, though not banished, from its modern scientific form. There is now an excellent historical literature exploring the complexities of bacteriology's advent, and these emphasise the continuities between germ theory and earlier aetiological concepts, as well as between microbe control and long-established medical, surgical and public health practices,[8] so the sustained currency of the language of sanitation, of which its pejorative form was but one instance, should not surprise us. The logic of sanitation, a kind of cleaning up based in long-standing ideas of health, illness, and dirt, continued to inform strategies of disease control throughout the early twentieth century. I suggest that this was the case even for quintessential 'microbe-hunting' public health policies, especially the identification, isolation and disinfection of healthy 'carriers' of disease, of the interwar years.

Pasteurisation and immunisation did not work on this sanitary 'cleaning up' model. Two strategies among the heterogeneous practices of infectious disease control, they constituted a gradual shift in public health, which marked the imprecise decline of the language and logic of sanitation. Understanding the introduction of pasteurisation and immunisation means tracking movements in the meaning of danger and risk and their correlates in approaches to self-government and state regulation. Pasteurisation and immunisation threatened the moral framework of sanitation. They marked the *failure* of microbe hunting and a consequent breakdown of the sanitary logic. They were called into play only when it became obvious that the public health strategies designed to control the unpredictable danger of disease transmission would never be successful. Microbe-hunting public health was based on controlling danger: preventing disease that lay latent in apparently healthy, hence almost undetectable, sources, such as the milk supply or child diphtheria carriers. Pasteurisation and mass immunisation were blanket techniques which made locating danger almost irrelevant. They shifted the notion of prevention from a focus on treating particular dangerous people and places to a focus on social defence. They represent capitulation to a fully modern public health characterised by risk reduction and central government intervention.

In making this argument I build on the work of Foucauldian scholars interested in ideas of 'risk' and their relation to government.[9] For Robert Castel 'risk society' is characterised by forms of intervention based on the calculation of abstract factors rather than direct relationships between experts and clients. He traces a shift in the form of governmentality from the nineteenth-century concern, identified by Foucault, with 'dangerous individuals', to late twentieth-century risk management. Castel argues that nineteenth-century reformers identified populations 'at risk' of illness by correlating disease with a range of living conditions (including housing, malnutrition, alcoholism and promiscuity), but their intervention was limited to the identification, isolation and disinfection of dangerous individuals. Such techniques have an inbuilt logistical limitation in that the diagnosis of dangerousness is always fallible, and can only be carried out on individuals one by one. The central problem is how to prevent the actualisation of a risk without having to confine the dangerous person. Castel claims this occurred after 1945, when the notion of risk became autonomous from that of danger through the techniques of factor calculation. While I would argue that what counted as 'danger' and what as 'risk' need a much more rigorous historical examination, in this chapter I agree with Castel's central thesis that it was the limitations of nineteenth-century techniques used to locate and neutralise danger that effected a transfer to considerations of risk. In this sense pasteurisation and immunisation resemble their contemporary policy, eugenics – they were protections *imposed* at the level of population – rather than the complex *self-surveillance* techniques of modern 'risk management' in which Castel is primarily interested.[10]

This study illuminates the particular social, ideological and administrative factors through which pasteurisation and immunisation became acceptable, then widespread in Australia. Certainly neither pasteurisation nor immunisation were the rational, logical consequence of early twentieth-century scientific medicine, nor did they immediately cause a stunning drop in disease incidence, as was claimed by their champions.[11] Both have only been widespread in Australia since the 1950s, following thirty years of piecemeal introduction, during which time their efficacy was consistently challenged. Advocated by officials for years, their introduction was frequently part of an immediate, emotional reaction by a local community to the experience of epidemic disease. Both were first used in metropolitan centres in the mid-1920s, gradually adopted in local districts in the 1930s, then increased exponentially between 1939 and 1950, when they became common practice as public health policy moved towards the centre of Australia's three-tiered governmental structure.[12] There were local, regional and State differences in their implementation.[13] Such differences remind us of the crucial importance of the local and particular in public health history. For example, my argument concerning the logic by which pasteurisation and immunisation operated applies to the UK, Canada and the USA and was, indeed, explicitly enunciated in them. In all these nations the protective logic of pasteurisation and immunisation required a shift from local to central government in directing public health activity.[14] Yet the time and circumstances of their use differed enormously: both pasteurisation and mass immunisation were well established in metropolitan North America by 1920, while neither was established in Britain until after the Second World War.[15]

The transmission of both diseases and ideas requires a suitable medium. Here I explore pasteurisation and immunisation through an event in which they were linked and which directly resulted in the first Milk Pasteurisation Act in Australia (State of Victoria, 1943): an epidemic of milk-borne typhoid fever in Moorabbin, Victoria. The first large outbreak of typhoid in decades,[16] the Moorabbin epidemic was shocking and dramatic. It was treated with great seriousness in the public health literature, and the Health Department's journal, the *Health Bulletin*, took the unprecedented step of separately printing and distributing the report of the officer in charge of the situation, Dr Frank Merrillees. In responding to the outbreak, Merrillees's *Report on the Outbreak of Typhoid Fever at Moorabbin* (hereafter 'the Report'), considered a range of public health instruments from notification, sanitation, disinfection and personal hygiene to carrier control and immunisation, thus exposing the gamut of public health thinking of his day. Above all, the outbreak was explicitly used by Merrillees, public health officials and by the public to demand the compulsory pasteurisation of milk.

Typhoid fever at Moorabbin: sanitation, epidemic disease and the milk supply

Between 1 March and 1 August 1943, 439 cases of typhoid fever (200 in the first two weeks), resulting in twenty-three deaths, were notified in the City of Moorabbin.[17] Justified by the imperative of wartime, the State Department of Health appointed Merrillees to control the situation. Within twenty-four hours, Merrillees had gathered the evidence showing that the epidemic was milk-borne and was caused by a single faecal carrier on a single farm. In his Report, he pointed out that Moorabbin (with the exception of one milk bar) was supplied by a single 'dairy' (milk depot), which pooled the milk supplied to it from a number of different farms. The effects of one instance of contamination were thus magnified into an explosive outbreak. The dairy sold no pasteurised milk to the public, a situation that was not unusual in 1943 but which left consumers unwillingly vulnerable to infected milk.

Because typhoid symbolised 'filth', Merrillees's Report meticulously examined the sanitary state of the town, an action which emphasised the continued centrality of classic sanitary public health measures in daily life. The Report began by outlining faulty aspects of Moorabbin's waste disposal and water systems. Much of the city was unsewered and the disposal of nightsoil from closet pans was unsatisfactory. '[P]ans frequently were left unchanged, or emptied into another and replaced without being washed (topping). What was even worse was that to make room for this topping the liquid portion of the nightsoil was often poured away into the street or yard.'[18] The Report also discussed the range of sanitary actions taken in response to the outbreak of typhoid fever. These actions emphasised systems of disinfection and isolation, purifying both individuals and their environment. Leaflets and advertisements were issued warning of the epidemic and advising the public to boil all milk, exclude flies and dust from food, and to take various precautions against faecal and other contaminants; sanitary pans from infected houses were removed to the depot and marked with red paint to indicate that more careful disposal and washing were necessary; a system of sanitary inspection of residential premises was established; instructions were issued concerning the disposal of excreta, the cleansing of bedding and utensils, the uses of disinfectants, the dangers of flies and water closets; and advice was given on avoiding further infection.[19]

These responses to typhoid at Moorabbin were standard practice. Each technique was designed to fulfil a particular function in the ultimate goal of locating, and then 'cleaning up', all instances of disease, and all possible locations of its transmission. The difference between treatment and prevention was indistinct, since any treatment would also prevent the spread of disease via new (and thus unidentified) sources created in the epidemic. If, as Merrillees argued, it must be assumed that a single typhoid bacillus could cause an outbreak under the right circumstances,[20] then every microbe had to be located and removed. The sanitary strategies used to achieve this came from health powers grounded in localism, where community control was secured through local representation, while the judgement of what measures were appropriate in each individual situation were deemed to be best made by those with the specific knowledge of where and what action was required. Although Public Health Acts of the 1880s and 1890s laid the legislative and institutional framework for the increasing centralisation of public health government (increased with the rise of bacteriology, as bureaucracy which managed tests and statistics was managed at State government level), the administration of public health remained in local hands.[21] The sanitary utilities which managed the rhythms of daily life, such as waste disposal and the provision of a clean water supply, were the major component of public health work at local government level. Sanitary measures depended on the rational, responsible actions of local authorities, physicians and all members of the local community.

Introduced in the 1880s and 1890s, notification was regarded and used as the primary and initial response to epidemic disease.[22] Notification joined the new diagnostic certainty of bacteriology with an assumed ongoing commitment to sanitation. It brought disease within the purview of governmental intervention by making it officially visible. This visibility was *consequentially* expected to lead to action which would limit its spread. Notification, according to one practitioner, was expected to render steps for control of a disease possible, to aid discovery of the source of infection, to help provide efficient treatment for the ill, to give local authorities information about the local history of the disease, to educate the community concerning its spread and to allow judgement of preventive measures.[23] Notification bound together a whole community through the processes of government, involving the coordinated efforts of local Medical Officers of Health, local Council, local physicians, the patient and their family and contacts, and the local community in general. Although vested in central government power, notification was designed primarily to facilitate local action.

As at Moorabbin, local action involved isolation and disinfection measures, ranging from reorganising nightsoil services, closing schools and disinfecting water supplies, to practices centred on the patient, their environment, and their family or other contacts.[24] Many of the latter techniques were ultimately reliant on the responsible self-government of individuals and their acquiescence to official directives. The broader goal of social change through education was therefore intrinsic to the logic of notification: it worked on the assumption that the public would be taught preventive practices. This in turn was founded on a construction of the public by physicians and public health officials as generally compliant and amenable to education, though also irrational and unreliable, requiring guidance and management. Merrillees was typical in joining placation to strategic management. For example, he commented candidly that: 'it was early decided that any attempt at germicidal effect by chemicals was too uncertain a matter to be entrusted to lay people. It was therefore decided that the chief function sought in any disinfectant in this outbreak would be the psychic effect of something smelling of cresol together with the really important property of fly repulsion.'[25]

The milk supply was frequently implicated in outbreaks of epidemic disease. At Moorabbin, the Report followed common practice in examining the milk supply system and, as with the other services, it found the present system inadequate. It identified several 'weak points' where the milk supply could be contaminated or bacterial growth encouraged: the milk was 'some hours' on the road between farms and the dairy, which allowed it to warm; the cleansing of milk cans depended on the personal habits of each individual workman; can lids could remain unsteamed or become soiled; and the milk was sold 'loose', that is dipped from a hand-can, the handle of which, soiled by the driver's hand, could infect the whole of the can's contents, a risk increased by the lack of sanitary conveniences and washing facilities. The Report reflected the necessity for the minute surveillance of milk production and distribution in a sanitary framework designed not merely to safeguard it from bacterial contamination, but to ensure its cleanliness, freshness and purity.

Because milk symbolised the essence of health, the milk supply was regarded as a public utility requiring sanitary regulation.[26] The dairy industry was also one of the nation's largest primary industries, and its financial regulation was important for economic security. The sanitary control of milk was therefore imbricated with market-oriented regulations: the grades established to fix prices also functioned to manage milk quality. The primary criterion for milk grades was butterfat content but included sanitary regimes as well, including sedimentation and acidity tests to detect contamination and adulteration.[27] Milk sanitation was built into dairy industry legislation passed by most State governments between 1890 and 1910, roughly contemporaneous with other sanitary public health measures. Rhetorically, milk control was built on the moral terms of sanitation: cleanliness, wholesomeness and freshness. The principal instrument used to secure sanitary compliance was the licensing system which operated on a parallel logic to notification. The system encouraged sanitary practice on each individual dairy by bringing it under official surveillance. To receive a licence, farmers, dairies, creameries, suppliers, distributors and vendors were required to comply with detailed regulations specifying herd management, feeding, premises design and care, milking, cooling, storage, care òf containers, transportation, separation, grading, distribution, and sale of milk. These specifications defined practices of cleanliness at every level with a minute thoroughness. The licensing system brought together economic, sanitary and social control. As its official history put it, 'it is through these provisions that the [NSW Milk] Board controls the numbers and types of persons who may be allowed to engage in the business of the milk industry'.[28]

Dangerousness: the carriers of disease

Merrillees's aim in his meticulous report was to *exclude* sanitary conditions as a cause of the outbreak. Those sections of the Report were designed to demonstrate conclusively that the epidemic was solely and entirely milk-borne and unequivocally traceable to a particular carrier on a particular farm. After his survey of sanitation, he uncoupled the connection between environmental 'filth' and typhoid fever, in direct refutation of public beliefs. He argued that the drop in typhoid fever incidence in the 1890s was *not* due to the contemporaneous construction of sewage systems. Instead, he claimed that the crucial factor was alteration in personal hygiene practices.[29] Merrillees used the familiar opposition between the 'old' view of typhoid as a 'filth' disease, to be controlled chiefly through sewering and waste disposal, and the 'true' conception of it as contagious, which underpinned his search for the 'carrier' whom he hypothesised as the cause of the outbreak. This was polemical in intent rather than descriptive of public health practice. As we have seen, Merrillees's executive actions and his Report continued to emphasise the traditional forms of sanitary response to infectious disease, and to imbricate them with the hygienic practices that identified and constrained infected individuals. Merrillees emphasised this: '[t]his chapter is not against sewerage in any way . . . The insanitary conditions which are usually abolished when sewerage is introduced are undoubtedly a cause of spread, but not of an outbreak, of typhoid such as this present one.'[30] The Report emphasised that it was the unsuspected transmitters of disease, like fresh milk or a healthy carrier, that were truly dangerous, rather than locations predictable by their filthiness, which merely facilitated disease after its occurrence.

The identification and monitoring of healthy 'carriers' was the central, though hardly the sole, policy in preventing certain diseases, chiefly diphtheria, in a very specific time period in Australia (roughly 1916 to 1936).[31] The policy rested on the medical fantasy that bacteriological techniques could render disease permanently visible, and thus monitored, or even eradicated. Widespread application of the techniques was therefore envisaged. As pioneering Australian bacteriologist Dr Thomas Cherry wrote of diphtheria in 1895, 'In the city of New York, all sore throats are examined bacteriologically by the Department of Health.'[32] In the early twentieth century, bacteriological identification of individuals as the nodes of infection, as at Moorabbin – Merrillees located his 'carrier' through a blood antibody test, the Widal, after faecal tests of all dairy personnel were returned negative – was also prominent in controlling other infectious diseases, including typhoid fever and tuberculosis. These techniques placed the 'carrier' at the centre of public health concern.

The carrier control policies confronted the problem of hidden menace explored by Foucault,[33] who argued that nineteenth-century criminology shifted its focus from the *event* of a crime to its *cause*. Psychiatry and law were much exercised over the problem of monstrous crimes committed by apparently normal people who previously exhibited no signs of their capacity for criminality. Their peculiar dangerousness resided in their near undetectability (experts might identify them by subtle signs) and ignorance of their own insanity, an insanity that was thought somehow to inhere in the individual. Foucault argued that the concept of *dangerousness* – a quality defined by future potential, and by reference to those threatened by it – emerged from questions of responsibility for these crimes. Because these crimes were motiveless, therefore unreasoned, it was argued that those who committed them must be insane, and so not responsible for their actions. Later criminal law incorporated the notion of 'no fault responsibility' with a range of measures (from elimination and exclusion to therapeutics) designed to manage the danger posed by the insane.

These notions of dangerousness and responsibility apply equally well to early twentieth-century constructions of the healthy carrier and the control of the danger they posed. The healthy carrier, like the homicidal maniac, was asymptomatic, and thus invisible to the community. Disease, like crime, could erupt from someone who displayed no sign of their infectivity. Identification of the carrier could only be made by an expert, in this case, the bacteriologist. As with the insane criminal, the carrier who caused an outbreak of disease could not be construed as at fault, since they were ignorant of their own dangerousness.[34] This was especially the case with child carriers, by definition not responsible for their actions.[35] Defined through the impersonal instrument of the laboratory, carrier status, arbitrary and temporary, was distinctively different from previous constructions of disease-causing individuals as dirty or immoral. In much medical literature the carrier was 'not responsible' in both legal and moral terms for outbreaks of disease.

Yet as Judith Walzer Leavitt has engagingly pointed out with respect to the most celebrated of carriers, 'Typhoid Mary', the nominally morally exempt 'scientific' category of the carrier *was* in fact constructed through ideas of morality and responsibility which were slippery, ambivalent and inconsistent in their application.[36] Unlike the insane criminal, the carrier was a rational actor, capable of exercising free choice in the government of his or her own actions. Carrier control policies made identified carriers responsible for containing the danger they posed to the community. Proliferating legal regulations were developed for carriers to manage their behaviour hygienically, including prohibiting carriers (especially of typhoid fever) from working in the dairy industry or with food. Failure to comply, as in the case of Mary Mallon, was thus deemed irresponsible, immoral, even criminal, behaviour. There was a tension in the medical literature between a sense that this bacteriological dangerousness was somehow inherent in particular individuals and the observation that in the majority of cases, the carrier state was temporary.[37] The carrier tended to be pathologised in the medical literature. Biological status was linked with behaviour, often causally: the child carrier was associated with stupidity and delinquency,[38] and Dr F. V. Scholes, a noted physician and public health officer, noted in his Foreword to the Report on Moorabbin that the carrier responsible was typical of such outbreaks: a woman, dirty in her habits.[39] Besides the danger posed to neighbours and contacts who might become infected, in some views the pathologised carrier endangered the biological status of the entire population. Ambiguously placed between illness and immunity, the carrier was depicted as inherently weak and sickly, and thus even 'unfit' according to eugenic criteria of the day.[40]

The institution of carrier control as disease prevention policy depended on the specific attitudes and administrative capacities of governments. Physicians in Australia were aware of the role of carriers in disease transmission from the 1890s,[41] but for the next twenty years disease control was vested in local strategies of isolation, disinfection and treatment in response to local outbreaks of disease. Carrier control became the premier organised policy in the prevention of diphtheria and typhoid fever in civilian populations in Australia during and after the First World War, one of the first mass strategies applied by a centralised public health administration.[42] These mass campaigns saw testing and isolation carried out across entire townships.[43] Carrier control was similar to other sanitary policies in that the central aim was the identification and cleansing of infected persons, and in that these policies had an intrinsic, albeit unstable and contested, moral valency. The localised, sanitary control of disease rested on the relevance of all 'cleaning up' procedures and the moral obligation to pursue them. They could only work if people effectively self-regulated their behaviour, by accepting testing and by complying with minute behavioural specifications if they were identified as carriers – as 'dangerous'.

The failure of sanitation: immunisation and the transition from clean to 'safe' milk

At Moorabbin the anxious general public demanded both practices that identified and eliminated dangers and those that protected from danger, specifically, immunisation. Merrillees was surprised by the overwhelming request by the public for a mass immunisation campaign. In fact, Merrillees did *not* advocate mass immunisation – his primary objection was that it might heighten the severity of incubating cases – but felt he had to justify this decision publicly, 'since', as he wrote, 'few will dispute the protection value of inoculation even to the individual and certainly in mass'.[44] Instead he advocated a policy of selective immunisation based on susceptibility. The population was categorised according to differentials of risk. For newcomers who had been in the district less than a week; for families with a member already a patient, after allowing incubation time to elapse; and for persons continually at risk through exposure (such as sanitary personnel), inoculation was advised without waiting, as the risk of contracting typhoid was considered to be greater than that of exacerbating any incubating cases. Everyone else was advised against inoculation unless 'necessary for some social reason, such as allaying the fears of customers or neighbours'.[45] The option of private immunisation was in fact taken up in large numbers and Merrillees's fears justified by the occurrence of coincident typhoid cases.

Merrillees's comment that few would dispute the protection value of inoculation *even to the individual and certainly in mass* indicates that immunisation was understood primarily as a blanket technique in contrast to local/individual strategies. This conception arose from the increasing use of epidemiological techniques which focused attention on macrosocial patterns of disease incidence and morbidity.[46] Using immunisation as a public health policy relied on a crucial shift in focus from the control of dangerous individuals to the minimisation of risk – based on the failure of the former. Carrier control policy manifestly failed to impact at the population level. In the early 1920s, it became increasingly clear that despite the enormous swabbing and isolation campaigns carried out to control diphtheria, its incidence was continuing to rise.[47] Diphtheria presented the threat of epidemic illness characterised by unpredictable cycles of virulence unleashed on a vulnerable community despite local and individual amelioration through antitoxin treatment and carrier isolation. In the late 1920s, public health officials instead began to consider 'prevention' in terms of the protection of the population as a whole through immunisation. The relationship between individual and population was reconstructed in terms of immunity and susceptibility. Instead of locating the carriers of diphtheria, mass immunisation was pursued by first locating all the 'susceptibles' by the Schick test. Where the carrier was 'dangerous', the susceptible was 'at risk'. Individuals were treated according to their immune status. Those who were non-susceptible and non-infected were to be ignored; those who were non-susceptible but infectious, isolated; those who were susceptible and infected, isolated and treated with antitoxin; and those who were susceptible but not infected, immunised.[48] Aside from the biological property of immunity, the policy made absolutely no social distinctions at all. Instead, immunisation was the first truly population-level policy. It aimed to achieve a single biological standard across the entire population. Focused on each individual, it sought a goal for the whole social body. By creating a unitary biological standard at the level of population, the eugenic threat posed by the sickly carrier disappeared.

The move from carrier control to immunisation paralleled the contemporaneous transition from policies aimed at securing *clean* milk to those guaranteeing 'safe' milk. The flourishing polemic mobilised in its promotion made 'safety' and 'pasteurisation' explicitly interchangeable terms: 'the first two of these factors [the health of the cows and hygienic practice in production] are aimed at the production of a clean milk supply, the last [pasteurisation] seeks to ensure a safe supply.'[49] Like the threat of increased virulence in diphtheria, the growing preoccupation with milk-borne illness as a public health problem following the First World War was a key factor in this transition. Most prominently, sanitary regulation of the milk supply was central to the widespread anti-tuberculosis campaigns of the early twentieth century. Large-scale tuberculin testing of dairy herds, requiring regular tuberculin testing of all dairy herds, the location of all bovine carriers of the disease, and the destruction of these animals, whatever their state of health, paralleled carrier control policies.[50] The control of tuberculosis was so much identified with the sanitary regulation of milk that 'clean' milk explicitly and significantly designated tubercle-free milk.[51] Other milk-borne illnesses were also of concern, including diphtheria, scarlet fever and whooping cough, cases of 'undulant fever' (the recently identified human form of *brucella abortus*, or contagious abortion of cattle), and non-pulmonary tuberculosis in young children.[52] Infantile diarrhoea, an iconic issue of the time, was correlated with unsanitary milk.[53] Finally, milk was an important vector for the enteric diseases, above all typhoid fever, by far the most common epidemic disease to result from milk-borne infection.[54]

The failure of anti-tuberculosis campaigns to control the disease gave impetus to the call for pasteurisation in the early 1930s. In any case, milk certified as tubercle-free did not ensure its freedom from other forms of pathogenic bacteria. 'Has not certified milk produced undulant fever and septic sore throat?' asked the editors of the *Health Bulletin*.[55] Pasteurisation was a simple bulk procedure, making milk safety independent of the myriad local factors which could affect the milk supply, from unsanitary maintenance of milking machines to the health of dairy cattle or dairy workers. It set a single standard of safety across the entire milk market, reducing risk in a known and identifiable way. The editors approvingly quoted the English *Report of the Reorganisation Commission for Milk*: 'It is evident that the closest attention should be given to the question of setting up a hygienic standard capable of application to a large proportion of the total supply of milk offered to the liquid market.'[56] The defence of economic security (from the sale of a substandard product, which might jeopardise the entire industry) here mirrored the defence of the population (from disease).[57] Thus when the Milk Board of NSW was established in 1930, it conflated threats to morality, economic security, and health by observing that unsatisfactory persons, whose sanitary habits were difficult to control, had taken advantage of the depression to become unlicensed milk vendors.[58] Blanket pasteurisation of the metropolitan milk supply offered a single, complete standard of safety not reliant on the hygienic condition of individual animals, farms, dairies or vendors as was the licensing system. 'There is nothing sacrosanct about certified milk and its pasteurisation will do it good . . . It is the best insurance, for the industry and for the consumer, and the simplest, cheapest, least objectionable, and most trustworthy method of rendering infected milk safe,' Professor Milton Rosenau was quoted by the *Health Bulletin*.[59]

The introduction of pasteurisation and immunisation was explicitly based on the *failure* of disease control through sanitary practices. This failure was partly logistic: it was not possible to make visible *all* bacteria *all* of the time. In 1918, the editors of the *Medical Journal of Australia* considered that 'if one could find and isolate all carriers, [the] disease would die out'.[60] By the early 1920s, it was clear that this was an impossible fantasy. Arguing for compulsory pasteurisation, writers for the *Health Bulletin* pointed out that no matter how frequently tuberculin testing and exclusion was carried out in herds, the sale and movement of animals, the passage of tuberculosis across species (for example, porcine tuberculosis resulting from feeding skim milk to pigs), incubation periods, human corruption or error and the occasional failures of the test itself made even certified milk ultimately unreliable: 'Tuberculosis is so insidious and easily propagated, cleanliness is so difficult to maintain, and men capable of supervising dairy herds are so scarce, that for years to come the idea of a pure source over the whole country remains an ideal.'[61] Danger could never be reliably isolated and removed. Rather, pasteurisation and immunisation were deployed as constant protection across the population: 'Raw milk is apt to be dangerous milk, and our only protection against these particular dangers is through pasteurisation.'[62] Instead of the *cause* of illness, they focused on the *defence* of the population by reducing risk. 'Parents with young children will not be satisfied with an assurance that on any particular day the odds are slightly less than sixty to one that the milk their children drink is not infected with the tubercle bacillus.'[63] Pasteurisation and immunisation diminished risk as close as possible to zero.

The failure of carrier control and other sanitary policies lay partly in the unreliability of the public, figured individually and collectively, to be sufficiently self-regulating. Pasteurisation and immunisation governed not through the hygienic conduct of individuals, but through impersonal, non-discriminating, normalising instruments of state regulation. The continuing incidence of milk-borne typhoid fever epidemics above all testified to the failure of policies which ultimately relied on the responsible self-government of the individual. There would always be occasions when the ignorance or negligence of a carrier would result in an outbreak such as that at Moorabbin. Doctors noted that the isolation of diphtheria carriers was more of a 'pious hope' or 'farce' than a reality. Similarly, a proposal to ensure milk safety by teaching all consumers to boil their milk was regarded as 'a method of desperation'.[64]

The admission of failure made by advocates of pasteurisation and immunisation testifies to the reluctance with which the social aspects of sanitary policies were abandoned. Notification of disease had made local factors of all kinds – judging the dirty habits of individuals, inducing Councils to reform waste disposal practices, educating the public – crucial to control and prevention. The use of mass immunisation made them irrelevant. Sanitary policies, where possible, were always preferred because of their social effects. '[The method] of ensuring the health of the herd and the cleanliness of the milk ... is the ideal one, but at the present time it presents so many difficulties as to be incapable of general application throughout the country ... the ideal of a pure milk source over the whole country remains an ideal.'[65] On the basis that 'diphtheria is not a sanitary matter, and it is useless to call the sanitary inspector', mass immunisation was first implemented against diphtheria in the early 1920s.[66] However, it was specifically *not* advocated against typhoid fever despite successful use during the First World War. Instead, it was explicitly stated that since typhoid fever was apparently controllable through sanitary measures, it was always preferable to use these instead of immunisation.[67] The demand for immunisation at Moorabbin signals an important change of attitude. In Merrillees's Report judgement of individual conduct took second place to pragmatic defensive measures. Once identified, the woman who caused the outbreak at Moorabbin was scarcely mentioned. Instead, the fact of her existence was used as a key argument for the need for pasteurisation: 'The great lesson of the outbreak is that it is not safe to drink raw milk.'[68] Since child carriers (from their irresponsibility) and housewives (from their food preparation) posed problems for self-regulation, it was decided simply to make immunisation of all members of the household a condition of hospital release for new carriers at Moorabbin.[69] Education of individuals was giving way to prevention at a population level.

Both pasteurisation and immunisation were intended to be, and depended for their effectiveness on being, blanket policies applied across the milk supply and population respectively; they created unitary standards. Their introduction centred on negotiations between new centralising and older local forms of public health administration, between coercive policy and liberal commitments to individual choice and autonomy. This negotiation was all the more important because of the clamorously vocal opposition to both practices.[70] Immunisation was both sign and facilitator of the increasing role of central government in initiating and directing Australian public health, reducing the role of local authorities to implementation. Mass immunisation campaigns (against diphtheria) were first encouraged by State Departments of Health in the late 1920s, and left to the voluntary implementation of local Councils, very few of which took up the strategy until the late 1930s however.[71] The widespread use and success of immunisation required a much more interventionist approach from central government, a condition facilitated first by the advent of war. Wholesale immunisation only became routine from the 1950s, when it was virtually demanded by State governments that each municipality would undertake a campaign biannually, furnishing the central authority with records of every child's immune status.

As with immunisation, the introduction of pasteurisation was local, pragmatic and piecemeal, little taken up until after the Second World War despite encouragement from government officials. Its history in Australia demonstrates the importance of local administrative factors in shaping industry practice. In the 1920s and 1930s, policy-makers expected dairies to voluntarily install pasteurisation plants because they would be profitable. Incentives to pasteurise were built into existing economic regulatory schemas. In New South Wales, pasteurisation was added to specifications for milk grades in 1929. It was anticipated that most dairies would switch to the production of high-grade milk, driven by demand from educated and responsible consumers. The strategy was reasonably successful: close to 90 per cent of Sydney's milk was pasteurised by 1949.[72] In Victoria, where pasteurisation was not a determinant of milk grades, the percentage of pasteurised milk was much lower until well after the outbreak at Moorabbin brought pasteurisation within the rubric of law.[73]

Central government management was necessary but not sufficient for the implementation of pasteurisation and immunisation. The two practices only became common through their interpretation and acceptance at the public level. According to the letter of the law, both were always voluntary practices, though strategically directed and managed by central government through a variety of incentives, punitive measures and propaganda. Consent was negotiated by continuing to manage the policies through local authorities and local institutions. Immunisation campaigns were always instituted by municipal Councils, and parents were required to sign consent forms for the procedure. Similarly, according to the terms of the 1943 and 1949 Victorian Milk Pasteurisation Acts, each municipal Council had the responsibility of declaring itself a 'pasteurisation zone', and requiring (backed by State legal powers) that all milk sold in the locality be pasteurised. Placing the onus for using pasteurisation and immunisation on municipal authorities made public demand and reaction a significant driving force in their introduction. Increasingly familiar, both were frequently demanded by a frightened local community following an outbreak of disease. The people of Moorabbin were paradigmatic in this respect.

Sanitary practices and beliefs were not removed by risk-reduction techniques like immunisation and pasteurisation. Rather, immunisation and pasteurisation were conceived and implemented in a framework which incorporated sanitation. Both public and professional response to epidemics continued to insist on the importance of local sanitary action as well as personal and domestic hygiene models, the importance of cause as well as protection. For example, a local Member of Parliament (for Berrigan, NSW) wrote to the Minister for Health in response to an outbreak of diphtheria in 1937:

> We admit that provision has been made for free injections of anatoxin as a protection *against* the disease, but feel that this is only one side of the question . . . the other side is finding the seat of the cause, and when it is fully appreciated what are the really insanitary conditions prevailing in Berrigan, the cause surely could be located . . . With the lack of a garbage collection service, we feel that the ever increasing amount of debris . . . is inimical to the health of the community.[74]

Similarly, the sanitary regulation of milk continued to be considered important. Pasteurisation became necessary because sanitation failed, but that did not make sanitary practice irrelevant, as objectors to pasteurisation feared. The reiterated fact that clean milk was not necessarily safe milk was matched by the equally common reminder that pasteurisation could not make 'dirty' milk 'clean'.[75] While milk 'safety' (pasteurisation) simply neutralised bacterial contamination from any source, milk 'cleanliness', its freshness and wholesome qualities, required perpetually vigilant sanitation. Those who thought that pasteurisation would lead to careless and unhygienic practices in the industry were assured that the continuing use of bacterial counts before and after milk was pasteurised would actually better reveal unsanitary practice or unsatisfactory pasteurisation.[76] Pasteurisation was to be accompanied by a continued commitment to ideals of education and responsibility. As was noted in the *Health Bulletin*: 'after the completion of pasteurisation, milk has still to be carefully handled . . . Education – not regulation – is the only means by which the care of milk in the home can be improved.'[77] In his Introduction to Merrillees's Report, Scholes commented piously: 'there should be washbasins and towels at or adjacent to every closet, urinal, or lavatory in every establishment where preparation, handling and distribution of food are carried out . . . There should be inculcated habits of personal cleanliness in every detail of the daily work. One cleanly habit begets another.'[78] Rosenau was again quoted: 'Pasteurization does not claim to replace sanitation and common decency. It cannot atone for filth, and should not be used as a redemption process.'[79]

Conclusion

Pasteurisation and immunisation were two of the earliest preventive policies based explicitly on a logic of risk reduction. They were strategies introduced as a result of the perceived failure of the sanitary model of preventive medicine which centred on locating and controlling dangerous things – individuals, animals, practices or places. Both were blanket, protective practices applied at population level, which operated by reducing risk as close as possible to zero. They worked by making individual actions more or less irrelevant. As such, their logic stands in sharp contrast to contemporary theories of modern risk-based public health and points to the importance of the careful historicising of such concepts as dangerousness and risk and their significance for differing public health policies. Scholars have typically located a shift from dangerousness to risk only towards the close of the twentieth century. For most theorists risk-based public health is characterised by health promotion and education measures which define the maintenance of public health as a matter of individual, rather than state, responsibility. Recent risk-based public health is centred on the self-reflexive, responsible actions of individual citizens, who are expected to identify and alter actions which place them at 'high risk' of an infinitude of possible pains.[80] The introduction of pasteurisation and immunisation marked the beginnings of an explicitly risk-based public health focused on effects most visible at the level of population rather than on individual instances. But this was a public health firmly grounded in state responsibility and individual unreliability: the normalisation of these practices occurred contemporaneously with the passage of national medical insurance legislation.[81] It was the very success of pasteurisation and immunisation which, in making a range of formerly devastating diseases virtually unknown, facilitated the transfer of attention to 'lifestyle' choices as the key to public health policy and the emergence of multiple strategies of risk management. Normalised only over the course of several decades, pasteurisation and immunisation call attention to the complex alterations in twentieth-century logics of disease prevention by which long-standing sanitary ideas gave way to those centred on risk.

Notes

1 'Immunisation', 'inoculation' and 'vaccination' were terms with different technical meanings in the nineteenth and early twentieth centuries, although they were also used interchangeably. Immunisation, associated above all with diphtheria, must be seen as an early twentieth-century public health policy quite different to nineteenth-century vaccination (against smallpox). See Bashford's discussion in this volume and C. Hooker, 'Diphtheria, Immunisation and the Bundaberg Tragedy: A Study in Public Health in Australia', *Health and History*, 2000, pp. 52–78.
2 It is important to keep these distinctions in mind, however, especially given the precise technical and cultural histories of their evolution. See e.g. the discussion of antisepsis and asepsis in A. Bashford, *Purity and Pollution: Gender, Embodiment and Victorian Medicine*, London, Macmillan, 1998, pp. 128–32, 138–9.
3 *The Compact Edition of the Oxford English Dictionary*, Oxford, Oxford University Press, 1971, vol. 2, p. 2637.
4 D. Armstrong, 'Public Health Spaces and the Fabrication of Identity', *Sociology*, 1993, vol. 27, p. 401.
5 A. Petersen and D. Lupton, *The New Public Health: Health and Self in the Age of Risk*, Sydney, Allen and Unwin, 1996.
6 N. Tomes, *The Gospel of Germs: Women, Men and the Microbe in American Life*, Cambridge, Mass., Harvard University Press, 1998, pp. 237–56.
7 See e.g. D. Porter, *Health, Civilisation and the State: A History of Public Health from Ancient to Modern Times*, London, Routledge, 1999, pp. 111–28. She terms Chadwick's reforms 'the sanitary idea', and sees this as succeeded by a period of

'state medicine', which covered preventative and palliative techniques specifically including the isolation and disinfection of individuals and the regulation of foods.
8 See e.g. among many others, A. Hardy, 'On the Cusp: Epidemiology and Bacteriology at the Local Government Board, 1890–1905', *Medical History*, 1998, vol. 42, pp. 328–9; *Bulletin of the History of Medicine and Allied Sciences*, 1997, vol. 42, N. Tomes and J. H. Warner (eds), *Special Issue on Rethinking the Reception of the Germ Theory of Disease: Comparative Perspectives*; and A. Cunningham and P. Williams (eds), *The Laboratory Revolution in Medicine*, New York, Cambridge University Press,1992.
9 I understand 'governmentality' to mean the multiplicity of practices, disciplines and regulations, by individuals, social institutions and the State, through which populations are managed. See R. Castel, 'From Dangerousness to Risk', in G. Burchell, C. Gordon and P. Miller (eds), *The Foucault Effect: Studies in Governmentality*, Chicago, University of Chicago Press, 1991, pp. 281–99; see also F. Ewald, 'Insurance and Risk', ibid., pp. 197–211; D. Lupton, *Risk*, London and New York, Routledge, 1999; A. Petersen, 'Risk, Governance and the New Public Health', in A. Petersen and R. Bunton (eds), *Foucault, Health and Medicine*, London and New York, Routledge, 1997; and M. Dean, *Governmentality: Power and Rule in Modern Society*, London, Sage, 1999.
10 Of particular interest is a quotation from 1914 in which vaccination (against smallpox) was compared with sterilisation of the unfit, in Castel, 'From Dangerousness to Risk', p. 285.
11 See e.g. J. H. L. Cumpston, *Health and Disease in Australia: A History* (Milton Lewis, ed.), Canberra, Australian Government Printing Service, 1989; H. J. Parish, *Victory with Vaccines: The Story of Immunization*, Edinburgh, E. and S. Livingstone, 1968; N. Gobold, *Cream of the Country: A History of Victorian Dairying*, Melbourne, Dairy Industry Association of Victoria, 1989. Although the advent of bacteriology did profoundly alter public health strategies, the Australian experience was different to that of the UK or Canada. For example, bacteriology was not *successive* to sanitation because the classic 'sanitary' strategies – sewering, garbage disposal, and so on – were only implemented in the 1890s, when bacteriological ideas were also taken up.
12 Composed of: Federal government, formed in 1901, and only beginning to expand into health, education and other social services by 1920; State governments; and local or municipal Councils.
13 Pasteurisation was more widespread in Sydney than Melbourne during the 1930s, thanks to the vigorous policies of the State of New South Wales Milk Board. See W. Murphy, *Milk Board of NSW: An Outline of its Origin and Development*, Sydney, The Milk Board of New South Wales, 1949. On the other hand, mass immunisation (against diphtheria), stimulated by proactive local Councils in Melbourne and Bendigo, was far more common in the State of Victoria than in New South Wales until after the war. See C. Hooker, 'Diphtheria, Immunisation and the Bundaberg Tragedy'.
14 J. Lewis, 'The Prevention of Diphtheria in Canada and Britain 1914–1945', *Journal of Social History*, 1986, vol. 20, pp. 163–76; E. Hammond, *Childhood's Deadly Scourge: The Campaign to Control Diphtheria in New York City, 1880–1930*, Baltimore, Johns Hopkins University Press, 1999.
15 J. Phillips and M. French, 'State Regulation and the Hazards of Milk, 1900–1939', *Social History of Medicine*, 1999, vol. 12, pp. 371–89; P. J. Atkins, 'White Poison? The Social Consequences of Milk Consumption, 1850–1930', *Social History of Medicine*, 1992, vol. 5, pp. 216–18.
16 Cumpston, *Health and Disease*, pp. 234–7.
17 F. Merrillees, *Report on Typhoid Fever in the City of Moorabbin, 1943*, Melbourne, Victorian Department of Public Health, 1943, p. 24.

18 Ibid., p. 10.
19 Ibid., p. 20.
20 Ibid., p. 35.
21 Cumpston, *Health and Disease*; J. H. L. Cumpston, *Health of the People: A Study in Federalism*, Canberra, Roebuck, 1978.
22 F. Hone, 'Notification or Prevention?', *Report of the Eighteenth Meeting of the Australasian Association for the Advancement of Science*, 1926, pp. 675–93; for a discussion of early infectious disease control techniques in Australia see A. Bashford, 'Quarantine and the Imagining of the Australian Nation', *Health*, 1998, vol. 2, pp. 387–402, and 'Epidemic and Governmentality: Smallpox in Sydney, 1881', *Critical Public Health*, 1999, vol. 9, pp. 301–16; P. Curzon, *Times of Crisis: Epidemics in Sydney, 1788–1900*, Sydney, Sydney University Press, 1985.
23 T. W. Sinclair, 'General Measures for the Control of Diphtheria, Including Legal Control and Disinfection', *Medical Journal of Australia*, 10 May 1924, pp. 300–4.
24 For a discussion of these different techniques in response to diphtheria, see C. Hooker and A. Bashford, 'Diphtheria and Australian Public Health: Bacteriology and its Complex Applications, *c*.1890–1930', *Medical History* (forthcoming, 2002).
25 Merrillees, *Report*, p. 22.
26 'The provision of an adequate supply of milk of good quality is a matter of major importance to the community and the milk supply is a public health utility.' Quoted in Murphy, *Milk Board of NSW*, p. 18.
27 Murphy, *Milk Board of NSW*; especially pp. 92–109; M. Lewis, 'Milk, Mothers and Infant Welfare', in J. Roe (ed.), *Twentieth Century Sydney: Studies in Urban and Social History*, Sydney, Hale and Iremonger, 1980, pp. 193–207.
28 Murphy, *Milk Board of NSW*, p. 90.
29 Merrillees, *Report*, pp. 16–19.
30 Ibid., p. 17.
31 Hooker and Bashford, 'Diphtheria and Australian Public Health'.
32 T. Cherry, 'Diphtheria Antitoxin', 20 Mar. 1895, *Medical Journal of Australia*, 17, pp. 101–6.
33 M. Foucault, 'About the Concept of the "Dangerous Individual" in Nineteenth Century Legal Psychiatry', in D. Weisstub (ed.), *Law and Psychiatry*, New York and Toronto, Pergamon Press, 1977, pp. 1–18.
34 In fact, carrier control and milk sanitary regulation bore a close affinity with the forms of civil law Foucault mentions in the same article. He raises the notion of 'risk' rather than 'danger' with respect to civil law. These terms will require more precise historicising.
35 See Hooker and Bashford, 'Diphtheria and Australian Public Health'; Hooker, 'Diphtheria, Immunisation and the Bundaberg Tragedy'; A. Hardy, *The Epidemic Streets: Infectious Disease and the Rise of Preventive Medicine, 1856–1900*, Oxford, Clarendon Press, 1993; T. Ziporyn, *Disease in the Popular American Press: The Case of Diphtheria, Typhoid Fever and Syphilis, 1870–1920*, New York, Greenwood Press, 1988.
36 J. Walzer Leavitt, *Typhoid Mary: Captive to the Public's Health*, Boston, Mass., Beacon Press, 1996 and J. Walzer Leavitt, ' "Typhoid Mary" Strikes Back: Bacteriological Theory and Practice in Early Twentieth Century Public Health', *Isis*, 1992, vol. 83, pp. 608–29.
37 Thus, although the majority of carriers were found to be temporary, some carriers would continue to 'harbour' bacteria for weeks, months or years – in the case of typhoid, carrier status was not infrequently found to be lifelong.
38 Hooker and Bashford, 'Diphtheria and Public Health'.
39 F. V. Scholes, 'Foreword', in Merrillees, *Report*, p. 3.

40 Foucault too argued that the danger the insane posed was not merely to themselves and their contemporaries but to future generations through the idea of 'degeneration'. There is however a significant difference between the notion of degeneration – which could be utilised in constructing the danger of the carrier, although this was rare – and the understandings of threatened population immunity or susceptibility of the time. Foucault, 'Dangerous Individual'.

41 The concept of the healthy carrier was first elucidated with respect to diphtheria. See Hardy, *Epidemic Streets*; C. Hooker, 'Community and Medicine: Diphtheria Management and Public Health in Australia, 1858–1895', *Occasional Papers in Medical History*, 1999, no. 9; F. B. Smith, 'Comprehending Diphtheria', *Health and History: Bulletin of the Australian Society of the History of Medicine*, 1999, vol. 1, pp. 138–61; Hooker and Bashford, 'Diphtheria and Public Health'.

42 Hooker and Bashford, 'Diphtheria and Public Health'. I note here that mass immunisation against typhoid fever was used for the armed services during the war but was not applied to civilian populations.

43 In 1918, 7,500 tests for diphtheria in Bendigo resulted in the isolation of over 500 carriers for periods of one week to not infrequently more than a month. See Hooker and Bashford, 'Diphtheria and Public Health'.

44 Merrillees, *Report*, p. 46.

45 Ibid., p. 47.

46 J. H. L. Cumpston pioneered the use of epidemiological measurements as the basis for public health strategies after the First World War. Immunisation and risk management can be viewed as 'produced' by such instruments just as swabbing campaigns had earlier 'produced' the 'carrier' as the fundamental problem of disease management.

47 Hooker, 'Diphtheria, Immunisation and the Bundaberg Tragedy'.

48 F. V. Scholes, 'Scarlet Fever and Diphtheria: Present Day Problems', *Australian Medical Congress: Transactions*, 1929, pp. 26–30.

49 'Milk in Relation to Public Health', *Victorian Communications in Public Health: Health Bulletin* [hereafter *Health Bulletin*], 119, 1958, p. 18. As the Chairman of the Milk Pasteurisation Committee said, 'there is now indisputable evidence that "safety" can be conferred by pasteurisation'. T. M. Jensen, *Pasteurization of Milk: Guide to Premises and Equipment for Pasteurizing Dairies*, Department of Agriculture, Victoria, 1950, p. 1.

50 The comparison is both real and representative, for example: 'The cow then becomes a "carrier" of the human type of bacillus.' In 'Milk and its Relation to Public Health', *Health Bulletin*, 1932, p. 985.

51 'The danger of raw milk (even so-called clean milk) ...' quoted in 'Milk in Relation to Public Health', *Health Bulletin*, 1943, p. 3. See also 'The production of clean milk' in 'Milk and its Relation to Public Health', 1932, p. 989; Murphy, *Milk Board of NSW*, p. 98.

52 These last two were particularly important, controversial issues in the 1920s and early 1930s. See 'Milk and its Relation to Public Health', 1932, pp. 984–6; 'Milk in Relation to Public Health', 1943, pp. 9–15.

53 Lewis, 'Milk, Mothers and Infant Welfare'; see also D. Dwork, *War is Good for Babies and Other Young Children: A History of the Infant and Child Welfare Movement in England, 1898–1918*, London, Tavistock, 1987.

54 'Milk and its Relation to Public Health', 1932, p. 980. This article cited statistics from Australia, America and Canada to show the importance of outbreaks of milk-borne typhoid fever.

55 Ibid., p. 998.

56 Ibid., p. 978. The potential and necessity for *universal* pasteurisation was frequently emphasised, see for example 'Milk in Relation to Public Health', 1943, p. 27.

57 A symmetry which Foucault argued was central to the era of governmentality. See Foucault, 'Governmentality', pp. 87–105.
58 Murphy, *Milk Board of NSW*, p. 11.
59 'Milk and its Relation to Public Health', 1932, p. 999.
60 'The Prevention of Diphtheria', *Medical Journal of Australia*, 2 Feb. 1918, pp. 90–1.
61 'Milk and its Relation to Public Health', 1932, p. 999. See also 'Milk in Relation to Public Health', 1943, p. 14; 'Milk and its Relation to Public Health', 1932, pp. 979, 983–4, as for example this quotation: 'No raw milk can be guaranteed as absolutely safe, the means of infection are so numerous, and the presence of carriers and "missed cases" undetectable.'
62 Ibid., p. 985.
63 Ibid., p. 983.
64 Ibid., p. 999.
65 Ibid.
66 'The Prevention of Diphtheria', *Medical Journal of Australia*, 8 Oct. 1921, p. 291.
67 J. Dale, 'The Prevention and Control of Diphtheria and Scarlet Fever', *Australian Medical Congress: Transactions*, 1929, pp. 32–41.
68 Scholes, 'Foreword', p. v; Merrillees, *Report*, pp. 50–3.
69 Merrillees, *Report*, p. 52.
70 For opposition to immunisation, see Hooker, 'Diphtheria, Immunisation and the Bundaberg Tragedy'. For opposition to pasteurisation see 'Milk and its Relation to Public Health', 1932, pp. 995–7; 'Milk in Relation to Public Health' 1943, pp. 14–41; Scholes, 'Foreword', pp. ii–iv; and Bibby, *The Case Against Pasteurization of Milk*.
71 See Hooker, 'Diphtheria, Immunisation and the Bundaberg Tragedy'.
72 Murphy, *Milk Board of NSW*, p. 99.
73 In 1949, the 'toothless' Act passed in 1943 was replaced by the Victorian government with a more stringent and directive Milk Pasteurisation Act.
74 Letter from R. I. Ball, Member of the Legislative Assembly, to the Department of Health, NSW, 21 Jan. 1937. Health Department: No. 8, State Archives of NSW, K 12/921.
75 'Milk in Relation to Public Health', 1943, p. 30; 'Milk and its Relation to Public Health', 1932, pp. 994, 998; Scholes, 'Foreword', p. v.
76 'Milk and its Relation to Public Health', 1932, p. 995.
77 Ibid., p. 995.
78 Scholes, 'Foreword', p. v.
79 'Milk in Relation to Public Health', 1943, p. 30.
80 P. Higgs and G. Scambler (eds), *Modernity, Medicine and Health: Medical Sociology Towards 2000*, London, Routledge, 1998.
81 See discussions in J. Roe (ed.), *Social Policy in Australia: Some Perspectives, 1901–1975*, Sydney, Cassell, 1976.

Part 2
Contaminating capacities in postmodernity

7 Vulnerable bodies and ontological contamination

Margrit Shildrick

Finding myself in Dublin some time ago, I visited the highly regarded Gallery of Photography to see a new exhibition by Karl Grimes. At the time I was engaged in an archival trawl of 'monster' texts, and had become deeply interested in the richness of representational forms of the monstrous. *Still Life* records the chance visit by Grimes to the specimen room of an Italian hospital at which he was working on a different project. The exhibition comprised a couple of dozen large photographic portraits of late foetal and neonatal infant bodies with gross congenital deformities, most of whom were preserved in vast glass containers, in some cases after partial dissection (see Figure 7.1). There were several concorporate twins, bodies with hydrocephalus, exposed spines, or other gaping orifices, their corporeal borders dis-integrated. In clinical terms they are monsters, in lay terms freaks. The collection was deeply disturbing; it touched those who saw it. As might be expected, some of the press reviews constructed *Still Life* as exploitative, voyeuristic, something that should not be put on public show. It was as though the bodies' aw(e)ful vulnerability put us, the viewers, at risk; as though they could contaminate. But that is to miss the point. The encounter with the others who define our own boundaries of normality must inevitably disturb for they are both irreducibly strange and disconcertingly familiar, both opaque and reflective. They enable us to recognise ourselves, they are our own abject. As Grimes himself notes, 'Images of what we have denied turn towards us.'[1] And once the initial shock of confronting what is usually excluded had passed, I found myself not repulsed, but moved to tears by the unaccountable beauty of the bodies. Beyond the marks of a violent and violating science that were evident in their confinement, both materially to specimen jars, and discursively to the category of abnormality, it was possible to acknowledge a siblingship which claims us.

How, then, can I theorise these autobiographical moments in the context of contagion and vulnerability? Among the several meanings of the word 'contagion' – all of which are deeply negative in their import – is the notion of a disease process spread by touch, or even by proximity. We understand that a contaminated object is one to be avoided or kept

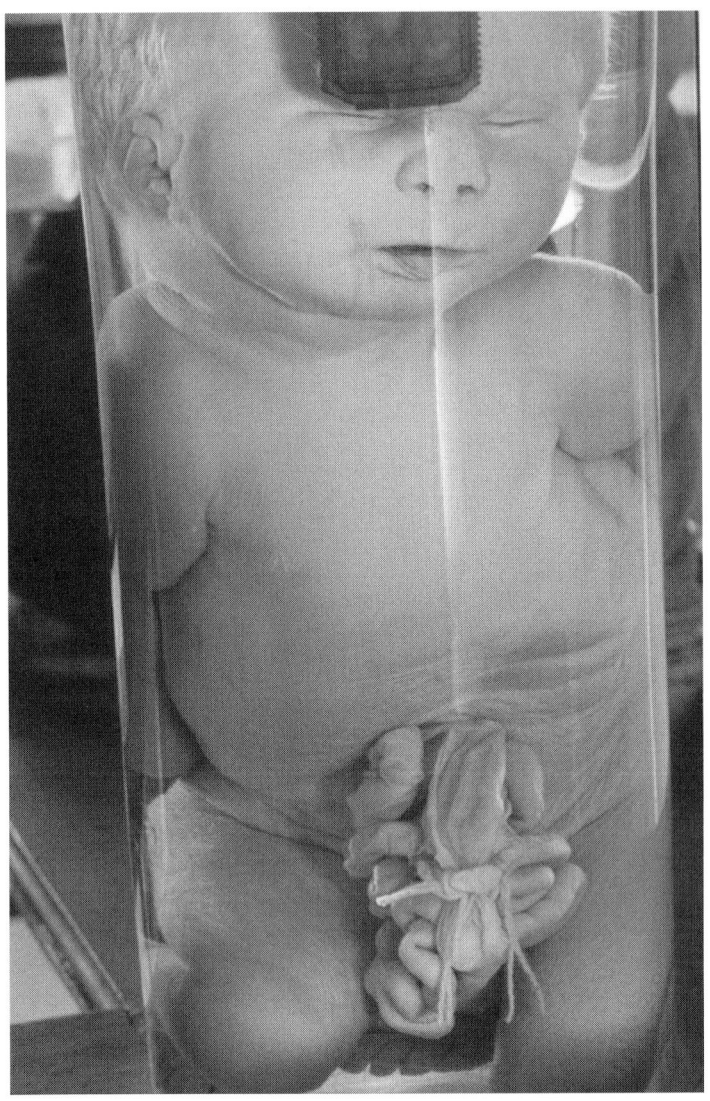

Figure 7.1 Karl Grimes, *Still Life*, 1997, chromogenic print, 72 × 48 in. Courtesy of the artist and Gallery of Photography, Dublin.

at a safe distance, lest we too become affected, our bodies opened up to the forces of disintegration. Our well-being, our very lives, are dependent then on the maintenance of a self-protective detachment, an interval not only between ourselves and evidently dangerous others – be they microbes, parasites, or infected human bodies – but also between ourselves and the mere potential of risk. Contagion is a familiar term in medical discourse; public health, for example, relies, in large part, on the success of epidemiological measures designed not simply to control, but also to avoid the threat of an other that would expose our underlying vulnerability to bodily degeneration. Thus the prophylactic strategies of, for example, the vaccination of children, anti-malarial drug regimes for travellers, or the practice of safe sex for us all, make good sense. The probability that any one threat might materialise may be extremely low, but nonetheless our well-being is seen to be enhanced by the erection of protective barriers. There is nothing particularly contentious in any of this, except perhaps in the calculation of risk, but I want to move away from the descriptive to explore more closely how the vulnerability of human bodies, and indeed of human being, is denied in the more general sense.

My argument is that in western discourse, the notion of the diseased, the unclean or the contaminated is never just an empirical or supposedly neutral descriptor, but carries the weight of all that stands against – and of course paradoxically secures – the normative categories of ontology and epistemology. In short, as the realisation of a contaminatory threat, contagion can figure any transgression of the categories of sameness and difference, any breach in the unity of the embodied self. As postmodernist theory makes clear, the self's clean and proper body – to use Julia Kristeva's phrase – is not a given, but instead an unstable construct under constant threat.[2] On the one hand there is the potential of internal leakage and loss of form, while on the other, it is at risk from the circulation of all those dangerous bodies – of women, of racial others, of the sick, of the monstrous – who both occupy the place of the other and serve to define by difference the self's own parameters. In this paper, I shall look in particular at the condition of disability. Quite deliberately, I use the term broadly, because although there are multiple ways in which it is experienced, those specific categories of disability are collapsed, in conventional discourse, into a generalised icon of improper embodiment. What is at issue is the way in which disability is positioned as the site of modernist discourses that figure the human body – or at least the white male body – as ideally closed and invulnerable. From historical archival material through to present day research into the genetic manipulation of potential congenital abnormalities, the stress throughout has been on controlling or eliminating the conditions of vulnerability as though science could settle ontology. But what, precisely, is at stake in the western imaginary with its dream of containment, and what marks the disabled body as a threat, as though it could contaminate? By using the notion of contagion as a model for relationship in western society, my concern is to suggest new ways of conceptualising disability. And what my postmodernist perspective demands and facilitates is a deconstruction of existing ethical parameters in the light of an always already present vulnerability as the disavowed condition of all bodies.

I want first to set out the ground on which, in western modernity at least, vulnerability is figured as a shortcoming, an impending failure both of form and function; a predicate that marks its subject as potentially beyond normative standards of being. It is not exactly that vulnerability is denied in and by the normative subject, but that the 'proper' unfolding of human life is taken to overcome such dangers. Those who too readily admit or who succumb to vulnerability are either weak or unfortunate, beset by either or both moral and material failure. Although the heroic narrative of individual transcendence over corporeal adversity – the triumph of mind over matter – is highly familiar, and constitutes the greater part of auto/biographical accounts of illness and disability,[3] its claim to our admiration exists alongside contrary tendencies. More usually vulnerability is feared as a condition of both mind and body, an ontological as well as physical state, an embodied being in which those familiar mind/body distinctions enacted by post-Enlightenment thought may not be made. Instead, the compromised body may invite the assumption of intellectual insufficiency – those with physical, and particularly congenital, disabilities are all too commonly denied access to standard education as children and find themselves spoken for as adults – or alternatively the outward appearance of an ailing body may be taken as the sign of an inner deficiency of will, or prior moral dereliction.[4] And while the first of those more negative responses might be evidence of the unsettling dis-ease occasioned by the non-normative body such that engagement is avoided, the latter speaks to a sense of danger.

That unusual bodily form has a long history of provoking both fear and condemnation is widely evidenced in a variety of texts. I'm not suggesting that it is the only response, but rather that whatever other explanations and interests are predominant at any particular time and cultural location, there seems to be a continuous thread of anxiety. The elision of ethical and physical affronts to the norms of human being has its roots in classical antiquity. If Aristotelian virtue is that which strikes the harmonious balance between the vices of excess and deficiency, the very same characteristics by which he defines monstrosity, then it is a simple step to corporeal disorder inviting moral condemnation. Transhistorically, the most widely accepted definition of the physically monstrous cites excess, deficiency or displacement as sufficient properties – and we might note in passing that for Aristotle, the female form was an intrinsic deformity.[5] And although Aristotle didn't advocate the destruction of female newborns, or indeed other deviant forms, there is nevertheless a long tradition in which corporeal difference invoked institutional erasure. In his history of the so-called monstrous races, for example, John Block Friedman cites customary Roman Law which states: 'A father shall immediately put to death a son recently born, who is a monster, or who has a form different from that of members of the human race.'[6] For medieval Christianity with its belief in human descent from the perfection of the single prelapsarian man, bodily difference represented the corruption of the species either by miscegenation, or as a result of divine punishment for a variety of other sins. The same beliefs in divine retribution for misdeeds already past – or alternatively in heavenly warnings or omens of evils yet to come – provided the most common explanatory models of monstrosity until the early modern period. And although a subsequent turn towards more scientific forms of knowledge is evident, those exist alongside a persistent belief that non-normative bodies of all kinds are marked by moral deficiency. In contemporary society, the inference that disabled people are paying for sins in a past life is clearly evident in the initial widespread public reception of AIDS as figuring a gay plague from which blameless heterosexuals were exempt.

It is not my claim that our response to disabling conditions is always as crude, or sets up so blatant a division between the 'normal' category – the whole-bodied – and the others – those whose bodily boundaries have in some way been breached or distorted. Nor are 'healthy' bodies seen as uniformly invulnerable: for infants and children whose bodily well-being is largely dependent on others, for older people facing the finitude of death and bodily decay, and for women whose intrinsic leakiness marks a body that is always already breached, the ideal of a closed, powerful and self-defined corporeal schema is already compromised. Nonetheless, at the beginning of a century in which evermore detailed biomedical accounts of the body are passing into lay usage, and in which we are invited to marvel at the capacities of biomedical technologies to remake the body, as in gene therapy, organ transplants, or even cloning, reminders of uncontrolled corporeal vulnerability are highly unwelcome. The cultural theorist Rosemarie Garland Thomson recounts her own shock at being given a copy of Robert Bogdan's scholarly study *Freak Show*: '"Freak" disturbingly summarized the accusation I had most dreaded my entire life', and she goes on to describe how owning her own very visible physical disability was akin to coming out. She adds:

> Indeed, pressures to deny, ignore, normalize, and remain silent about one's own disability are both compelling and seductive in a social order intolerant of deviations from the bodily standards enforced by a quotidian matrix of economic, social and political forces.[7]

What I would want to add to Thomson's matrix is the power of psychic and ontological anxiety that must itself be denied.

Where the fully self-present sovereignty of the modernist subject is taken for granted, there is an expectation, and indeed biomedical discourse encourages us to believe, that our bodies are similarly under control, predictable, determinate, and above all independent in form and function. The mapping of the human genome, which promises both a measure of individual uniqueness and a template for enhanced control and manipulation, signals that the perfect body, marked by its consistency and self-transparency is available to all. Such a standard serves to deny corporeal vulnerability, and, as many commentators have already pointed out, further strengthens the othering of those whose bodies fall short. The more we believe that we can control our bodies, the greater the anxiety that is generated by the evidence of vulnerability, whether as the result of the accident of disabling conditions, both chronic and acute, or in the form of those routine biological processes of change in which the feminine is over-determined. And it's somewhat ironic, as Susan Wendell points out, that in contesting the traditional link between women and their unruly bodies, feminism too displays a certain somatophobia, having little to say about certain forms of anomalous embodiment.[8] The noticeable paucity of academic interest, both there and elsewhere, in disability studies may look like indifference, but I suggest it plays into the wider issue of our perception of non-normative corporeality.[9] The disabled body, the body that resists the conscious control of the will, that is effectively out of control, may carry no infectious agents, and yet is treated as though it is contaminatory.

Although such a potentially dangerous entity must be kept at a distance, beyond the capacity to touch, it is nonetheless a privileged object of the gaze. What is evoked at worst is a kind of revulsion and dehumanisation, characterised historically by the public display of human 'monsters' – both dead and alive – as, for example, in the freak shows of the nineteenth and early twentieth century, or today, as Andrea Dennett suggests, by the enfreakment of corporeal extremes – especially of the 'fattest' or 'heaviest' variety – on many American television day-time talk shows.[10] What is striking about such spectacles, however, is that they may elicit the contradictory responses both of horrified disengagement, and of fascination and recognition. The present day staging of disability may seek to avoid the offensive excesses of the past under a banner of education or social concern, but the invitation – like the freak show barker's pitch – appeals, more or less explicitly, to the model of the abnormal viewed from a safe distance. In his fascinating analysis of US charity telethons in aid of various illnesses and disabilities, for example, Paul K. Longmore demonstrates both the distancing effect of the gaze, and the way in which the apparently altruistic structure of the events authorises the contemporary equivalent of finger pointing.[11] In such orgies of public 'compassion', Longmore sees as the prime motivation the conspicuous display, not of links of sameness, but of boundaries of difference. Although agreeing with the outlines of his analysis, I believe the relationships are more complicated than Longmore allows. Where he would see vulnerability – which he characterises primarily in terms of dependency – as fixed by the gaze as the property of the differentiated other, the underlying anxiety of the encounter with the corporeal anomaly needs further explanation.

It is of course precisely the failure of the monstrous body to observe a material and metaphorical cordon sanitaire, its failure wholly to occupy the place of the other, that grounds anxiety. Thinking, for example, of the negative responses to the pictures in the *Still Life* exhibition, it is evident that the triple confinement of the unruly foetuses, in death, in glass containers, and in the photographic image, was nonetheless insufficient to allay the uncomfortable feeling that they could reach out and contaminate. Clearly the artist was well aware of the power of his images, which were intended to breach the immunity of the gaze, but nonetheless, the gallery was constrained to give a written warning to visitors that they might be disturbed. So powerful is the impulse to avoid actual contact with anomalous bodies, that as Rosemarie Garland Thomson reminds us in *Extraordinary Bodies*, the so-called 'ugly laws' effective in the United States during part of the nineteenth and twentieth centuries actually banned those with visible disabilities from appearing in certain public places.[12] Even when at best there may be compassion and an attempt at empathy with the corporeally deviant, that empathy is about trying to smooth out differences, to find the grounds of sameness, but it is clearly not about opening oneself – becoming vulnerable – to an encounter with irreducible strangeness. Indeed, insofar as the gaze remains operative, we might say that no real encounter takes place, for the emphasis is not on exchange in which mutual transformation might occur, but precisely on forestalling such a move. Monstrously embodied selves are, then, fundamentally disturbing in that they cannot be accounted for within the binary parameters of sameness and difference, in which the latter is measured in terms of the former. Instead, they transgress boundaries in being simultaneously too close, threatening merging and indifference, *and* in being excessive, in being irreducibly other to the binary itself.

Before going on to theorise that in more clearly postmodernist terms, I want to trace the aporias within modernism itself. What is really unsettling about non-normative embodiment is not simply the reminder of the empirical instability of all bodies, but the intuition that despite the privileging of mind in western discourse, our embodied selfhood is a matter of complex interweaving. Far from maintaining a Cartesian belief that our selves remain unchanged by the vicissitudes of the flesh, we are obsessed with our bodies, particularly as they deviate from normative ideals. Whenever the body is at risk, it is the stability of the self that is threatened. In short, corporeal and ontological anxiety are inseparable. From a phenomenological point of view this is hardly surprising, for there the structure of the self is fully imbricated with its corporeal capacities. But although the *transcendent* split between mind and body may be problematised by our phenomenological experience of being-in-the-world, we do still see our bodies almost as though they were suits of armour protecting a core self. We are unsurprised by references to the 'real me' inside. Any breach in the ideal impregnability of the surface flesh signals potential contamination, an openness to the assault of the other. Moreover, the post-Enlightenment ideal of autonomous subjectivity and agency relies on a spacing, an interval between self and other that covers over the putative threat of engulfment by the other. As we know too well, the transhistorical hostility towards the feminine expresses a fear of, and revulsion for, bodies that appear unable to maintain the distinction and definition required by the sovereign self.

As we would anticipate, the dominant systems of western ethics, and I'm thinking here particularly of bioethics, reflect that ideal of distinction and separation and characterise individual bodies primarily as the property of autonomous selves. The rights I hold in my own body are both protective and must be protected against the incursions of others. In such a system the interaction between such subjects is mediated by implicit contract which assumes the independence of each. Medical law is quite clear on the point, as is evident in a seminal judgement of the 1960s: 'Anglo-American law starts with the premise of thoroughgoing self-determination. It follows that each man is considered to be master of his own body.'[13] As a corollary of such formulations, vulnerability is positioned not as an existential state, but as a contingent physical dependency, that is taken to justify temporary paternalism towards those in ill-health.[14] It is only those others – pregnant women, those who are mentally sick, people with congenital disabilities – all who are deemed incapable of fully autonomous agency, for whom vulnerability appears intrinsic. Yet paradoxically, alongside a mainstream bio/ethical discourse saturated with the vulnerability of the other, where vulnerability signals dependency (and in ethical terms a claim on the duties of beneficence and non-maleficence), both biomedical and lay discourse see embodied selves as vulnerable to contamination by proximity to those same others. Clearly, what is characterised as disability as opposed to disease is not in itself literally contagious. The desire, then, to deter the approach – through limiting access, and through isolation and silencing – of those who are thus marked as disabled is an indication of a simultaneous denial and fear of vulnerability. It is not my purpose, however, to investigate here the oppositional, social model of disability which insists that disabling effects are produced by society rather than being the property of individuals;[15] nor to explore the claim that we are all just temporarily able bodied (TAB) in the sense that disabling illness, accident and old age are the possible or certain fate of all. What will concern me rather is that the positivist model of the body assumed by the preceding account may itself be disturbed by reading it through a postconventional perspective.

As I've already outlined, the tendency is to understand vulnerability as some kind of falling short which is attributed to others, in one major ethical strand, by virtue of their devalued embodiment. Accordingly the dominant ethical response is to suppose that those who are in any degree unable to fulfil normative standards of self-care, may for that reason have special claims for care from others. But for A's interests and needs to depend on B, means that A is vulnerable to B. As Robert Goodin puts it: 'You are always vulnerable to, and dependent upon, some individual or group who have it within their power to help or harm you in some respect(s)',[16] and although Goodin goes on to acknowledge some degree of vulnerability in us all, he nevertheless has in mind an intrinsically asymmetrical model in which some are called upon to protect the vulnerability of others. It is precisely the kind of binary thinking that I want to unsettle, which, as Megan Boler recognises, is based on power relations. Boler herself turns to a consideration of whether an empathy with the other, a kind of caring for the other by the effort of putting oneself in her place, is an improvement.[17] Unlike many other feminist ethicists who work within a liberal humanist frame and see such responses very positively, Boler concludes that empathetic identification remains trapped within a self/other binary that ultimately consumes and annihilates the other. Instead she prefers a testimonial response that requires the encounter *with* vulnerability to rest on an openness to the unpredictably strange and excessive, an openness that renders the self vulnerable. This seems to me an altogether more fruitful approach that acknowledges both that the self and the other are mutually engaged, and yet irreducible the one to the other.

What meaning, then, would vulnerability have if we stepped back from the relentless binaries of western epistemology that set health against illness, conformity against disparity, the perfect against the imperfect, the self against the other? What would it mean in other words to address the issue of vulnerability not *without* recourse to normative standards, but with a critique that exposed not simply the limits set by the cultural specificity of normativity – as opposed to the claim of a general if not universal validity – but more radically yet that the dichotomous structure is itself unstable? One immediate effect would be to place less emphasis on vulnerability as the dependency of others, and more on the notion of vulnerability as the risk of ontological uncertainty for all of us. And what if the question of contagion, of contamination, were found to reside not in the supposed materialities of bodies, but in the structure of discourse itself? I propose to reread the body as a discursive construction, by now a widely familiar move to poststructuralists, but one that still often seems to stymie those who work in the health care disciplines. The problem is that aside from a thoroughgoing deconstruction of the discourses of sexuality, such as Judith Butler's work on queer bodies, and a relatively small number of specific studies like Catherine Waldby's book on AIDS or some of my own previous work with Janet Price on disability, it is hard to find many postmodernist texts that address not just the body as a concept, but the body as it is lived, in pain as well as pleasure.[18] What is called for is a rethinking that challenges the conventional opposition of the material to the discursive, and marks them as fundamentally intertwined.[19] The importance of the move, for me, is not just whether we can successfully retheorise the taken-for-grantedness of bodies, for clearly feminist theory in particular has generated many such reconfigurations, but whether those can be carried forward to make a difference in practice. The project is, I think, ultimately an ethical one of being enabled to act differently because we can also think differently.

But how does this all relate to bodies, and more particularly to disabled bodies? Where the convention insists that some bodies are or become vulnerable by default, the postmodernist understanding of discursive instability speaks to the intrinsic vulnerability of all bodies and indeed all embodied selves. Moreover the corpus to which I have been referring as though it were a given materiality, is more properly a body schema, a psychic construction of wholeness, that – in most cases – belies its own precariousness and vulnerability. I want to look fairly briefly, then, at two psychoanalytic models before turning to consider the implications of a linguistic approach. In Lacan's account of the mirror stage in infant development, it is clear that the emergent sense of embodied and bounded selfhood is phantasmatic to the extent that the infant's actual experience of 'motor incapacity and nursling dependency' is covered over. This is how Lacan characterises it:

> The *mirror stage* is a drama ... which manufactures for the subject, caught up in the lure of spatial identification, the succession of phantasies that extends from a fragmented body-image to a form of its totality ... and lastly to the assumption of the armour of an alienating identity, which will mark with its rigid structure the subject's entire mental development.[20]

The stability and distinction of normative embodiment relies then, from the first, on a re/suppression of the dis-integration which belongs to the subject as embodied, and, indeed, precedes the subject as such. What this suggests is that any body which manifests signs of insecurity may become the repository of both corporeal and ontological anxiety. In the encounter with the disabled or damaged body, the shock is not that of the unknown or unfamiliar, but rather of the pyschic evocation of a primal lack of unity as the condition of all. But as something unacknowleged and unacknowledgeable, that vulnerability is projected onto the other, who must then be avoided for fear of contamination.

At a similar level of analysis of the psychic constitution of the subject, Julia Kristeva's concept of the abject offers perhaps an even clearer explanatory model of the contaminatory potential of non-self materiality. For Kristeva, the abject is the term for all those things which a subject must disavow in the attempt to secure 'the self's clean and proper body', most notably those sticky, viscous, or amorphous things which are associated primarily with the female, and most particularly with the maternal body.[21] In being expelled, the abject is properly neither subject nor object in the binary sense, but occupies the place between where it partakes of both. In other words it never really leaves the subject-body, but remains as both reminder of, and threat to, the precarious status of the closed and unified self. As Kristeva puts it:

> It is something rejected from which one does not part, from which one does not protect oneself as from an object. Imaginary uncanniness and real threat, it beckons to us and ends up engulfing us.[22]

In her long discussion of the abject in biblical texts, Kristeva makes clear that while it is not lack of health itself that 'causes' abjection, but rather 'what disturbs identity, system, order',[23] nonetheless the disabled body is, by virtue of its corporeal nonconformity, among those things which may represent abjection. In marking its debt to nature – the supposedly violent tearing away from the maternal insides – on its own flesh, such a body cannot be proper, that is it cannot be wholly one's own. And if as Kristeva indicates, it is the disavowed trace of the maternal body that grounds the concept of the abject, then it becomes clear why disabled bodies should threaten contamination.

Compelling though I find such psychoanalytic accounts which seem to resonate with a wide variety of cultural practices and beliefs, whilst giving due regard to their specificity, I want to push the argument into territory which breaks entirely with biologistic explanation. I am thinking in terms of the linguistic register, and particularly of the analytic offered by Jacques Derrida and the way in which it has been taken up in Judith Butler's more recent work. As critics of both are all too ready to claim, the level of theorisation involved often makes it difficult to see where or how their abstract insights could be applied to lives as they are lived. If, however, we take seriously, as postmodernists surely must, the claim that bodies and subjects are discursively constructed – materialised rather than material, as Butler has it – then the problematic of language cannot be ignored.[24] What seems to me to warrant further thought in particular is the structure of iterability. Iterability is the process of resaying. It functions not simply as the repetition that seeks to authorise and sediment meaning by repeated reference to a prior context, but as the moment of slippage inherent in repetition that destabilises meaning even as it establishes it. It is, in other words, the rearticulation that introduces the interval of transformation. My question is what difference does a consideration of iterability make to our understanding of contamination and vulnerability? But first I want to recall briefly what the primary moves of the deconstructive approach already entail.

In contradistinction to the binary system that seeks to divide self from other so completely that each may have mutually exclusive properties, one major insight of poststructuralism is that each term is fundamentally reliant on the other for its definition, in the sense both of meaning and outline. Presence defines itself against absence, good against evil, unified against fragmented, able-bodied against disabled, and so on. In place of the closed and complete boundaries that ostensibly mark difference and separation as absolute, the move of deconstruction has been to demonstrate that both primary and marked term are mutually dependent, and measured against a single standard in terms respectively of wholeness and lack. Each term is as Spivak puts it, 'an accomplice of the other',[25] or to put it more materially they are opened up to one another. But what that description misses perhaps is that because the constitutive interdependency – that is, the trace of the one in the other – is overlain in western discourse by a binary structure of sameness and difference, a more appropriate expression of the relationship might be that each term is contaminated by the other. The relationship is one of what Derrida calls *différance*, whereby the necessary operation of the trace of the other within means that for every term 'the presumed interiority of meaning is already worked upon by its own exteriority'.[26] In short, *différance* defers and detours meaning, destabilising all claims to purity. Can we not claim then, as I have suggested elsewhere, that the inherent leakiness of meaning in the logos is paralleled by a necessary uncertainty about bodies, as themselves discursive constructions?[27] Among the many synonyms of *différance*, Derrida proposes the term *pharmakon* which can denote both poison and cure.[28] And can we not see that very same undecidability in the *pharmakos*, the figure of the scapegoat, that both cleanses and is cast out by the community as the nominated carrier of contamination? Not surprisingly Kristeva marks the scapegoat as a figure of abjection.[29]

In understanding how the deconstructive move operates, then, we are already alerted to a certain anxiety at the borders of both concepts and bodies. As Judith Butler reminds us in a much quoted phrase, it is the very process of exclusion that 'produces a constitutive outside to the subject, an abjected outside, which is after all, "inside" the subject as its own founding repudiation'.[30] And moreover, insofar as the constitution of the subject and the materialisation of the body are performative, the process is never complete, but must be repeated constantly: it must be re-iterated. There is in consequence no way of securing the purity of the subject, not least because in the mode of becoming, in the iterative structure itself, there is always slippage such that the 'standard' effects its own internal othering. In other words, iteration is not simply the repetition that 'fixes' what is performed, but the scene of its difference from itself. As Derrida insists: 'Iterability alters, contaminating parasitically what it identifies and enables to repeat "itself".'[31] Now although Derrida here and Butler in her later work *Excitable Speech*[32] are concerned primarily with the analytic of the speech act, it seems to me that the very same trajectory is at work in bodies. However much we speak our being in the body as closed and secure, the ideal invulnerability that we intend to perform is breached in the very repetition. Derrida again:

> (iterability) limits what it makes possible, while rendering its rigour and purity impossible. What is at work here is something like a law of undecidable contamination.[33]

The implication that Derrida later spells out is that iterability 'troubles the binary and hierarchical oppositions that authorize the very principle of "distinction"', and he is explicit that this is as true of common parlance as of philosophical discourse.[34] Yet again, what is at stake is the instability of the boundaries that divide 'whole' bodies from 'broken' ones.

As should now be established, what is at issue, for me, is a radical undoing of the very notion of embodied being as something secure and distinct from its others. Although the post-Enlightenment standard of a wholly autonomous body and mind can be critiqued for its failure both to accommodate at very least the patina of a functional or emotional vulnerability due to us all, and to recognise the interrelatedness of social life, the western imaginary is remarkably resilient. Even within that tradition, Martha Nussbaum's observation that '(t)he peculiar beauty of human excellence just is its vulnerability'[35] – a remark, note, that preserves the subject – is a rare insight indeed. In contrast, my purpose is to reconfigure vulnerability, not as an intrinsic quality of an existing subject, but as an inalienable condition of becoming. The deconstructive enterprise does not of course aim to change things in and of itself, but to provide a critique which gives some account of the violence with which the process of othering different forms of bodyliness is conducted. That violence, it is worth noting, operates both on a discursive and metaphorical level – as the violent hierarchies of the binary system that Derrida refers to, and as material violence to which the eugenic programmes of sterilisation or even extermination of the feeble-minded and feeble-bodied stand witness. And clearly, similar fears of the contamination of a notional purity are operative in the response to racial others. All this poststructuralism understands, and in a telling phrase, Gayatri Spivak refers to deconstruction 'as a radical acceptance of vulnerability'.[36] Her insight does not supplant that of Nussbaum, but gives it rather more depth and urgency.

Such perceptions should not be taken as mere abstractions, but as insights that help further to explain my own face-to-face responses to the images of the *Still Life* presentation. Although persisting at one level as the objects of my gaze, those radically disordered bodies in all their undefended openness crossed the boundaries of otherness and touched my own sense of self. It was not a moment of identity as such, for their difference remained unassimilable, but a recognition of commonality that exposed the fragility and contingency of the protective shell of the embodied self. The threat of contamination is illusory, for each of us was, and is, already

166 *Margrit Shildrick*

vulnerable, without unity or closure. The notion of an irreducible vulnerability as the very possibility of a fully corporeal becoming, of ourselves and always with others, shatters the ideal of the self's clean and proper body; and it calls finally for the willingness to engage in an ethics of risk.

Notes

1 K. Grimes, *Artist's Statement. Still Life*, Dublin, Gallery of Photography, 1998.
2 J. Kristeva, *Powers of Horror*, New York, Columbia University Press, 1982, p. 71.
3 See e.g. T. Couser's account of disability narratives in T. G. Couser, *Recovering Bodies: Illness, Disability and Life Writing*, Madison, Wis., University of Wisconsin Press, 1997.
4 P. K. Longmore, 'Conspicuous Contribution and American Cultural Dilemmas: Telethon Rituals of Cleansing and Renewal', in D. T. Mitchell and S. L. Snyder (eds), *The Body and Physical Difference: Discourses of Disability*, Ann Arbor, Mich., University of Michigan Press, 1997, pp. 134–60.
5 Aristotle, *De Generatione Animalium*, trans. A. L. Peck, London, Heinemann, 1953, 728a 18; 737a 27.
6 J. B. Friedman, *The Monstrous Races in Medieval Art and Literature*, Cambridge, Mass., Harvard University Press, 1981, p. 179.
7 R. G. Thomson (ed.), *Freakery: Cultural Spectacles of the Extraordinary Body*, New York, New York University Press, 1997, p. xvii.
8 S. Wendell, *The Rejected Body: Feminist Philosophical Reflections on Disability*, New York, Routledge, 1996.
9 It is not that disability studies are non-existent, but rather that they are largely seen as the responsibility of academics who themselves have disabilities. As with feminist studies, their limited impact may in part reflect a certain self-policing of boundaries, of who is and who is not entitled to speak, teach or research, but that only serves to confirm the binary thinking at institutional level.
10 A. S. Dennett, 'The Dime Museum Freak Show Reconfigured as Talk Show', in Thomson, *Freakery*, pp. 315–26.
11 Longmore, 'Conspicuous Contribution and American Cultural Dilemmas'.
12 R. G. Thomson, *Extraordinary Bodies: Figuring Physical Disability in American Culture and Literature*, New York, Columbia University Press, 1997, p. 35.
13 *Natanson v. Kline*, 1960, 186 Kan. 393.
14 By paternalism I mean making decisions on behalf of others, or acting in their supposed interests, without their fully informed consent.
15 For examples, see M. Oliver, *Understanding Disability: From Theory to Practice*, London, Macmillan Press, 1996, and T. Shakespeare and N. Watson, 'Defending the Social Model', *Disability and Society*, 1997, vol. 12, pp. 293–300. The implication is that a 'real' self is frustrated by the attribution of an *improper* status.
16 R. E. Goodin, 'Vulnerabilities and Responsibilities: An Ethical Defence of the Welfare State', in G. Brock (ed.), *Necessary Goods*, Lanham, Md., Rowman and Littlefield, 1998, pp. 73–94.
17 M. Boler, 'The Risks of Empathy', *Cultural Studies*, 1997, vol. 11, pp. 253–73.
18 J. Butler, *Bodies that Matter. On the Discursive Limits of 'Sex'*, London, Routledge, 1993; C. Waldby, *AIDS and the Body Politic: Biomedicine and Sexual Difference*, London, Routledge, 1996; M. Shildrick and J. Price, 'Breaking the Boundaries of the Broken Body', *Body & Society*, 1996, vol. 2, pp. 93–113; J. Price and M. Shildrick, 'Uncertain Thoughts on the Dis/abled Body', in M. Shildrick and J. Price (eds), *Vital Signs: Feminist Reconfigurations of the Bio/logical Body*, Edinburgh, Edinburgh University Press, 1998, pp. 224–49.

19 M. Shildrick, *Leaky Bodies and Boundaries: Feminism, Postmodernism and (Bio)ethics*, London, Routledge, 1997.
20 J. Lacan, 'The Mirror Stage as Formative of the Function of the I', in *Ecrits*, trans. A. Sheridan, London, W. W. Norton, 1977, p. 4.
21 Kristeva, *Powers of Horror*, p. 71.
22 Ibid., p. 4.
23 Ibid.
24 Butler, *Bodies that Matter*.
25 G. C. Spivak, 'Introduction' to J. Derrida, *Of Grammatology*, Baltimore, Md., Johns Hopkins University Press, 1976, p. lxviii.
26 J. Derrida, *Positions*, trans. Alan Bass, London, Athlone Press, 1981, p. 33.
27 Shildrick, *Leaky Bodies*.
28 J. Derrida, 'Plato's Pharmacy', in *Dissemination*, trans. Barbara Johnson, Chicago, University of Chicago Press, 1981.
29 Kristeva, *Powers of Horror*.
30 Butler, *Bodies that Matter*, p. 3.
31 J. Derrida, *Limited Inc*, Evanston, Ill., Northwestern University Press, 1988, p. 62.
32 J. Butler, *Excitable Speech: A Politics of the Performative*, London, Routledge, 1997.
33 Derrida, *Limited Inc*, p. 59.
34 Ibid., p. 127.
35 M. Nussbaum, *The Fragility of Goodness: Luck and Ethics in Greek Tragedy and Philosophy*, Cambridge, Cambridge University Press, 1986, p. 86.
36 G. C. Spivak, *The Postcolonial Critic*, London, Routledge, 1990, p. 18.

8 A pig's tale

Porcine viruses and species boundaries

Marsha Rosengarten

The first pig's tale that I want to recount here is that of Babe, from the film of the same name.[1] At the centre of the narrative is a pig who, having been raised by a border collie sheep-dog, believes his task in life is to round up sheep for his 'boss', a farmer who has the capacity to recognise and value this identity shift in his pig. The play on species boundaries is signalled at the very outset when the pig first comes to the farmer's notice and the narrator, in voice over, states: 'Something passed between them: the faintest hint of a common destiny.' The predetermined events, signalled in a strangely ominous tone, rely strongly on an imaginative play with identity. It is a play not entirely dissimilar from what could be said of the making of another tale about pig destiny, a tale already under way in the realms of medical science and one in which the threat of contagion looms large. I am referring here to the practice of xenotransplantation, the use of animal organs and/or cells in place of human matter for transplantation.

There is one very poignant scene in *Babe* that captures, in a rather tangential way, the sort of stakes evident in the challenge to the species divide posed by xenotransplantation. The night before Babe is to perform alongside the farmer in an important sheep rounding up competition, the farm cat tells Babe that the other animals are laughing at him for behaving like a dog and, more importantly, for not knowing what he is really for. Babe enquires, 'What are any of us here for?' The cat begins to list the farm animals and their varying purposes including the cows for milking and herself for being beautiful and affectionate. Pigs, like ducks, are then claimed to have no purpose. But, soon after, she reworks her rejoinder and, in a catty sort of way, states: 'Animals that don't have a purpose actually have a noble purpose. They are for eating.' Babe is highly disturbed by this information. He returns to his 'mother' the border collie sheep-dog and asks if it is true that humans eat pigs. A series of affirmative responses by the sheep-dog confirm that this is true even of 'the boss', and that is what happened to Babe's 'real' mother, father, brothers and sisters. The scene is a truly confronting and appallingly distressing one for Babe, so cleverly characterised as the embodiment of innocence.

The anthropomorphising of Babe gives emphasis, in a rather saddening way, to the usual destiny of pigs that also makes possible their use as a source of replacement parts for human survival. But also pertinent in the scene that I have described is the suggestion that all creatures have their rightful place. As pigs and humans come to share a common destiny, in the sense that their matter becomes fused through new and developing medical technologies, the grounds of difference, on which the species divide is lived, may be brought into question. Assumptions of rightful place, contingent as they may be on what is imagined as human and non-human animal identity, may no longer hold. Participating in the making of this precariousness is the threat of contagion or, more accurately, what it is that we recognise as contagion. Although I have found it difficult to settle on a precise definition of contagion, it is most surely based on a presumption of at least two distinct bodies, in some way self-identical in themselves and different from each other (with the exception of blood, organs within the same body are rarely, if ever, understood to infect each other). Further, within the space that distinguishes the objects as different to each other, some movement of substance or influence from one to the other must occur.

Locating contagion

My interest in pigs, porcine viruses, and species boundaries, as a site of potential contagion, has evolved from prior work on the way in which organ transplantation, of the human to human kind, poses a challenge to the integrity of the imbricated human body and subject.[2] Here I shall review these challenges through the lens of contagion. The territory of intra-species transplantation provides fertile ground for thinking contagion at the inter-species divide, particularly as medical science moves to address the shortage of donor human organs and tissue through the use of non-human animal matter.[3] Prohibiting this move, however, is the fear of transferring a relatively ineffective virus across the animal/human species divide, possibly to induce all sorts of unknown and incurable disease effects at the level of a pandemic.[4] Since most of this interest is in the use of pigs, concern centres on the risk of contagion by endogenous porcine viruses transferred to human individuals who may then pass them on to others through the exchange of bodily fluids. While this risk has, to date, not been proven in scientific terms, it is, no doubt, already informed by current evidence that the human immunodeficiency virus (HIV) originated from primates.[5] Evidence of other viruses jumping the species barrier also contributes to speculation of potential contagion. Historically, influenza epidemics have been attributed to an avian virus crossing species boundaries. For instance, the 'bird flu' outbreak in Hong Kong in 1999 was traced to the virus A(H5N1) and is understood to have jumped directly from chickens to humans.

Throughout my inquiry, organ transplantation – human to human and animal to human – will be treated as an empirical set of medical practices constituted by, as well as constitutive of, a play of meanings in the imagination stakes of newly medicalised destinies. This will serve a twofold purpose. On the one hand, it will test an argument by Paul Rabinow that 'it is not the newness of contemporary technology that leaves us culturally unprepared. It is also the effacement of "the oldness" of so many of the background assumptions and practices that lurk unexamined at the edges in these cases which contextualise the technology and frame our questions and responses.'[6] On the other, it will enable an assessment of how these assumptions, which I understand as prior modes of conceptualising the who and what of humanness, might also be brought into question by the effects of contemporary medical technologies. This assessment has been framed bearing in mind recent criticism of cultural analyses of the body for their tendency, in effect, to occlude the question of matter. Here I shall place what is read from, as well as into, matter at the centre of my discussion. The empirical findings of medical intervention in the body will be examined for what they reveal of prior cultural assumptions. But they will also be considered for challenges they pose to these cultural assumptions and conceptions of embodiment.[7]

Underpinning the background assumptions and practices referred to by Rabinow, may well be a certain sort of thinking beyond which it is difficult to imagine. This is an argument made in the early work of Michel Foucault that provides a cue for an inquiry concerned with the role of contagion in a seemingly self-evident species divide. In the preface to the *Order of Things*, Foucault cites a taxonomy of animals, listed by Borges, from a Chinese encyclopaedia. The taxonomy includes 'tame', 'stray dogs', 'sirens', 'sucking pigs', 'embalmed', 'frenzied', 'fabulous', 'drawn with a very fine camel hair brush'. He says of it: 'In the wonderment of this taxonomy, the thing we apprehend in one great leap, the thing that, by means of the fable, is demonstrated as the exotic charm of another system of thought, is the limitation of our own, the stark impossibility of thinking *that*.' Nevertheless, he goes on to explain, the entities do have very precise meanings and a demonstrated content. They can all be included because each is contained by a category of its own. The containment by category, Foucault states, 'localises their power of contagion'. For, although some are real and some reside solely in the imagination, there is no confusing of the distinction.[8]

While Foucault's usage of contagion could be interpreted as referring to the passing on of symbolic meaning, my own approach here will endeavour to traverse the distinction between the symbolic, as in *influence* (including emotions), and that of physical disease.[9] In doing so, I shall seek to show how troublesome and limiting an insistence on this distinction may be. I have no intention of denying that disease occurs outside the symbolic, nor do I want to imply that its presence is knowable without the ascribing of meaning. The distinction relies on a fallacy that the real or the material is available outside the effects of the modes of comprehension. To put this another way, it presumes that materiality has been able and continues to escape the contagious effects of our thinking. As many writers have now shown, despite a sense of self-evidency that we might have about the matter of our human form, this knowledge and at least some of our experience of embodiment, may be brought into question as an effect of culture.[10] Donna Haraway, taking a lead from the almost canonic claim of the French feminist Simone de Beauvoir, states, 'bodies are not born but made'. For Haraway 'biological bodies emerge at the intersection of biological research, writing and publishing; medical and other business practices; cultural productions of all kinds, including available metaphors and narratives; and technology'.[11] It is this type of argument that underpins Judith Butler's claim that the body is not 'an independent materiality that is invested with power relations external to it, but is that for which materialisation and investiture are coextensive'.[12] This latter point gives emphasis to the differential designating of objects that takes place in the making of their intelligibility.

Contagious effects

In the following section I shall outline some of the effects of organ transplantation. While there is a considerable array of bioethical issues arising in response to transplantation,[13] my focus will be oriented towards those areas that highlight the potential operations of contagion. The two areas of challenge that I shall focus on are, in medical terms, organ or tissue rejection and, in relation to human-to-human transplantation, psychological difficulty with integrating the new organ or tissue.

The sub-discipline of immunology features strongly in the problem of what is understood as physiological rejection. One of the concepts most frequently used to describe the human immune system is that of 'self' as opposed to 'non-self' or 'foreign'.[14] The 'self' at the centre of immunological description is often spoken of as an entity actively defending its boundaries against foreign invasion, the body's natural defence against contagion. It is figured as a central player within a scenario described through metaphors of military warfare and the complex operation of high tech surveillance systems. As Catherine Waldby argues, this engagement of cultural concepts and metaphors in biomedical representations of the real, 'makes the real mean [sic] in particular ways'.[15] Waldby's approach, following that of Haraway and to some extent Butler's, situates biomedicine within, rather than alongside or as superior to, the cultural definition of what is understood to constitute human identity. This type of textual reading of the productive workings of medical science makes evident the way in which materiality is represented through prior concepts, since the very notion of re-presentation no longer holds. Moreover, it highlights the way in which cultural concepts infiltrate the imaginary endeavours of those struggling to come to grips with what is already determined as 'the immune system'. By doing so, it reveals the ways through which meaning makes the material knowable.[16] The empirical material of medicine, however, provides for a further claim. In the following discussion, of both the science and the experiential of organ transplantation, it will become evident that cultural concepts not only inform or inscribe bodily identity. Cultural concepts also come unstuck as the matter to which they are presumed to represent (the referent) is revealed as different.

To illustrate what I mean here by culture coming unstuck in light of the newly evident, yet still culturally inscribed, empirical of medical science, I want to turn briefly to the site of bone marrow transplantation, the source of red blood cell generation. In other instances of transplantation it is the host that potentially may, in the language style of immunology, identify and attack the donated foreign matter. In bone marrow transplantation it is the donated matter that rejects the host.[17] This places the transplant recipient at risk of attack and likely death rather than the organ/tissue. Bone marrow, unlike other forms of transplantation, suggests the 'self' of immunological language is located in the donor rather than the host. The shift of 'self' through bone marrow transplantation also hypothetically shifts the source of threat of contagion. In a different manner, a challenge to, or contagion of, sexed identity might also be read from the bone marrow scenario. Since the red blood cells produced from the transplanted cells carry the genetic identity of the donor, the recipient's sexual identity may not be consistent with his or her blood.[18] This inclusion of sex-determining chromosomes from another 'self', within a host body, may not pose a challenge to sexual identity in the knowledge framework of biology. Nor is the presence of a second set of sex-determining chromosomes a threat to viability in the more nuanced framework of biogenetics and immunology. Nevertheless, the outcome of DNA testing on the host's blood would offer a different 'truth' of identity to that of other tissue taken from the same body.

Psychiatric literature in this area provides highly provocative accounts of how organ transplantation challenges the way in which the internal space of the body is identified. It also shows how the body may become differentiated according to existing or, as Rabinow might say, 'older' cultural notions of identity. According to Dubovsky et al., 'difficulties with the internalization process have been said to result primarily from an inability to identify with the donor and to imbue the transplant (and by extension, the donor) with the qualities of a positive or benevolent introject, which can be successfully integrated with existing introjects'.[19] Integration, it seems, requires a gradual process of psychological internalisation whereby the patient comes to view the implanted organ as part of his or her self rather than as a 'foreign body'.[20] In addition to the concept of self, or assisting in the inscribing of 'foreignness', are the concepts of sexual and racial difference. In one case documented by Dubovsky *et al.*, it was stated: 'A black man who distrusted whites fantasized that he had received a kidney transplant donated by a white woman and was afraid the organ hated him and would reject him.'[21] Included in the same article is a discussion that suggests gendered notions of a new organ may be a causal factor in cases where males, upon receipt of a kidney from a female donor, experience impotence. The gendering of organs is, possibly, also facilitated by surgeons who have been found to refer, on occasion, to an organ as 'she' or 'he' based on knowledge of the donor's gender. However, the most striking rupture to identity, which I have found within this literature, is the case of a Ku Klux Klan Grand Dragon who, as Owen S. Surman reports, 'joined the National Association for the Advancement of Colored People after learning that his new kidney came from the cadaver of a black person'.[22]

Although the above case study accounts may appear extreme, the use of cultural concepts, such as sexuality and race as identifiers, is not unlike immunological sense-making. The psychiatric material can be read as evidence of a type of sense-making in the context of an experience understood to involve the insertion or grafting of something other, or different, into a space culturally inscribed as an individual self. If, as the above accounts show, the donated matter is inscribed as non-self, it can challenge an individual's sense of self-sameness. In other words, at some level there is the potential here for an experiential sense of contagion if the latter is understood as an alteration to what has come before and an alteration that involves the inclusion of something from an 'other'. Contagion could be argued to occur because of change produced in what is already understood as a distinct host. As a result of the inclusion of matter from an other, the host might no longer be considered the same. The experiential outcomes are contingent, however, on a prior sense of self – unified or otherwise – as well as a variety of ways of identifying one's self against another self. They also appear to be structured according to a mind/body split as are, not surprisingly, the psychiatric analyses of the accounts.

Clare Sylvia, in her autobiographical account of being a heart recipient, cites a range of experiences by organ recipients, including her own, which indicate a changed self revealed in dietary and clothing preferences as well as memory. The changes are reported to bear close resemblance to aspects of the deceased donor, of which the recipient had no socially obtained knowledge. For instance, Sylvia says she took to eating chicken nuggets and drinking beer after receiving a new heart. These were things she then found her donor used to do. She also cites the case of a heart transplant recipient who found he was bothered by the clicking sound of the windscreen wipers on his car. He learnt later that his heart had come from a man who had been killed in a car accident. The deceased donor had been driving on a rainy night with his girlfriend in the car. The two had an argument after which they drove in silence with, according to the girlfriend, only the sound of the windscreen wipers until the accident. While the anecdotes are not unlike the stuff of science fiction and are certainly reminiscent of urban myth, the book provides quotes by members of the scientific community seeking to explain the experiences through reference to the notion of cellular memory.[23] If the accounts are taken at face value, or at least not dismissed for failing to fit an existing order of thinking, such as a mind/body split, they could be read as suggestive of a type of carrying over of qualities that exceeds the usual bounds of what is understood to be at risk in a medicalised context of contagion.

Organ transplantation may assist with quality and longevity of life. But, by incurring a profound rupture to the integrity of the imbricated human subject and body, it also produces new questions about the very basis of what and how we know. Importantly, in light of Rabinow's argument, there is considerable evidence here to suggest that increasing medical alterations to the human body pose a challenge to the very concepts and presuppositions on which medical intervention depends. The medical and psychological ruptures, outlined above, point to the way in which current notions of identity may falter within the very space that has historically given legitimacy and authority to such concepts.

Humanising pigs

In this section I shall outline some of the key issues now under debate in relation to the practice of xenotransplantation, particularly as attention has turned to the use of pigs. Initially there was considerable interest in non-human primates. This was because non-human primates are regarded as more similar to humans. After all, they are of the same order in a taxonomy of animate creatures. And, in keeping with this classification, their intra order-based resemblance is understood to pose less risk of severe rejection by a human host's immune system than non-primate animals, those that fall into a broader system of classification.[24] Nevertheless, the 'same order' classification has not turned out to be a necessarily favourable factor for transplant suitability. It is possible that the similarity or immunocompatibility of non-human primates may increase the risk of contagion.[25] But it is not the risk of contagion that rules out their use as replacement parts for humans. It is another apparent similarity that makes primates ethically unacceptable for transplant purposes. This similarity is read from their capacity to exhibit human type character traits, as illustrated in the UK Advisory Group on the Ethics of Xenotransplantation ruling that primates cannot be used for transplant purposes because they 'would be exposed to too much suffering'.[26]

Since pigs, in contrast to primates and as the cat points out, are already bred for the explicit purpose of slaughter and human consumption, they are more ethically acceptable within a classificatory system that organises suffering according to a western anthropocentric system. Their ignoble purpose – as fit for eating – also means they are in ready supply. Important, though, is what one medical journal article notes as 'a remarkable anatomical and physiological similarity between pig and human organs', a point I shall return to.[27] But the use of pigs poses its own problems. Porcine organs are rejected by a process called hyperacute rejection (HAR) that may occur within minutes after transplantation. According to Dorling *et al.*, this response is the hallmark of rejection in discordant species combinations. Interestingly, while on its own HAR provides strong evidence to support existing species classification systems, it is not necessarily absent from concordant species combining. By concordant species, I understand they are referring to creatures, such as primates, who are understood as higher up the evolutionary scale (and therefore close to humans) than creatures who make up the broader category 'mammals'. For instance, baboon organs transplanted into human beings will be hyperacutely rejected if unmatched for blood group, even though they are technically concordant species. Furthermore, different organs show differing degrees of susceptibility to HAR, with livers and lungs being relatively resistant.[28] Rejection cannot, therefore, be taken as the absolute or essential grounds for a taxonomy, informally termed the species distinction.

It is in efforts to prevent HAR that contagion becomes a critical issue. If a virus, even a relatively harmless one, is present in the source species, it may have a greater chance of survival, replication and destruction, when transplanted or grafted into a therapeutically suppressed immune system.[29] This risk of contagion through transmission of a virus across the species boundary, has been suggested as the inverse of immunisation. Whereas immunisation is intended to protect the population at the risk of the occasional individual adverse reaction, xenotransplantation offers the potential benefit to the individual while putting the population at risk.[30] Bach *et al.*, state that the clinical practice of xenotransplantation may therefore require not just the surveillance of patients/recipients as possible sites of contagion, but also those with whom they are in close proximity. Further, although perhaps of a lesser concern, there is the possibility that the development of a new infectious agent with altered pathogenicity arising within the xenograft recipient may represent a danger to the pig population.[31]

To counter the risk of rejection, the source matter may be genetically altered.[32] The UK advisory committee cited earlier, recommends that the use of pigs as sources of tissue is ethically acceptable providing appropriate conditions of animal welfare are met.[33] Transgenic (genetically altered) pigs are said to be acceptable sources providing 'the pig neither suffers unduly nor ceases recognisably to be a pig'.[34] An almost 'tongue-in-cheek' response to this decision is provided in the editorial of the journal in which the discussion on bioethics is reported. The proviso on use of transgenic pigs, the editorial claims, suggests the surreal prospect of the head of the committee, an archbishop and his authority given by

God, determining when a transgenic pig is still a pig.[35] Interesting in this debate, and highlighted by the editorial, is the presumption of a core identity that must be preserved. It is a stance mounted, not in response to a fear of contagious disease, but in response to altering the very order of species-being and differentiation. It is not surprising that the grounds on which the restriction is to be imposed remain unclear and very much open to interpretation. For the very notion of a pig is contingent not on empiricist observation but, rather, on the way in which the matter of this creature is understood and essentialised as 'a pig'. Before elaborating this point, I want briefly to address what I would argue is the relational notion of risk of contagion as it, too, is contingent on what is understood to be 'a pig'.

Despite the obvious ethical challenges posed by the genetic alteration of pigs, the latter should not be confused here with a strategy of preventing contagion. All vertebrates, including humans, contain thousands of retroviral elements. And, while most of the elements seem defective, some, including proviruses present in mice, cats, and chickens, can give rise to infectious retroviruses. In pigs these viruses are widely distributed in different breeds and expressed in different tissues, including spleen, kidney, and heart.[36] Because of the way retroviral elements are inherited in pigs, they will be virtually impossible to eliminate from source herds.[37] Further there is evidence of porcine viruses developing in vitro. To date, in-vitro replication of two pig retroviruses, PERV A and PERV B, has taken place in certain human cell lines. But there is still no guarantee that viral transmission from pigs to humans would occur in a transplantation and, if so, whether it would result in a pandemic. The in-vitro situation is not an exact replication of the conditions found in vivo. Porcine viruses may be able to develop in a petri dish in the absence of a human immune system. But they might not survive within a human body in which the immune system is understood to attack and eliminate 'foreign' matter.[38]

Mythical creatures or modern chimeras

Underpinning the concerns arising in relation to transplantation is the difference between same and other. There is one particular instance of the use of pig matter that may provide a clue as to how same and other might be thought differently, or reworked to suggest something beyond a clearly bounded distinction between (in)compatible matter. Insulin dependent diabetes is understood to be a disease of the autoimmune system. The body is understood to kill off its own pancreatic cells needed for producing insulin. Foetal pig pancreatic cells are suitable replacements, in the first instance, because the anatomical similarity of pigs and humans, in contrast to cows for instance, includes a very similar digestive system. And, in contrast with organs from mice or chickens, pig organs are much larger and therefore afford a greater number of cells. In the second instance, and crucial to the success of using foetal pig cells, with limited pharmacological immunosuppression, they are not recognised by the human body's immune system as same or different, either of which leads to their being killed off, even by an immunosuppressed system. In this space of seeming non-recognition, they are able to develop into and then survive as insulin-producing cells. Further, as yet no evidence of infection with porcine endogenous retrovirus has been found. One study of ten immunosuppressed recipients of porcine islet-ell xenografts, found no signs of infection four to seven years after the transplant.[39]

The possibilities promised by the foetal pig cell grafting appears, in part, to arise from their inability to be organised according to the categories of same and other, self and non-self, or even what might be assumed to constitute the species divide, if we are to rely on immunology. It is the outcome of something taking place that cannot be explained according to a simple same/other binary based on a species divide. For in the clinical context of insulin dependent diabetes, the space of same is already differentiated and acted upon, within, as other. In a conceptually similar manner, in the human-to-human bone marrow transplant scenario, human foetal cells have also been found to evade an assumed human defence system. Cord blood, blood cells extracted from the umbilical cord, requires less matching than bone marrow for transplantation. This is explained by the notion that cord cells are immunologically naive. They have not acquired the array of antigens on their surface that makes them identifiable as foreign and dangerous.[40] Both sets of foetal cells – pig and human – appear to be less differentiated than cells with a longer history. While I am wary of slipping into an acceptance of a symbolic/material distinction, I do find it fascinating that there is a coming together here of the two. Moreover, in this coming together, it seems that a Foucauldian analysis, committed to recognising the workings of history on the body, is borne out in the empirical domain.

The possibility that we 'humans' might be threatened by a retrovirus transferred through xenotransplantation or xenografting brings into relief some of the presuppositions on which we base the species boundary of human/animal. It also brings into relief how the perceived risk of contagion may be one of the mainstays of differentiating species as well as differentiating within species. What may be overlooked in this act of differentiation is, however, the historical nature of matter as much as the historical nature of its intelligibility.

In a discussion on the Human Genome Project, Rabinow points out that the genomes of non-human organisms provide model systems for mapping because most genes are found across species.[41] For Waldby, this potential for another species to stand in for humans constitutes a tacit acknowledgment that 'all organisms are open systems which engage in transversal and intraspecies genetic exchanges as well as filial, species-specific genetic lineages'. Her observation is based on an argument made by Keith Ansell Pearson that biology has resisted acknowledging that the evolution of species has taken place through viral cross-infection and other kinds of non-sexual, trans-species forms of genetic exchange. Evidence of this exchange challenges the more orthodox notion that organisms are discrete genetic entities.[42]

Making pig's tales

The story of a newly medicalised pig, soon to become incorporated within human flesh, in contrast to the lesser purpose of food for consumption, is, like *Babe*, a product of a western imaginary. It has been developed with the aid of taxonomy, immunology, and even psychology, with the effect of now posing a fabulously complex and fraught medical tale. Without the aid of these knowledges that differentiate pigs from primates, the story might be very different. Research on attitudes to the use of pigs for transplant purposes reflects something of the way pigs are culturally invested as low-level creatures and an anxiety about the sort of characteristics that might be passed on through their incorporation in the space of a previously fully 'human body'. A study of one hundred transplant recipients found twenty-four thought a xenograft would change their appearance, personality, or eating or sexual habits.[43] Another surveyed 113 patients awaiting or having received an organ transplant on the question of transplantation. All were generally supportive of cadaveric organ donation; most were prepared to accept an organ from a living donor. However, only 48 per cent believed it appropriate to breed animals to provide organs and only 42 per cent were prepared to accept an animal organ.[44]

The decision about the use of pigs for human part replacement is a difficult one and may require consideration of issues outside those raised by medical and associated ethical debates. These notwithstanding, it is also worth reflecting on whether the assessment of risk of contagion is shaped, in some way, by the way in which pigs are already a product of an anthropocentric differential designation of difference. Stallybrass and White, in *The Politics and Poetics of Transgression*, point out that pig-loathing is in no sense a cultural given, there are cultures where pigs are celebrated. Within Papua New Guinea, for instance, one anthropological study reports that pigs are treated as members of the family. Piglets are petted, talked to, and fed choice morsels. Moreover, 'the climax of pig love is the incorporation of the pig as flesh into the flesh of the human host and of the pig as spirit into the spirit of the ancestors'.[45] Consumption is, it seems, the ultimate embracing of this valued creature.

The outcomes of medical research as well as psychological responses to organ transplantation are influenced or infected by prior cultural modes of inscription. If, therefore, immunology relies on existing concepts of identity (for example, a unified self, foreign or non-self, gendered self and metaphors of military warfare), it is not unrealistic to question the meaning making of pigs as an activity that contributes to, as well as now being effected by, research. Nor, given the way in which transplant recipients may make sense of the identity of their medically acquired organ, is it unlikely that cultural notions of pigs will have some significance; rather, we should expect this. To put this another way, if pigs were not an object of scorn, as illustrated in references to police, chauvinists and fascists as pigs, would this produce a very different set of attitudes? And, in turn, would this different set of attitudes be reflected in a differently shaped medical tale? Further, would it give rise to a different sort of experiential effect of living with a transplanted graft or organ?

The rupturing of identity concepts within the space of organ transplantation reveals the precariousness of our understanding of humanness. What may be presumed self-same, as opposed to other-different, is not only specific to particular knowledges of the body, it gives rise to specific understandings of contagion as an effect of these knowledges and the empirical evidence they yield. This is not to deny that there is much that can be established about the risk of contagion across what is construed as a species boundary between human and pig. It is, however, to recognise that there is a need to think beyond the confines of a distinction that assumes the matter of species being is outside or not already contaminated by prior cultural concepts. Further, as I have shown, the possibility for making such a recognition is already well evident within the very field of their legitimacy. Paradoxically, science is the very area that has, since the Enlightenment, been assumed to provide the stable ground for what it is that we can know. Yet, in the story of pigs, porcine viruses, and species boundaries, there is a vast amount of matter that provides highly provocative material for bringing such presumptions into question and thus provides a valuable source material for thinking differently.

Notes

This essay has benefited from discussions with Carla Drago, Kane Race, Gary Smith, Elizabeth Wilson and Catherine Waldby. I would also like to thank Sue Kippax, Director of the National Centre in HIV Social Research for granting me the time to write it.

1 The film *Babe* was directed by George Miller in 1995. It was based on the book *The Sheep-Pig* by Dick King-Smith.
2 M. Rosengarten, 'Transmigrating Organs: Gilguls, Politics and Medical Intervention in the Israel/Palestine Divide', in J. Docker and G. Fischer (eds), *Adventures of Identity: Constructing Multicultural Identities*, Tübingen, Stauffenburg Verlag, forthcoming.
3 Unless otherwise indicated, the term species is used here in a colloquial/ informal sense. This is the usage illustrated in the medical literature cited here.
4 A. Dorling, K. Riesbeck, A. Warrens and R. Lechler, 'Clinical Xenotransplantation of Solid Organs', *The Lancet*, 1997, vol. 349, pp. 867–71.
5 HIV-I has, for some time, been thought to come from primates. There is now strong evidence that it came from a sub-species of chimpanzee in Africa in

180 *Marsha Rosengarten*

which it has no serious effects. See C. Yang, B. C. Dash, F. Simon, G. Van der Groen, D. Pieniazek, F. Gao, B. H. Hahn and R. B. Lal, 'Detection of Diverse Variants of HIV-1 Groups M, N, and O and Simian Immunodeficiency Viruses from Chimpanzees Using Generic *pol* and *env* Primer Pairs', paper presented at '7th Conference on Retroviruses and Opportunistic Infections', sponsored by the Foundation for Retrovirology and Human Health, 30 Jan.–2 Feb. 2000.

6 P. Rabinow, 'Severing the Rites: Fragmentation and Dignity in Late Modernity', *Knowledge and Society: The Anthropology of Science and Technology*, 1992, vol. 9, pp. 169–87 at 170.

7 Elizabeth Wilson states that a determination by feminist work to refute biological reductionism has had the effect of excluding the biological from consideration altogether. See E. Wilson, 'Somatic Compliance – Feminism, Biology and Science', *Australian Feminist Studies*, 1999, vol. 14, no. 29, pp. 7–18, p. 8. A similar concern is expressed by Katherine Hayles about the erasure of embodiment in work on the posthuman as a result of treating human beings as mere inscriptions. This erasure of embodiment is also identified as a problem in liberal humanism. According to liberalism, the subject is understood to possess a body rather than being a body. See K. Hayles, 'The Posthuman Body: Inscription and Incorporation in Galatea 2.2 and Snow Crash', *Configurations*, 1997, no. 5, pp. 241–66.

8 M. Foucault, *The Order of Things*, London and New York, Routledge, 1974, p. xv.

9 The *Oxford Shorter English Dictionary* gives an account of both and allows for the former to take a good or neutral sense.

10 I am using 'knowledge' here in the restricted sense of acquired through a conscious process and not in the possibly also appropriate sense of affects. While I would not exclude affects from a consideration of the effects of transplantation, it will not be covered in the scope of this essay.

11 D. Haraway, 'The Biopolitics of Postmodern Bodies: Determinations of Self in Immune System Discourse', *Differences*, 1989, vol. 1, Winter, pp. 3–42, at 12.

12 J. Butler, *Bodies That Matter*, London and New York, Routledge, 1993, p. 35.

13 For a summary of these see L. Sharp 'Organ Transplantation as a Transformative Experience: Anthropological Insights into the Restructuring of the Self', *Medical Anthropology Quarterly*, 1995, vol. 9, pp. 357–89.

14 See e.g. A. I. Tauber, 'The Immune Self: Theory or Metaphor?' *Immunology Today*, 1994, vol. 15, pp. 134–6.

15 C. Waldby, *AIDS and the Body Politic*, London and New York, Routledge, 1996.

16 Dr Polly Matzinger, immunologist with the US National Institutes of Health, in an interview on 'The Health Report', ABC Radio National, 15 Dec. 1997, made the claim that understandings of the immune system are locked in an old mindset. In place of a model based on a discrimination of self and non-self, she proposes a system that defines things that do damage: 'it's a conversation between every tissue. Where tissues find themselves with the damage activate [*sic*] the local presenting cells of the immune system, that's what starts an immune response.'

17 There are numerous articles discussing the issues raised by graft versus host disease in medical science journals. W. D. Shlomchik, M. S Couzens, C. Bi Tang, J. McNiff, M. E. Robert, J. Liu, M. J. Shlomchhik and S. G Emerson, 'Prevention of Graft Versus Host Disease by Inactivation of Host-Antigen-Presenting Cells', *Science*, 1999, vol. 285, pp. 412–15, state: 'Graft versus host disease, an alloimmune attack on host tissues mounted by donor T cells, is the most important toxicity of allogeneic bone marrow transplantation. The mechanism by which allogeneic T cells are initially stimulated is unknown', p. 412.

18 M. J. van Toh, R. Langlois van den Bergh, W. Mersker, M. C. Ouwerkerk-van Velzen, J. M. Vossen and H. J. Tanke, 'Simultaneous Detection of X and Y Chromosomes by Two-Colour Fluorescence in situ Hybridization in Combination with Immunophenotyping of Single Cells to Document Chimaerism after Sex-Mismatched Bone Marrow Transplantation', in *Bone Marrow Transplantation*, 1998, vol. 21, pp. 497–503.
19 S. L. Dubovsky, J. L. Metzner and R. B. Warner, 'Problems with Internalisation of a Transplanted Liver', *American Journal of Psychiatry*, 1979, vol. 36, pp. 1090–1.
20 Ibid.
21 Ibid.
22 O. S. Surman, 'Psychiatric Aspects of Organ Transplantation', *American Journal of Psychiatry*, 1989, vol. 146, pp. 972–82.
23 C. Sylvia and W. Novak, *A Change of Heart*, London, Little Brown, 1997, see pp. 217–18.
24 A. Dorling et al., 'Clinical Xenotransplantation'.
25 F. H. Bach, J. A. Fishman, N. Daniels, J. Proimos, B. Anderson, C. B. Carpenter, L. Forrow, S. C. Robson and H. V. Fineberg, 'Uncertainty in Xenotransplantation: Individual Benefit Versus Collective Risk', *Nature Medicine*, 1998, vol. 4, pp. 141–4 at 141.
26 Editorial, *The Lancet*, 1997, vol. 349, p. 219.
27 C. Groth, 'The Viral Issue' [Review 1998: Xenotransplantation] *The Lancet*, 1998, vol. 352, suppl. IV, p. 26SIV.
28 The term used to describe the immune system response is hyperacute rejection. 'The pathology of hyperacutely rejected organs is typical of vascular rejection, the prominent features being haemorrhage, oedema, and infarction of interstitial tissues, with thrombosis of xenogeneic vessels.' See Dorling et al., 'Clinical Xenotransplantation'.
29 Organ recipients are given immunosuppressant drugs to prevent organ rejection.
30 F. H. Bach et al., 'Uncertainty in Xenotransplantation'.
31 Ibid.
32 Genetic altering would aim to produce a pig that is homozygous for a human complement regulatory factor gene (decay-accelerating factor or membrane cofactor protein). See K. Morris 'No Early Rejection of Animal Organs in UK', *The Lancet*, 1997, vol. 349, p. 257. Pig hearts 'humanised' in this way by UK biotechnology group, Imutran, have been transplanted into monkeys without development of HAR.
33 Ibid.
34 Ibid.
35 Editorial, *The Lancet*, 1997, vol. 349, p. 219.
36 C. Patience, Y. Takeuchi and R. A. Weiss, 'Infection of Human Cells by an Endogenous Retrovirus of Pigs', *Nature Medicine*, 1997, vol. 3, pp. 282–6.
37 J. D. Boeke and J. P. Stoye, 'Retrotransposons, Endogenous Retroviruses, and the Evolution of Retroelements', in J. M. Coffin, S. H. Hughes and H. E. Varmus (eds) *Retroviruses*, Cold Spring Harbor, NY, Cold Spring Harbor Press, 1997, pp. 343–435.
38 U. Martin, V. Kiessig, A. Haverich, T. Herden, G. Steinhoff, J. H. Blusch and K. von der Helm, 'Expression of Pig Endogenous Retrovirus by Primary Porcine Endothelial Cells and Infection of Human Cells', *The Lancet*, 1998, vol. 352, pp. 692–4.
39 W. Heneine, A. Tibell, W. M. Switzer, P. Sandstrom, G. V. Rosales, A. Mathews, O. Korsgren, L. E. Chapman, M. Thomas and C. G. Groth, 'No Evidence of Infection with Porcine Endogenous Retrovirus in Recipients of Porcine Islet-Cell Xenografts', *The Lancet*, 1998, vol. 352, pp. 695–9.

40 For a medical scientific account of the benefits of cord blood see: E. Gluckman, V. Rocha and C. Chastang, 'Cord Blood Stem Cell Transplantation', *Baillieres Clinical Haematology*, 1999, vol. 12, pp. 279–92.
41 P. Rabinow, 'Artificiality and Enlightenment: From Sociobiology to Biosociality', *Essays on the Anthropology of Reason*, Princeton, NJ, Princeton University Press, 1996, pp. 97, 98.
42 K. A. Pearson, cited in C. Waldby, *The Visible Human Project: Informatic Bodies and Posthuman Medicine*, New York and London, Routledge, 2000.
43 K. L. Coffman, L. Sher, A. Hoffman, S. Rojter, P. Folk, D. V. Cramer, J. Vierling, F. Villamel, L. Podesta, A. Demetriou and L. Makowka, 'Survey Result of Transplant Patients' Attitudes on Xenografting', *Psychosomatics*, 1998, vol. 39, pp. 379–83.
44 P. J. Mohacsi, J. F. Thompson, J. K. Nicholson and D. J. Tiller, 'Patients' Attitudes to Xenotransplantation', *Lancet*, 1997, vol. 349, p. 1031.
45 This last point is made by Rappaport cited in P. Stallybrass and A. White, *The Politics & Poetics of Transgression*, Ithaca, NY, Cornell University Press, 1986.

9 Taking the HIV test

Self-surveillance and the making of heterosexuality

Lisa Adkins

In analyses of the discursive and administrative techniques associated with HIV antibody testing, it is often suggested that such techniques may be understood as part of the general social drive to identify the homosexual.[1] But what such arguments tend to overlook is the ways in which HIV testing is increasingly being sought by heterosexuals. While Waldby, for example, has suggested that the techniques of testing figure the category of heterosexuality as immune in relation to HIV/AIDS,[2] others have suggested that representations of heterosexuals as at risk in relation to HIV transmission (for example, in health promotion campaigns) constitutes anxiety and fear amongst heterosexuals and has led to increases in heterosexual testing.[3] Both medical and social researchers have tended to define such heterosexual testing as 'low risk' testing, and it is sometimes understood in terms of boundary maintenance in regard to sexuality. For instance, Lupton *et al.* have suggested such testing often concerns 'a strong need to re-establish subjectivity in the face of their exposure to "contaminating" Others'.[4] However, in this chapter I suggest that heterosexual testing concerns not so much an anxious response to health promotion campaigns in which heterosexuals are represented as at risk in regard to HIV/AIDS, but rather a figuring of heterosexuality in terms of voluntary self-governance and self-control. In particular, I consider the ways testing makes available techniques of the self through which heterosexuality may be performed not only as immune from contagion, but also as self-regulating and 'responsibilised'. In this sense I suggest that heterosexual testing should not be understood as an issue of 'low-risk testing', but rather that testing figures the category of heterosexuality as low risk. Moreover, I suggest that testing makes self-reflexivity only fully available to the category of heterosexuality, and thus constitutes new self–other relations in regard to sexuality, in particular, hetero-reflexive selves and non-hetero, non-reflexive others.

Risk culture and reflexivity

A range of commentators have noted the increasing cultural significance of risk as an organising principle of contemporary life.[5] Beck, for example, has argued that we are currently in the midst of a transition from industrial to risk society. For Beck, risk society is post-traditional where social position and conflicts are defined not by a logic of the distribution of goods, but by the distribution of risks, hazards and insecurities which themselves have been produced by the successes of industrialism.[6] In risk society the threats produced by industrial society therefore predominate and there is an increasing identification, awareness and concern of and with risks. Indeed, risks are the axial principle of social organisation. But for Beck risk society is also understood to involve increasing reflexivity. First, risk society is reflexive since it involves a confrontation of industrial society with itself, where modernisation processes 'produce threats which call into question and eventually destroy the foundations of industrial society'.[7] Risk society is therefore understood to be constituted by industrial society turning back in on itself and reflecting on itself, where modernisation is confronted and undermined by its own limits and consequences. Second, in risk society reflexivity arises in the attempt to deal with contemporary risks, where risks make us aware of a new reflexive self-determination. In particular, the recognition of the unpredictability of threats 'necessitates self-reflection on the foundations of social cohesion and the examination of prevailing conventions and foundations of "rationality"'.[8] In risk society there is therefore a reflexive monitoring of risk, involving attempts at assessing, defining and regulating risks. However, such reflexivity is intensified by the ways in which in risk issues no one and everyone is an expert.

This proliferation of knowledges regarding risk and of 'risks' themselves means risk society is also one characterised by uncertainty, doubt and ambivalence. As the certainties of industrial society dissolve and people are expected to live with a broad variety of different global and personal risks they are therefore 'now expected to master ... "risky opportunities", without being able, owing to the complexity of modern society, to make the necessary decisions on a well-founded ... basis'.[9] This leads to a reflexive conduct of life, a planning of one's own biography, where the untying of individuals from the norms and expectations of industrial society compel people not only to create and invent their own certainties, forms of authority and regulation, but also to create and invent their own self-identities. In risk society the standard biography becomes a do-it-yourself, reflexive biography mediated by categories of risk. For Beck, self-reflexivity is therefore understood to be an *effect* of risk culture: a reflexive project of self-monitoring, self-regulation and self-building becomes a necessity because of the break up of old certainties (such as those of nation, class, status, gender, sexuality) in the move to risk culture.[10]

Surveillance, risk and reflexivity

While Beck's analysis of risk society focuses predominantly on environmental hazards in relation to the proliferation of risks, uncertainty and reflexivity, nevertheless a range of commentators have noted the ways in which more and more areas of social life are coming to be defined in terms of risk.[11] Higgs, for example, has considered the ways social and health policy is increasingly organised in terms of a logic of risk identification and risk assessment.[12] Here risk is defined not only as environmental, but also as the result of lifestyle choices made by individuals, a logic which results in health promotion strategies aimed at changing behaviours. Higgs points, for instance, to the ways in which a 'Salience of Lifestyle' index has come to be used as a diagnostic measure in Britain in the targeting of health promotion towards those most vulnerable to strokes. Using this measure individuals are categorised as 'lifestylist' or 'fatalist', where 'fatalists' are defined as less amenable to health promotion and therefore more at risk of strokes. Higgs notes that what is important in the adoption of such measures is that rather than a matter of government responsibility, the pursuit of public health comes to be defined as a matter of individual action, where primary responsibility is located with the individual who is expected to adopt certain lifestyle choices. An ideal of a choosing, self-monitoring, self-regulating, self-forming subject, who makes use of his/her own agency to govern his/her self is therefore being figured through and by social and health policy newly arranged in terms of risk.

This figuring of a self-reflexive subject in relation to risk is also at issue in Armstrong's influential analysis of the rise of surveillance medicine, a form of medicine which he suggests emerged from the early twentieth century onwards alongside the then hegemonic hospital medicine, but which is now dominant. Armstrong argues that one of the characteristics of surveillance medicine is its concern not with the ill patient (as was the case in hospital medicine) but with the surveillance of 'normal', healthy populations. A central feature of surveillance medicine is therefore the targeting and monitoring of everyone, a monitoring which takes place through techniques of testing, surveys and health promotion. Armstrong suggests the main expansion in such techniques occurred after the Second World War 'when an emphasis on comprehensive health care, and primary and community care, underpinned the deployment of explicit surveillance surveys such as screening and health promotion'.[13] But a further feature of surveillance medicine is that responsibility for surveillance is given to, and taken up by, populations themselves. In health promotion, for example,

> concerns with diet, exercise, stress, sex, etc. become the vehicles for encouraging the community to survey itself. The ultimate triumph of Surveillance Medicine would be its internalization by all the population.[14]

The techniques of surveillance medicine therefore involve the constitution of self-monitoring and self-regulating subjects in relation to health.

Armstrong argues further that the shift to this framework also involved a fundamental reordering of the spatialisation of illness. In hospital medicine a symptom was linked to the findings of a clinical examination (the signs) to indicate the presence of a hidden pathological lesion. In surveillance medicine however, the relations between symptom, sign and illness are reconfigured. Specifically, instead of working through a linkage based on surface and depth 'all become components in a more general arrangement of predictive factors'.[15] While in hospital medicine symptoms were understood to be produced by hidden lesions and were used to infer both the existence and nature of disease, in surveillance medicine symptom, sign and disease are reconfigured as contingent *risk factors*, which point to, but do not necessarily produce, future illness. Moreover, while in hospital medicine symptoms, signs and diseases were located in the body, in surveillance medicine risk factors concern any state or event from which a probability can be calculated. Surveillance medicine therefore,

> turns increasingly to an extracorporal space – often represented by the notion of lifestyle – to identify the precursors of future illness. Lack of exercise and a high fat diet therefore can be joined with angina, high blood cholesterol and diabetes as risk factors for heart disease.[16]

In surveillance medicine therefore 'the whole of the individual's life is subject to scrutiny for risky behaviours that might give rise to future health problems'.[17] Indeed so strong is this scrutinisation that surveillance medicine is understood by Armstrong to map a different form of identity: a new risk identity for the 'normal' and 'healthy'.

Surveillance medicine and HIV antibody testing

Armstrong's thesis regarding the rise of surveillance medicine as involving a new figuring of health in terms of risk and the creation of self-reflexive subjects has immediate purchase in relation to recent findings regarding HIV/AIDS. Analyses of HIV antibody testing, for example, suggest this diagnostic test may be understood as a technique of surveillance medicine involving as it does procedures of risk assessment, risk identification, (often) asymptomatic testing, and practices of subjection and subjectification. Indeed, Lupton has argued that discourses of health risk and diagnostic testing 'are highly interrelated' since the logic of testing involves the identification of those defined to be 'at risk'.[18] That is, testing involves the identification of those positioned as having a potential to develop a certain condition or disease, and an incitement of those defined to be at risk to test through a process of self-identification in relation to risk categories. In addition, if testing points to the potential of a future condition or disease, such knowledge will lead to appropriate forms of self-management and self-regulation in relation to health, including the self-disciplining of behaviour to ensure potential conditions or diseases are not passed on to others.

In a more extended analysis of the micro-politics of power involved in HIV antibody testing, Waldby expands on these themes. Along with other commentators she notes the ways in which HIV antibody testing represents a key technology in HIV policy for many 'first' world nations.[19] For example, Waldby argues that the general AIDS education strategy for Australia has 'involved asking every citizen to assess their own risk and decide accordingly whether to be tested'.[20] However, it is not only self-assessment and self-identification in relation to risk categories which Waldby shows to be at work in the techniques associated with HIV testing, for she also shows how HIV testing may also be understood as a technology of sex, as a 'constellation of administrative and discursive techniques whereby subjects are classified and socially ordered through a securing of a confession as to the "truth" of their sexuality'.[21] Thus Waldby describes the bio-administrative techniques involved in testing, including the taking of a blood sample, counselling, biochemical analysis of the sample, the reporting of results, and, if the test is positive, a confessional test for what she terms a transmission identity where,

> each seropositive subject is asked to provide a history of their sexuality, to review sexual practices for the probable 'mode of transmission' so that they can be positioned in the classificatory schemas of AIDS epidemiology as a transmission type, for instance homosexual, (male) bisexual or heterosexual transmission, and so on.[22]

The techniques and procedures of HIV testing which oblige subjects to 'know themselves as sexual identities and to make themselves available for sexual identification'[23] therefore not only work to position the virus in the particular body, to mark the positively tested with a sign of seropositivity, but also to mark the positively tested with a sign of a sexual 'transmission category', 'type', or identity. Indeed in this way Waldby argues that HIV testing is best understood as a technology through which the virus is *personified*, as diagnosing a type of person who is seropositive, a type of person who is often defined in terms of categories of sexual identity.[24]

Waldby also shows how such forms of marking render subjects visible within technologies of socio-medical surveillance into which they are inserted. For example, a positive result both makes the tested person visible in relation to public health surveillance, and inserts them into regimes of medical management, which may include in- and out-patient hospital services, regular monitoring, referrals to counsellors and invitations to volunteer for clinical trials and epidemiological cohort studies. Such forms of administration and regulation concern not just subjection but subjectification since they attempt 'to induce the internalisation of the self as dangerous, as infected, and hence to precipitate a new ethics of sexual practice and institutional deportment for the seropositive person'.[25] Thus the medical management of seropositivity involves both an incitement towards a permanent state of self-examination and self-regulation and an obligation to adopt disciplined sexual practices oriented towards the protection of others. In these ways Waldby suggests HIV testing must also be understood as a technology of the self, since testing 'not only compels subjects in certain ways but ... also induces the internalisation of new norms of identity and self-management, above all the management of one's health and one's sexual practices, in the interest of minimising illness and HIV transmission'.[26] But the administrative and discursive techniques of HIV testing make self-monitoring, self-regulation and 'responsibilisation' not just desirable but *obligatory* for the seropositive, and in these ways Waldby argues that HIV testing has severe implications for particular subjects.

In this account of HIV testing the self-monitoring, self-assessing subject central to Armstrong's analysis of surveillance medicine is highly visible. So too is the scrutiny of 'the whole of the individual's life' for 'risky' behaviours evidenced, for instance, in the 'confessional' elements of testing. Also apparent is the invention of new categories of risk identity which Armstrong suggests is a further feature of surveillance medicine. But, as Waldby shows through her analysis of HIV testing as a technology of sex, the risk, exposure or transmission identities constituted through testing are defined predominantly in terms of sexuality. And she goes on to show, as indeed have others both in relation to testing and in relation to epidemiological, public health and health education discourses on HIV/AIDS more generally, that risk is defined not only in terms of sexual identity, but also that sexual identities are ordered hierarchically, with gay and bisexual men defined as high risk and heterosexuals as low risk.[27] Thus in terms of health education strategies which ask every citizen to assess their own risk and to decide whether or not to be tested, this hierarchicisation of sexual identities in relation to risk means,

> the demand for risk assessment is far more rigorous for certain groups than it is for others depending on what position their self-identified categories occupy in the hierarchy of infectiousness determined by epidemiology ... This category position will further determine the extent to which they are actively medicalised, sought out or 'targeted' by programmes designed to encourage testing.[28]

This has amounted, Waldby suggests, to a strong sense of obligation to be tested for gay-identified men (as well as for pregnant women).[29] Indeed, she suggests that the classificatory logic of the discursive and administrative techniques of testing is so powerful that it 'resembles the general social drive to identify the "homosexual" '.[30] This identificatory view of testing – as a drive to identify the 'homosexual' – is also supported by Treichler, who has argued that the ongoing fascination and fixation with HIV testing concerns an anxiety to put a stop to gay men's successful passing as straight. Indeed she argues that so strong is the identificatory logic of testing for gay-identified men, refusing to take the HIV test is culturally analogous to pleading the United States' Fifth Amendment, that is, exercising the constitutional right of refusing to answer questions in order to avoid incriminating oneself.[31]

The universalisation of HIV/AIDS risk: the 'responsibilisation' of heterosexuality

Despite the significance of such analyses, it is important to recognise that the discursive and administrative techniques of testing should not be read as entirely determinate of identity. In his study of the ways the identities of people with HIV/AIDS living in Britain are formed and shaped, Heaphy stresses that 'while people with AIDS/HIV are, in some senses, subject to dominant medico-moral and medico-scientific discourses on AIDS and HIV, they do draw on counter-discourses in making personal sense of the virus and syndrome, and do not accept dominant meanings uncritically'.[32] He examines the ways in which medical and other dominant knowledges on HIV/AIDS are mediated in various ways through, for example, the gay press, self-help groups and alternative medical manuals. Heaphy goes on to argue that the meaning of HIV/AIDS must therefore be understood as negotiated, and that people living with HIV/AIDS play an active role in the creation of their own identities. Similarly Bartos argues that while AIDS policy in Australia may be understood in terms of a framework of governmentality – where populations are rendered calculable in terms of risk and where success is measured in terms of the adoption of governmental objectives by the targets of government themselves – there are important sources of disruption of the governmentalisation of HIV/AIDS, sources which he terms 'the queer underside of government'.[33] He looks at the ways in which people living with and against HIV work to defy governmentalisation; for example gay-identified men who have expert knowledge about safe-sex practices may practise unprotected sex as a way of resisting governmentalisation, especially the tyranny of identification associated with AIDS policy. Indeed, it has also been noted that the identificatory logic of testing has been challenged through resistance to HIV testing itself by gay-identified men.[34]

While it is important to register that the classificatory and identificatory logic associated with HIV testing and other techniques of governance in relation to HIV/AIDS is sometimes disrupted, it is also necessary to stress that analyses which suggest that testing constitutes a drive to identify the homosexual, tend to overlook other evidence which suggests that HIV antibody testing is increasingly being sought by heterosexuals, or, in epidemiological terms, is increasingly being sought by 'the general population' or 'general community'. For example, in a 'community' studies-styled telephone survey of Sydney residents (aged 16–50) conducted in 1988, 71 per cent of 651 respondents said 'yes' to the question 'Have you ever considered having an AIDS [sic] test?'.[35] And in a repeat study in 1989, 80 per cent of 701 respondents answered in the affirmative to the same question.[36] In a large-scale study designed to overcome what the researchers term a neglect of 'large-scale surveys of HIV testing in the Australian population', which looked at testing rates and factors associated with testing amongst first year heterosexual tertiary students in Sydney, Van de Ven et al. found that of 2,759 surveyed over the period 1992–5 'almost one in five of the students reported that they had ever had an HIV antibody test'.[37] Moreover, the proportion tested was found to be significantly greater in later years of data collection. Thus in 1992 14.5 per cent of 926 students surveyed reported having had an HIV antibody test, and in 1995 20.3 per cent of 506 students surveyed reported testing.[38] While a number of the students cited various mandatory reasons for testing, for instance in cases of blood donations and for occupational, immigration or insurance requirements, the researchers found a broad group of what they termed 'voluntary' reasons for testing, including testing out of curiosity. Moreover, the researchers found 'that voluntary testing increased disproportionately over time'.[39] Such intensifications of testing over time are reflected in generally high rates of antibody testing in Australia, and in the significant rises in the number of tests each year since its availability. Since 1987 over 9 million HIV tests have been conducted with 700,000 tests performed in 1997.[40] In the Australian state of Victoria alone 50,000 tests were performed in 1987 and by 1993 this figure had more than doubled with 120,000 conducted.[41]

Some commentators have suggested that the intensification of HIV antibody testing is linked to the ways in which testing is increasingly understood as a routine health check. Willis, for example, has argued that HIV testing is moving from the unusual to the usual to be part of the routine of everyday medical science, much like any other screening test such as screening for blood pressure.[42] This view of testing is supported by the findings of Lupton, McCarthy and Chapman who, in a study of fifty adults concerning their decisions to have one or more HIV tests, found 'many of the respondents appeared not to discriminate between the HIV test and other tests; they are all medical tests, serving the function of providing "knowledge" of one's condition, and useful to undergo if offered as part of one's general maintenance of the body'.[43] However, the intensification of testing in Australia has also been widely linked to what is sometimes referred to as the 'degaying' of AIDS. Specifically, it has been argued that high rates of HIV testing are linked to health promotion campaigns and news media representations in the late 1980s which universalised risk in relation to HIV/AIDS, a universalisation which is often understood by AIDS researchers to have been constituted by the construction of heterosexuals as 'at risk' in relation to HIV/AIDS.[44] This supposedly caused 'panic, fear and anxiety' and led to demands for heterosexual HIV antibody testing.[45] Indeed it is widely suggested that mass media public health campaigns and/or intense news media coverage of the risk of heterosexual transmission of HIV are frequently followed by upsurges in rates of heterosexual testing.[46]

The construction of heterosexuals as 'at risk' in relation to HIV/AIDS, however, is considered to explain not only the growing demands for testing, but also low levels of seropositive tests. Both the high numbers of tests and the low proportion of positive tests in the state of Victoria (where the proportion of positive tests has remained at less than 1 per cent since 1988)[47] have been understood by medical researchers to 'reflect continued high demand for HIV testing by individuals not at high risk of HIV infection'.[48] Thus Thompson *et al.* report for the period 1991–3 that 'many of those being tested for HIV do not fall into ... identified personal "risk" categor[ies]', categories which the researchers report as 'homosexual', 'injecting drug user', and 'prostitute'.[49] For the latter they say 'less than 10% of tests [have been] undertaken on people identified as having personal risks for HIV'.[50] Moreover, they report the majority of 'low risk' individuals testing identify as heterosexual, indeed that the majority of testing was performed on those identified as heterosexual.[51]

The figuring of heterosexuality as 'low risk' and homosexuality as a 'risk category' in and by medical research clearly calls into question the argument that there has been a simple universalisation of risk in relation to HIV/AIDS, revealing as it does a hierarchy of risk in relation to sexual identities. But if, as Waldby and Treichler argue, the logic of the administrative and discursive techniques of testing constitutes a drive to identify the 'homosexual', what are we to make of heterosexuals seeking testing? As we have seen, part of Waldby's argument regarding the identificatory logic of testing rests on the claim that, while health education strategies ask every citizen to assess their own risk in relation to HIV/AIDS, the hierarchicisation of sexual identities in relation to risk means the demand for risk assessment is far more rigorous for certain groups than it is for others, especially for gay men, for whom as a result there is a strong sense of obligation to be tested.[52] Does this mean that heterosexuals are now in some way also 'obliged' to test? Some analyses suggest this may indeed be the case. Lupton has argued that the construction of heterosexuals as at risk in relation to HIV/AIDS has involved the creation of a new micro-politics of self-regulation in relation to HIV/AIDS for heterosexuals. She suggests that discourses of HIV/AIDS risk in relation to heterosexuality extended a micro-politics of self-surveillance to every individual, or 'responsibilised' every subject in terms of HIV/AIDS risk. Through emphasising individual behaviour change, all individuals therefore became responsible for minimising the transmission of HIV.[53] Moreover, Lupton argues such moves were 'legitimized by the pre-existing discourse of risk which dominates public health discourses', a discourse which she understands as serving as a panoptic agent of surveillance.[54] For Lupton increasing demands for heterosexual testing are therefore understood to be connected to a new politics of subjection and subjectification in relation to heterosexuality, involving 'responsibilisation' and the creation of self-managing, self-regulating heterosexual subjects in relation to HIV/AIDS. Similarly, in his analysis of governmentality and risk Turner agrees that HIV/AIDS discourses have led to such a 'generalised' micropolitics of self-surveillance. He comments,

> the notion of *generalised* risk in the environment may lead to greater surveillance and control through the promotion of preventative medicine. The AIDS 'epidemic' creates a political climate within which intervention and control are seen to be both necessary and benign. Individuals need, especially in the area of sexual etiquette, to become self-regulating and self-forming.[55]

Such analyses therefore seem to question Waldby's view that the administrative techniques and procedures of HIV testing simply concern the identification of the homosexual, since many of the techniques which Waldby associates with the drive towards the identification of the homosexual including subjection, subjectification and responsibilisation appear from these analyses also to be at issue in regard to heterosexuality. Indeed, it has been suggested that the universalisation of HIV/AIDS risk discourse involves not so much a drive to identify the homosexual but signals an important shift in relation to sexuality. Lupton, for instance, has argued that the extension of risk discourse in relation to HIV/AIDS to heterosexuals concerns a shift in representations of 'AIDS from a disease of the deviant and (primarily) homosexual Other to a disease of the heterosexual Self', that is, a kind of 'heterosexualisation' of HIV/AIDS.[56] Yet while she understands the universalisation of risk in relation to HIV/AIDS to signal a new kind of regulation in terms of subjection and subjectification for heterosexuals, which incites testing as one such self-regulative act, nevertheless, Lupton is curiously silent on the kind of heterosexual self being constituted in practices of self-surveillance in relation to HIV/AIDS risk.

Testing and making self-reflexivity

In what follows, however, I suggest that the universalisation of HIV risk and heterosexual reflexivity in relation to HIV/AIDS should not be understood simply as an issue of the heterosexualisation of HIV/AIDS. Specifically, and through a discussion of a range of secondary data on testing, in this section I will show that testing makes self-reflexivity only fully available to the category of heterosexuality, defining other sexual identities as non self-reflexive, that is deemed as incapable of voluntarily performing self-management and self-regulation and therefore in need of more obligatory *external* monitoring and checking in relation to HIV/AIDS. Thus, I suggest rather than a heterosexualisation of HIV/AIDS, heterosexual self-reflexivity in relation to HIV/AIDS concerns new self–other relations in relation to sexuality: hetero-reflexive-selves and non-hetero non-reflexive others. Let me begin with a brief discussion of the concept of 'low-risk' testing.

For medical researchers the intensification of heterosexual testing is often interpreted as unnecessary, excessive over-testing for a group defined as 'low risk'.[57] This concern has also informed social research concerned with heterosexual testing. For example, in discussing the findings of their large-scale survey of heterosexual students in Sydney, Van de Ven *et al.* ask, 'Do these findings support the assertion that current levels of testing in "low-risk" populations are excessive?'[58] In response they report, 'The heterosexual tertiary students in our sample would not generally be regarded as being at high risk of HIV infection. On the whole they would belong to the so-called low risk group.'[59] Nevertheless, Van de Ven *et al.* suggest that a great deal of testing was done for good reasons, including medical, occupational, personal or interpersonal considerations. Similarly, questions concerning 'low-risk' testing also informed Lupton, McCarthy and Chapman's study of fifty adults who had had one or more tests. In particular the ways in which testing patterns have been interpreted to mean that the majority of people being tested for HIV are 'low risk' led Lupton *et al.* to ask why heterosexuals seek testing. To approach this issue and for a sample of mostly heterosexual respondents who had recently had a test, they looked at the socio-cultural meanings of testing, and also at how people used the test result. From the point of view of my concerns here, especially those regarding the kind of heterosexual self constituted through testing, the findings of this study are of particular interest, especially since, on my reading, they make clear how testing makes self-reflexivity only fully available to the category of heterosexuality.

For a number of those interviewed by Lupton *et al.* in this study HIV testing represented a sign of responsibility, as testing was understood to show maturity and to demonstrate a concern for one's health. For instance, 'both sexes commonly used words such as "positive", "responsible", "sensible" and "right" to describe having the test'.[60] One young woman described the way in which having the test 'was a statement about the "responsible" nature of her character'.[61] But for these respondents testing also provided a way of establishing self-regulation. Thus in discussing their experiences of testing, narratives of self-regulation and self-care were performed. One respondent, for example, said 'I go for pap smears, I know [cervical cancer is preventable], so I go for those sorts of things. . . . It's something I can do something about, same with HIV, it's something I can do something about';[62] and another: 'I've monitored everything as far as my body is concerned . . . I do look after myself, check and everything.'[63] For these respondents HIV testing therefore made available particular narratives of the self, those of self-responsibility, self-regulation and self-care. Put another way, testing figured their 'selves' in these terms. And in this way it seems that doing the test – indeed testing itself – may be understood as a technology of the self constitutive of responsibilised, self-reflexive heterosexual subjects.

Du Gay has recently shown how the 'responsibilisation' of subjects involves a figuring of subjects as agents of themselves, that is as reflexive subjects who are continuously engaged in a project to shape their lives as autonomous, choosing individuals driven by the desire to optimise the worth of their existence through the constant building and rebuilding of their own resources.[64] And in this sense it is interesting to note as Lupton *et al.* do, that for their respondents the HIV test provides 'important social currency' or a 'bargaining tool' especially in the domain of intimacy and relationships.[65] In this sense it seems that HIV testing for these respondents may constitute a technology for 'enterprising up' the self, for constituting not only a 'responsibilised' and reflexive self, but also resources of the self which may be mobilised and exchanged.

In addition, the respondents in the Lupton *et al.* study reported that testing made them feel 'better', 'confident', 'safe', 'less anxious', 'sure', giving them a 'sense of reassurance'. One respondent commented on the practice of testing as 'just, for peace of mind – it's like any sort of test, you may be fairly certain that you haven't got it but you need a test anyway, just to make sure'; and another: 'in the back of my mind, I know I always practise safe-sex, but I'm a bit of a hypochondriac, so I tend to go for those things, you know, if I go to the doctor's you know, "Give me a test".'[66] These responses indicate that testing for these respondents may be a repetitive performance, and that the practice of testing constitutes not only an enterprising self, but also one figured in terms of notions of 'safety'. Indeed, in the context of the universalisation of risk in relation to HIV, Lupton *et al.* suggest that the ways in which the test allows 'safety' to be established may 'provide some explanation for the increasing numbers of HIV tests among anxious yet apparently "low risk" individuals'.[67]

In establishing their own safety through HIV testing however, a number of these respondents invoked 'other' categories of person to construct their own safety: 'impure', 'contaminating', out-of-control others who were deemed to be in need of external regulation and control. Indeed, Lupton *et al.* suggest the test serves as means of boundary maintenance against those deemed 'risky', especially since: 'those who felt at risk from HIV infection articulated feelings of extreme vulnerability and a strong need to re-establish subjectivity in the face of their exposure to "contaminating" Others.'[68] More than this, these 'contaminating Others' were understood to be particular categories of sexually defined person, for example the 'gay man', the 'bisexual man' and the 'female prostitute'.

Here then are practices of the personification of risk as categories of sexual identity which Waldby and others have identified to be at issue in relation to the administrative and discursive techniques of testing. But here it is not just that particular categories of sexually defined person are constructed as 'risky', but also that through the practice of testing, heterosexuality is imagined as 'safe' and 'low risk'. Indeed, Waldby's analysis of the techniques and procedures of testing shows that similar processes take place inside the biomedical techniques of testing. Specifically, she shows how such techniques personify or perform heterosexuality as 'low risk', since the techniques of testing work on an explicit assumption of the cleanliness of the heterosexual. For example, she shows how the interpretation and classification of test results work 'to make the heterosexual category the most residual, the least likely to be nominated as a "source" of infection'.[69] Rather, 'sources' of infection are represented as outside of the category. Hence it is assumed that heterosexuality is 'regulated', 'checked' and 'safe', that it may only be infected by the 'outside', by contaminating 'Others', that heterosexuality is at risk rather than risky, threatened rather than threatening.

On this kind of evidence it seems that HIV testing figures heterosexuality as internally checked and self-regulated and therefore as a 'safe', 'low-risk' sexual identity. Indeed, as I have illustrated the practice of testing made available such narratives of self-identity. Thus, on this evidence it seems that the universalisation of risk in relation to HIV/AIDS involves not a straightforward shift of 'AIDS from a disease of the homosexual Other to a disease of the heterosexual Self', but new self–other configurations. Specifically, it suggests that through testing heterosexuality is defined as a self-reflexive identity, while other sexual identities, for instance, homosexuality and bisexuality are defined as non self-reflexive and, as a consequence, in need of more 'coercive' 'external' monitoring rather than voluntary, self-regulative measures. Put another way testing creates a hierarchy of sexual identities defined in terms of reflexivity.[70]

This hierarchicisation of sexual identities in terms of reflexivity is also visible in other studies of the procedures of testing. For example, a study of post-test counselling found that in cases of negative results, gay men, injecting drug users and others classified as 'high risk' are often told 'that some people who test negative are actually infected and given advice on behaviours to limit the transmission of AIDS, i.e. limit the number of sex partners, limit body fluid exchange ... avoid intravenous drug use, and don't donate blood, plasma, organs or sperm. Some recommend a follow-up test after 6 months.'[71] Seronegatives defined as 'low risk' however, 'are told simply that their test results show they are not infected'.[72] While gay seronegative men and others are told to discipline themselves, especially in regard to sexual practices, and make themselves available for further medical surveillance, for seronegative heterosexuals no such measures are recommended. This hierarchy in terms of reflexivity is also visible in Bray and Chapman's two community studies-styled surveys. Here, while the overwhelming majority of respondents said they had considered having a voluntary HIV test, over half in both surveys said 'testing should be *compulsory* for certain groups',[73] the most common groups cited being homosexuals and prostitutes. Thus it seems, as Patton has argued in relation to HIV/AIDS education, that the administrative and discursive logics of testing constitutes the 'mainstream' as having a 'right to know, that is a right to protect *themselves*' and gay men and others with 'an *obligation* to know and act appropriately'.[74]

Conclusion

In these ways I suggest that HIV testing can be understood as a technology which serves not only to identify the 'homosexual' but one which is also constitutive of a heterosexuality figured in terms of self-reflexivity; that is, as a technology through which heterosexuality is constituted as a self-regulated, self-monitored, internally checked identity. It therefore comes as no surprise that Lupton *et al.* found that HIV testing offered a way of establishing a heterosexual subjectivity or identity based on self-responsibility and self-monitoring, for testing itself constitutes heterosexuality as a sexual identity which can only be understood in these terms. Thought through in this way, it is clear that the now often-asked research question in the social and medical sciences 'why are "low risk" groups – especially heterosexuals – increasingly opting for HIV testing?' misses the crucial point: testing precisely constitutes heterosexuality as self-regulating in relation to HIV/AIDS, as 'low risk', and 'safe'. Indeed, put like this, the dominant assumption which informs many of the analyses of 'risk' culture discussed throughout this chapter – that a generalised risk culture creates insecurity, uncertainty and doubt which then incites practices of self-reflexivity and a reflexive project of the self – becomes questionable. Specifically, it seems from the example of HIV testing, that the making of a self-reflexive identity cannot be assumed to be as straightforward in risk culture as many analyses of risk and AIDS claim. For, as the example of HIV testing suggests, the possession of such an identity cannot be taken for granted, indeed is an issue of cultural contestation. In addition, rather than assuming the meaning of risk in advance, I hope this chapter has illustrated the importance of opening up for question how categories and hierarchies of 'risk' are made up in everyday life. Here I have suggested, as Higgs has argued in regard to technologies of risk for social and health policy more generally,[75] that HIV antibody testing is a technology which serves not only to 'responsibilise' but also to define and identify so-called 'risky' groups, who are deemed incapable of adequately and voluntarily performing self-monitoring and self-management, that is of being self-reflexive.

A range of recent social and cultural theory foregrounds increasing tendencies towards self-reflexivity. More than this, the self-reflexive subject is increasingly emerging as an ideal subject across a range of fields. Thus, the voluntary governance of the self, involving demonstrations of capacities of self-control through the taking on of various technologies of the self increasingly constitutes what it currently means to be a citizen.[76] Yet if the very techniques and procedures of responsibilisation make self-reflexivity only available to the category of heterosexuality, indeed are constitutive of a hierarchy of sexualities, then a little more caution may need to be exercised than has so far been the case in asking and answering questions such as 'why are increasing numbers of heterosexuals having HIV tests?' Indeed, if ideal subjects are those who make use of their own agency to govern and invent themselves, then surely a politics of reflexivity may be in order. This may be especially important if the technologies of this ideal constitute particular subjects as lacking reflexivity, including self-knowledge, self-management and self-monitoring. It may also be pressing if, as Beck and others have argued, social position is increasingly determined by the distribution of 'risks'. I have suggested here that reflexivity is closely aligned to such distributions, where those who are able to claim self-reflexivity are also able to claim a 'safe' identity, while those defined as unable to adequately perform self-monitoring and self-management are deemed to be 'at risk' and 'risky'. If this is the case then the ability to politicise and contest current definitions of risk may need to involve a politicisation of the self-reflexive subject.

Notes

1 See e.g. P. Treichler, 'AIDS, Gender and Biomedical Discourse: Current Contests for Meaning', in E. Fee and D. Fox (eds), *AIDS: The Burdens of History*, Berkeley, Calif., University of California Press, 1988, pp. 190–266; C. Waldby, *AIDS and the Body Politic: Biomedicine and Sexual Difference*, London, Routledge, 1996.
2 Waldby, *AIDS and the Body Politic*.
3 See e.g. D. Lupton *et al.*, '"Doing the Right Thing": The Symbolic Meanings and Experiences of Having an HIV Antibody Test', *Social Science and Medicine*, 1995, vol. 41, pp. 173–80; D. Lupton *et al.*, '"Panic Bodies": Discourses on Risk and HIV Antibody Testing', *Sociology of Health and Illness*, 1995, vol. 17, pp. 89–108; S. Thompson *et al.*, 'A Profile of HIV Testing in Victoria to the End of 1993', *Australian and New Zealand Journal of Public Health*, 1996, no. 20, pp. 165–71.
4 Lupton *et al.*, '"Panic Bodies"', p. 106.
5 See e.g. U. Beck, *Risk Society: Towards a New Modernity*, London, Sage, 1992; U. Beck, 'The Reinvention of Politics: Towards a Theory of Reflexive Modernization', in U. Beck *et al.*, *Reflexive Modernization: Politics, Tradition and Aesthetics in the Modern Social Order*, Cambridge, Polity, 1994, pp. 1–55; S. Lash *et al.* (eds), *Risk, Environment and Modernity*, London, Sage, 1996; B. Turner, 'From Governmentality to Risk: Some Reflections on Foucault's Contribution to Medical Sociology', in A. Peterson and R. Brunton (eds), *Foucault, Health and Medicine*, London, Routledge, 1997, pp. ix–xxi.
6 Beck, *Risk Society*, p. 20; see also Beck, 'The Reinvention of Politics'.
7 Beck, 'The Reinvention of Politics', p. 6.
8 Ibid., p. 8.

9 Ibid.
10 Indeed, a range of social theory points to increasing tendencies towards self-reflection, self-regulation and self-monitoring for the making of identities in the context of the untying of individuals from the rules, norms and traditions of modernity. See e.g. U. Beck and E. Beck-Gernsheim, *The Normal Chaos of Love*, Cambridge, Polity, 1995; A. Giddens, *Modernity and Self-Identity: Self and Society in the Late Modern Age*, Cambridge, Polity, 1991; A. Giddens, *The Transformation of Intimacy: Sexuality, Love and Eroticism in Modern Societies*, Cambridge, Polity, 1992; A. Melucci, *The Playing Self: Person and Meaning in the Planetary Society*, Cambridge, Cambridge University Press, 1996.
11 See e.g. D. Lupton, *The Imperative of Health: Public Health and the Regulated Body*, London, Sage, 1995; S. Nettleton, 'Governing the Risky Self: How to Become Healthy, Wealthy and Wise', in Peterson and Brunton (eds), *Foucault, Health and Medicine*, pp. 207–22; A. Peterson, 'Risk, Governance and the New Public Health', in Peterson and Brunton (eds), *Foucault, Health and Medicine*, pp. 189–206; A. Peterson and D. Lupton, *The New Public Health: Health and Self in the Age of Risk*, St Leonards, UK, Allen and Unwin, 1996.
12 P. Higgs, 'Risk, Governmentality and the Reconceptualization of Citizenship', in G. Scambler and P. Higgs (eds), *Modernity, Medicine and Health: Medical Sociology Towards 2000*, London, Routledge, 1998, pp. 176–97.
13 D. Armstrong, 'The Rise of Surveillance Medicine', *Sociology of Health and Illness*, 1995, vol. 17, p. 398.
14 Ibid., pp. 399–400.
15 Ibid., p. 400.
16 Ibid., p. 401.
17 Higgs, 'Risk, Governmentality and the Reconceptualization of Citizenship', p. 189.
18 Lupton, *The Imperative of Health*, p. 104.
19 For discussions in relation to the United States and for a comparative analysis of Britain, Hungary and Sweden, see respectively, C. Patton, 'What Science Knows: Formations of AIDS Knowledges', in P. Aggelton *et al.* (eds), *AIDS: Individual, Cultural and Policy Dimensions*, London, Falmer, 1990, pp. 1–18; and R. Danziger, 'HIV Testing for HIV Prevention: A Comparative Analysis of Policies in Britain, Hungary and Sweden', *AIDS Care*, 1998, vol. 10, pp. 563–70.
20 Waldby, *AIDS and the Body Politic*, p. 114.
21 Ibid., p. 113.
22 Ibid.
23 Ibid., p. 120.
24 For a further discussion of practices of 'personification' in relation to the medical and counselling experiences of people with HIV/AIDS, see B. Heaphy, 'Medicalisation and Identity Formation: Identity and Strategy in the Context of AIDS and HIV', in J. Weeks and J. Holland (eds), *Sexual Cultures: Communities, Values and Intimacy*, Basingstoke, UK, Macmillan 1996, pp. 139–60.
25 Waldby, *AIDS and the Body Politic*, p. 124.
26 Ibid., p. 114.
27 See e.g. S. C. McCrombie 'The Cultural Impact of the "AIDS" Test: The American Experience', *Social Science and Medicine*, 1986, vol. 23, pp. 455–9; Patton, 'What Science Knows'; N. Schiller *et al.*, 'Risky Business: The Cultural Construction of Risk Groups', *Social Science and Medicine*, 1994, vol. 38, pp. 1337–46.
28 Waldby, *AIDS and the Body Politic*, p. 114.
29 See also C. Patton, *Inventing AIDS*, London, Routledge, 1990.
30 Waldby, *AIDS and the Body Politic*, p. 121.
31 Treichler, 'AIDS, Gender and Biomedical Discourse', p. 200.

32 Heaphy, 'Medicalisation and Identity Formation', p. 153.
33 M. Bartos, 'The Queer Excess of Public Health Policy', *Meanjin*, 1996, vol. 55, pp. 122–31 at 126; see also C. Patton, 'Tremble, Hetero Swine', in M. Warner (ed.), *Fear of a Queer Planet*, Minneapolis, University of Minnesota Press, 1993, pp. 143–77.
34 See e.g. N. D. Hunter, 'Censorship and Identity in the Age of AIDS' in M. Levine *et al.* (eds), *In Changing Times: Gay Men and Lesbians Encounter HIV/AIDS*, Chicago, University of Chicago Press, 1997, pp. 39–53.
35 The researchers used the term AIDS as piloting 'revealed that many people were unfamiliar with the term HIV', see F. Bray and S. Chapman, 'Community Knowledge, Attitudes and Media Recall About AIDS, Sydney 1988 and 1989', *Australian Journal of Public Health*, 1991, vol. 15, 1991, p. 107.
36 Bray and Chapman, 'Community Knowledge', p. 110.
37 P. Van de Ven *et al.*, 'HIV Testing Among Heterosexual Tertiary Students', *Venereology*, 1997, vol. 10, p. 27.
38 Ibid.
39 Ibid., p. 29.
40 Lupton *et al.*, '"Doing the Right Thing"'; L. Lamont, 'The Condom Generation Conquers Campus', *The Sydney Morning Herald*, 14 Nov. 1998, p. 3.
41 Thompson *et al.*, 'A Profile of HIV Testing', p. 166. The high levels of testing in Australia have been compared to those found in Sweden, which has one of the 'highest rates of HIV testing per capita in Europe. By 1996, 9.5 million tests had been carried out among Sweden's population of 8.5 million.' See Lupton *et al.*, '"Panic Bodies"'; Danziger, 'HIV Testing for HIV Prevention', p. 567.
42 E. Willis, 'The Social Relations of HIV Testing', in S. Scott *et al.* (eds), *Private Risks and Public Dangers*, Aldershot, UK, Avebury, 1992, pp. 168–83.
43 Lupton *et al.*, '"Doing the Right Thing"', p. 177.
44 See e.g. Lupton *et al.*, '"Panic Bodies"'; A. Morlet *et al.*, 'The Impact of the "Grim Reaper" National AIDS Educational Campaign on the Albion Street (AIDS) Centre and AIDS Hotline', *The Medical Journal of Australia*, 1988, no. 148, pp. 282–6; Thompson *et al.*, 'A Profile of HIV Testing'; J. Tulloch and D. Lupton, *Television, AIDS and Risk: A Cultural Studies Approach to Health Communication*, St Leonards, UK, Allen and Unwin, 1997.
45 D. Lupton, 'AIDS Risk and Heterosexuality in the Australian Press', *Discourse and Society*, 1993, vol. 4, p. 324; see also Lupton *et al.*, '"Doing the Right Thing"'; Lupton *et al.*, '"Panic Bodies"'; Morlet *et al.*, 'The Impact of the "Grim Reaper"'; Thompson *et al.*, 'A Profile of HIV Testing'.
46 Lupton *et al.*, '"Doing the Right Thing"', p. 174; see also Chippendale *et al.*, 'Reasons for HIV Antibody Testing: Plus ça Change?', *International Journal of STD and AIDS*, 1998, no. 9, pp. 219–22; Morlet *et al.*, 'The Impact of the "Grim Reaper"'.
47 For example, of 70,000 tests performed in Victoria in 1989 0.9 per cent of the specimens tested for antibody to HIV were reported seropositive and in 1993 of the more than 120,000 tests performed 0.7 per cent of the specimens were reported seropositive. See Thompson *et al.*, 'A Profile of HIV Testing', p. 166.
48 Thompson *et al.*, 'A Profile of HIV Testing', p. 168; see also Lupton *et al.*, '"Doing the Right Thing"'; Lupton *et al.*, '"Panic Bodies"'.
49 Thompson *et al.*, 'A Profile of HIV Testing', p. 167.
50 Ibid., p. 169.
51 Ibid.
52 Waldby, *AIDS and the Body Politic*.
53 Lupton, 'AIDS Risk and Heterosexuality in the Australian Press', p. 317; see also Lupton *et al.*, '"Doing the Right Thing"'; Lupton *et al.*, '"Panic Bodies"'.
54 Lupton, 'AIDS Risk and Heterosexuality in the Australian Press', pp. 324–5.

55 Turner, 'From Governmentality to Risk', p. xix, my emphasis; see also Peterson and Lupton, *The New Public Health*, pp. 69–70.
56 Lupton, 'AIDS Risk and Heterosexuality in the Australian Press', p. 324.
57 See e.g. Thompson *et al.*, 'A Profile of HIV Testing'.
58 Van de Ven *et al.*, 'HIV Testing', p. 10.
59 Ibid.
60 Lupton *et al.*, '"Doing the Right Thing"', p. 176.
61 Ibid.
62 Ibid., p. 177.
63 Lupton *et al.*, '"Panic Bodies"', p. 103
64 P. Du Gay, *Consumption and Identity at Work*, London, Sage, 1996, p. 181.
65 Lupton *et al.*, '"Doing the Right Thing"', p. 176; Lupton *et al.*, '"Panic Bodies"', p. 107; see also Van de Ven *et al.*, 'HIV Testing'.
66 Lupton *et al.*, '"Doing the Right Thing"', p. 177; Lupton *at al.*, '"Panic Bodies"', p. 94.
67 Lupton *et al.*, '"Panic Bodies"', p. 106.
68 Ibid.
69 Waldby, *AIDS and the Body Politic*, p. 126.
70 Some recent evidence suggests that heterosexual men are more likely to seek voluntary HIV testing than heterosexual women suggesting that testing may therefore figure male heterosexual sexual identities as the most charged in relation to self-reflexivity. See J. Meyrick *et al.*, 'To Test Or Not to Test, Could You Repeat the Question?', *International Journal of STDs and AIDS*, 1997, no. 8, pp. 36–9.
71 McCrombie, 'The Cultural Impact of the "AIDS" Test', p. 456.
72 Ibid.
73 Bray and Chapman, 'Community Knowledge', p. 110, my emphasis.
74 Patton, 'What Science Knows', p. 14, my emphases.
75 Higgs, 'Risk, Governmentality and the Reconceptualization of Citizenship'.
76 Ibid.

10 The promiscuous placenta

Crossing over

Jane-Maree Maher

The outline of the pregnant body preserves the visual contours of bodily integrity that underpin the unified subject.[1] The protrusion of the belly does not necessarily constitute a break in the integrity of the body. Instead, edges are retraced; pregnancy is a gradual transformation in a still-unified corporeal space. In this way, the pregnant body participates in the particular western requirements of subjective identity where it is the edges that delimit the subject.[2] While the pregnant body preserves its edges, it shifts them outwards and, in so doing, subverts and confounds the notion of the bounded body. In the pregnant body's expansive and malleable materiality, it accommodates and contains another thing. This body of the one is simultaneously the body of at least two. The possibility of bodily integrity and subjectivity is at once preserved and radically restructured as the edges of this body are defined across the figure of two. In what follows, I argue that the question of subjective intention and bodily instrumentation converge in the pregnant body in ways that confound and contaminate the bounded body as the location of, and instrument for, the subject. In particular, I locate the placenta as fundamental in understanding and reformulating the infectious activity and meaning of the pregnant body.

The process of contagion can be defined as the communication of disease from body to body. I argue that pregnancy operates as a performance of contagion where the 'disease' communicated can be understood as embodied subjectivity. The passage of fluid inside the pregnant body, backwards and forwards between the pregnant woman and the foetal entity, enacts the process of contagion as it constitutes the movement toward the moment of birth – the separation into two subjects with body boundaries appropriately restored. From the morphological confusion of pregnancy emerge two bounded subjects. But this process of contagion, a material communication between two entities in one pregnant body that allows for the putative constitution of these subjects, is scripted out of narratives of pregnancy. The emphasis on instrumentality, visual definitions and 'mother and child' at the site of pregnancy occludes the uncertain boundaries that construct the corporeal entity of the foetus and refigure the previously bounded body of the woman.

The placenta is the organ through which these fluid interactions occur. It is the materialisation of the necessary contagion of pregnancy in two ways. It is the point of communication between pregnant woman and foetal entity, allowing for and recognising their difference. The crossover occurs here. But it is not only the conduit of fluid, it is a materialisation of contagion itself. The placenta as organ belongs neither to the corporeal location of the pregnant woman nor that of the foetus. It offends and refigures bodily integrity and boundaries, it allows for at least two to work together at the site of one, while preventing against a collapse into singularity. The placenta operates as a border, but only a porous and provisional one. It enacts contamination and it insists that contamination, seepage and crossover are constitutive of embodied subjects, rather than threatening to them. This chapter foregrounds the function of the placenta in pregnancy in order to make explicit the processes of contamination that both construct the bounded body and subject in pregnancy and expose it as always already implicated in exchange and leakage.

But the potentially contagious fluidity of the placenta forms the basis of a broader argument that extends the physical into the theoretical. As well as impacting on how we envisage the pregnant body, the contaminating possibility of the placenta extends beyond the boundaries of the pregnant body itself. This transformation depends on an understanding of each body as produced in and through a placental framework of connection and fluid exchange. In the first instance, in the pregnant body that divides, multiplies and creates another entity out of and inside itself, the contagious capacity of functioning placenta can be characterised as the breakdown of the delimited self. The distinctions between mind and body and between differentiated mind/body entities are blurred and infected with the uncertainty of the placental boundary.

The coexistence of subjective uncertainties and physiological confusions means that the mind/body distinction carries a new meaning when mapped onto the pregnant body. Questions of intention, instrumentation and ownership are confused in the non-directed process of pregnancy. It forms part of my argument that this disturbing possibility is contained by the deployment of the visual field to separate the pregnant woman and the foetus and bestow subjectivity on the foetus. In my reading of the pregnant body, the mind/body distinction does not cease to have significance, but the terms on either side of the binary are complicated, contaminated and refigured by the existence of the other. This refiguration echoes in the morphological transformations of the body in pregnancy.

The second possibility of contagion turns on the notion of the placental economy raised in discussion between biologist Helene Rouch and Luce Irigaray to which I will return.[3] The initial crossover and division that is enacted in the development of the pregnant woman and the foetus in the pregnant body prefigures the possibility of crossing over other corporeal boundaries. The placenta operates as a precondition for the production of bodies. All bodies are formed in this process of division and split in the pregnant body. Each body that appears bounded comes to its boundaries through the interconnectedness of a pregnant body. Through the navel, they bear the trace of this connection as a function of their distinction. Each corporeal entity is thus caught in a contagious reconception of the body through its placental formation. For a woman's body that has passed through the process of pregnancy, this mark is revisited and intensified. In pregnancy, the endlessly communicative and transgressive nature of embodied subjectivity is exposed.

A turn to the functioning placenta as formulating new ways of understanding subjectivity necessarily incorporates all embodied subjectivities under this rubric. In what follows, the specificity of the placenta and its contagious activity is explored. The location of the placenta is understood as the point of connection for the maternal and foetal entities as well as signifying the point at which each embodied subject, despite its apparently bounded nature, is located in a relation of connection and interdependence through its origin. For a state of pregnancy to exist, there must be a placenta, either in place or developing. In this way, in biological and physiological terms, the placenta is essential for pregnancy. To this extent, it is universal and does not depend on the variations of experience, emotion, and physical circumstances that construct each woman's individual pregnancy. At the same time, the operation of the placenta itself is totally driven and determined by its location within the pregnant body, at the connection point of maternal and foetal entity. It has reference only to that particular embodied instance of pregnancy; it is constructed from the cells and products of each pregnant body in conjunction with the developing foetus. These multiplicities, where the placenta operates both as universal trope and highly specific element, underpin this chapter and also carry its connection to the central theme of contagion. The permeability and transmutability of the placenta in physiological terms allows for the passage of fluid within the pregnant body, commonly located as maternal–foetal transmission. In this chapter, this transmission is extended to include the possibility of a porous conception of subjectivity.

This chapter turns to the placenta to refigure subject/instrument through the process of contagion. In so doing, there are times when the placenta is offered a form of agency, discursively and materially, in order to describe its functioning within and its rupture of common subject schema. The discursive emphasis on all activity as being generated in and through subjective will, even undirected activity of the corporeal, is one of the frameworks with which this chapter engages. The anthropomorphic contamination of this project, where the placenta appears to be endowed with will in order to function, signals the impossibility of fully distinguishing the corporeal and the subjective realms. Instead, they continually cross over, with the corporeal activity of the placenta appearing to have will, while the pregnant subject is seemingly caught in the bodily project. Rather than discursively containing this difficulty, the anthropomorphic confusion stands inside the frame as a marker of the problematic this chapter is seeking to address.

There are three phases to this location of the placenta as a material form for rethinking the boundaries of pregnancy and embodied subjectivity. The first section of the chapter explores how pregnancy complicates and contaminates notions of mind and body in its multiple interactions. The second section, 'Perceiving placentas' investigates the matter and meaning of the placenta. It argues that the physiological activity of the placenta offers a way of understanding gestation outside the frames of 'mother' and 'child' through which the state of pregnancy is usually represented. Fluid exchange, the contagious process, is located as productive and positive. The third section, 'Do you see what I see?', examines how visual technologies are deployed to contain this inchoate body of pregnancy. Here, the impact of visual technologies in constructing distinct foetal and maternal bodies rather than illuminating the body of pregnancy is located in connection with anxieties of the seeping possibilities of the placental pregnant body. Rather than *look at* the pregnant body, I argue these technologies look away from the disturbing and contagious implications for embodied subjectivity that are materialised there. In the placental body that is open to both pregnant woman and foetus, that is partially governed by intent and partially outside government, I explore the possibility of a refigured subjectivity produced by contagious exchange, not threatened by it. The collision of competing meanings in the placental body; the sense of self and not self; the body as instrument *and* independent project manager, signals to this possibility of contamination. If bodies and subjective intent can shift, collide and even contradict as they do in a 'placental body', what boundaries are safe from this contagious understanding of the bounded subject as endlessly porous and of the mind/body distinction as a binary that no longer holds the line?

The non-instrumental self of pregnancy

The notion of the body as instrument is key to understanding the body/mind configuration that generally informs concepts of subjectivity. The body as instrument is understood to act in the service of the subject. The intentions of the subject to move and determine the action of its own body are seen as paramount for that subject's existence and meaning. Discourses as wide-ranging as Christianity, sporting motivation and sexual satisfaction promote the management of the body by the mind as the key to success and salvation. This chapter concerns itself with the pregnant body precisely because the pregnant body does not fit comfortably into these discourses. Physiological processes of becoming pregnant, maintaining and managing a pregnancy can be assisted by the subject's activity, but the subject cannot direct or control these processes. Unprotected sexual intercourse, for example, may allow for the possibility of pregnancy, but cannot ensure its commencement. Infertility, miscarriage, nausea, and placenta previa are some of the conditions which demonstrate that pregnancy resides outside the subject's control. While the subject may desire the pregnancy itself, that desire cannot contain or direct the embodied pregnancy experience.

In her groundbreaking essay, 'Pregnant Embodiment', Iris Marion Young describes the complication of subjectivity that occurs in the pregnant body. For Young, the pregnant subject is always mediated simultaneously through the double frame of self and other. 'It is always decentred, split or doubled . . . I move as if I could squeeze around chairs . . . only to find my way blocked by my own body sticking out in front of me . . . but yet not me, since I did not expect it to block my passage.'[4] Young's use of 'I' here is complicated by the 'not I' that the gestational body implies at the same moment. There is a confusion of activities. Young's movement through the door, the point where she engages her body as instrument, collides with the corporeal activity of gestation, which has continued, *without her subjective presence*, in her body. This proliferation of positions is one of the most significant aspects for a theorisation of the corporeality of pregnancy. In *the bodies of women*, Rosalyn Diprose suggests that self-conscious intentionality, a sense of the embodied 'I', 'arises after a *call-back* to the body from habitual engagement'.[5] Diprose argues that we become aware of our bodies at the point that they will not acquiesce in silence to our subjective demands. Drawing on the work of Merleau-Ponty and Drew Leder, she notes that the effacement of the body is usually ruptured in illness or pain, where the corporeal schema that enables bodily activity generally 'goes limp' and is unable to achieve its goals.[6] The subject becomes aware of its own bodily limits through its refusal of the subject's command. There is an inscription of the body on the conscious life of the subject. I use the term 'inscription' to indicate a process of marking out, and bringing to the subject's awareness, the terms and form of the subject's body.

In pregnancy, this inscription does not occur in the context of the failure of intention Diprose outlined above. The notion of the callback as representing a failure of intention is refuted and refigured. A pregnant subject, engaged in intentional and non-intentional corporeal activity, experiences this callback without necessary disruption to the corporeal schema. Young is able to make her way through the door, but her body grazes the edges of it, thus bringing that body to her mind. As Young describes it, the inscription of pregnancy on the body intervenes to mark out bodily edges, but does not necessarily prevent the achievement of the project. Instead, it makes explicit the conditions, or corporeal schema, through which the pregnant body is able to act. This body *can* connote bodily intentionality, but only ever as a partial representation of its self. This double meaning at the edges of the pregnant body space is a mirror for the doubled internal landscape of the gestating body.

The notion of a 'placental body' offers several strategic advantages in rethinking this instrumental focus. Viewing the placenta refigures the discrete images of 'mother' and 'baby' that are commonly represented on the site of the pregnant body and emphasises a dynamic and interactive body. It offers a sense of the body as productive, but not as an expression of the subject's will. Instead, the particular corporeal productivity of the pregnant body interrogates the concept of the instrumental body, as the subject can only partially control the process. The placenta is the central organ of transmission and development in this process. It is both the means of communication between the two bodies and the communication itself. This exchange forms the matter of contagion in pregnancy as the productive centre of the process.

In pregnancy, the capacity to cross the line, to transfer fluid with its contagious possibilities is the defining process. The exchange of fluid between the two entities of the pregnant body acts as a direct vector of contagion, a material way in which the pregnant body inevitably requires contamination to function. The nutrients and waste that cross back and forward between the pregnant body and the foetus across the placenta are the productive matter of pregnancy. The process of fluid exchange allows for foetal development and the continuation of the pregnancy. Significantly, these exchanges occur outside the subjective consciousness. They occur as part of the body project, rather than the subjective one, and, as such, confound notions of instrumentality and intention as the only sites of productivity for the body. But these exchanges also contest the notion of contagion as threatening to the body entity. In its productive move toward birth, the pregnant body must engage in processes that simultaneously enact and refigure notions of contagion. The negative possibilities of contamination through pregnancy are possible only through the positive and irreducible activity of contagious fluid exchange. These possibilities are the matter of the placenta.

Perceiving placentas

In considering this double face to the subject/body relation in pregnancy, the placenta offers itself as a useful construct both materially and theoretically. For the placenta operates with a double face also. The placenta stands at the nexus of the pregnant woman and the foetal entity. The pregnant body is conditioned by and responsive to a set of needs that cannot be situated within one subject or corporeal locus. The growing foetus places a series of demands on the woman's body, more or less onerous at certain times. Although the pregnant subject may empathise with and feel positively toward these needs and movements, she cannot determine or direct them. The illness, tiredness and hormonal fluctuations, kicks and pressures of this one body represent negotiations between two needy and productive corporeal sites. And these two corporeal entities have a complex relation, with a separate register of interests, as well as a common one.

This imbricated and diffuse relation is materially rendered in the placenta. It acts as the mediation point. This is where the crossover occurs – of blood, nourishment and waste. It is a *between* that is always already within. It is an organ that offends the concept of bodily integrity because it acts between the two. The development of the placenta, the distinction of placental cells and the engagement of the placenta between embryo and gestating woman occur outside the purview of the intentional self. One cannot mandate that the placenta does its work – it engages and mediates in and through the process of pregnancy without direction. After that, it is expelled becoming useless to both pregnant woman and foetus at the point at which they become – materially, figuratively, representationally – at least two bodies instead of one.

In an interview which Luce Irigaray conducted with Helene Rouch, a biologist, Rouch cited the placenta as the point of differentiation between the mother and child that exists before language.[7] Both Rouch and Irigaray argue that what they term 'the placental economy' confounds expectations and understandings of the masculine economy of meaning and self, since it is a point of separation *and* connection, a 'sort of negotiation between the mother's self and the other that is the embryo'.[8] This doubled face of placental activity is crucial for understanding the potential refiguration implicit in the placental body. Identity is not collapsed in this frame, rather the edges are reconstituted as fluid and provisional. Embodied subjectivity here cannot depend on the maintenance of rigid boundaries, but rather formulates itself across and through exchanges of matter and fluid.

The placenta inside the pregnant body is located outside the possibilities of intention and instrumentalisation. One cannot direct one's placenta to activity; one cannot regulate its location or feel its movement. Rather than accepting the body as instrumentalised, the pregnant body enacts the limits of intention as productive of both subject and body. It refuses the notion of an intentional subject in an instrumental body, instead allowing modes and moments of intentionality to coalesce and disperse on either side of this dualistic formation. In the process of gestating, the body continues to work, even when the subjective consciousness of the process disappears. This is the point at which Young's intending subject must necessarily run into the acting body in the doorway. The intent subject is re-embodied in the collision of subjective focus and active materiality. The multiplication of terms and positions elaborated in Young's progress through the door, the intermingling of subjective achievement and the simultaneous recognition of the on-going, extra-subjective body project of pregnancy, instantiates the porous and proliferating preconditions of pregnancy.

This organ, for all its 'betweenness' resists transferability or re-creation. Unlike the other parts involved in conceptive technology – ova, sperm, embryo – it cannot be extracted, re-routed or resituated. Mechanical constructions and biological additions cannot replicate the complexity of the placenta as both discrete organ and intercorporeal entity. The attempt to support foetuses through the replication of the placenta fails, usually after a period of days. Even attempts to keep the placenta operative in cases where the mother has died do not succeed. Instead, in scientific endeavours, this connective entity is refigured as a chamber, a container. Susan Squier notes that in 1993, patents were sought for a placental chamber that could bring reproductive medicine closer to Huxley's brave new world.[9] Thus, in this application, the placenta is literally and figuratively emptied of content. The transmogrification from organ to chamber that is manifest in the patent application provides a useful context for considering how the corporeal implications of the placenta are evacuated and reframed. In its refusal to be resituated, the placenta continues to insist on its location at the intersection between two corporeal sites sharing one bodily space, and it can only exist there for as long as this related corporeality continues. It connects them, but belongs to neither. For the purposes of this exploration and refiguration of the pregnant body, it is process made flesh, incorporated, represented.

In and of itself, the placenta marks a particular non-presence, which renders it significantly resistant to concrete definition. The 1984 Warnock Report undertaken in Britain suggested a fourteen-day limit for embryo experimentation.[10] The limit was set by scientific evidence that this was the point where foetal cells distinguished themselves from the placental cells and thus provided evidence of an individuated potential.[11] In the representational stills used by Lennart Nilsson in the now famous *Life* magazine foetal photo shoots, the placenta had to be removed in order that the view of the foetus could be obtained. Here the placenta must be excised in order that a requirement of visual codes of knowledge, a clear view, is satisfied.[12] Thus, the placenta functions as that which complicates the picture both physiologically and metonymically. It can be seen as the 'not I', the site of absence which authorises and defines presence. In its citation as non-originary material, or the other, the placenta is located in excess of the definitional boundaries.[13]

The significance of fluid for the placenta further pushes these boundaries of definition and delimitation. The primary role of the placenta is to facilitate the crossover of fluid between the pregnant woman and the foetus. As such, it is key for the development and maintenance of healthy pregnancies. It is a productive and necessary contagion that allows for the corporeal constitution of the foetus and the (re)constitution of the pregnant woman. But this potential, so necessary and fundamental, has been identified as a threat in discourses of foetal alcohol syndrome, ingestion of drugs, alcohol and other toxic substances while pregnant, and the Rh-blood flow where maternal antibodies can attack the foetus.[14] The double meaning and definition of the placenta's fluid nature can be read in several ways. Bodily fluid is often identified as problematic for Cartesian conceptions of the body/self relation: it attests 'to the permeability of the body, its necessary dependence on an outside, its liability to collapse into this outside ... [It is an] affront to the subject's aspirations ... [to] the "clean" and "proper"'.[15] In the development of a placental body, the pregnant body described and understood through the irreducible presence of the placenta within it, fluid exchange must be seen as the inherent and constitutive mode of that body. Philosopher Elizabeth Grosz's identification of fluid as an 'affront' to the subject's aspirations takes on a new possibility here as the fluidity of the placenta infects not one body site but at least two. Through its irreducibility, it gathers in all bodies as participants in these fluid processes. The attendant dangers, difficulties, productivities and contagious possibilities of bodily fluid and subjective fluidity are intensified in the 'bloody sieve' that is the placenta.[16]

The placenta marks the expansive and frightening power of fluid, since it carries the load of providing blood and dealing with waste products for much larger entities than itself. It has an enormous, complex, but materially finite, capacity and uniquely lacks the desire to preserve itself that Freud identified as the primary characteristic of the organ.[17] Instead, the placenta works toward its own obsolescence; each instance of its functioning adds strength to the inevitable separation of the two entities to which it is connected. As the foetus draws nourishment through the placenta, it moves toward its distinction from the pregnant body. This process of foetal development marks the pregnant body as transitory as well. The successful enactment of placental function is the redundancy of the placenta itself at the point of birth.

As the material marker and matrix of pregnancy, the placenta enacts and represents embodied connection and distinction. It inscribes the process of contagion as productive and irreducible for the construction of embodied subjectivities. The exchange of fluids, the enmeshed surfaces of the foetus and the pregnant woman, that occur in the placenta and also *are* the placenta, figure subjectivity as a process of contamination and seepage. The apparent differentiation of the bounded subject is produced in, marked by and is productively vulnerable to crossover. Common representations of gestation, however, show that this model of viewing the pregnant body is not conventionally deployed. As feminist theorists have argued, the routine use of visual technologies has resulted in the construction of the foetal subject and the erasure of the maternal subject.[18] What one sees is one body with a bulge. But through the use of images, stills, photos, drawings and medical technology, we are made to see in that embodied singularity, two separate bodies. While these representations of pregnancy abound, it is my contention that they represent a pregnant body in a non-functional frame. The irreducible activity of pregnancy; the development process; the interdependent exchange of fluid; the subjective and corporeal confusions, is not rendered in these images. The potential slippage that has capacity to engage and refigure the boundaries of all bodies, the implicitly contagious nature of the mind/body relation of pregnancy, cannot be viewed. Instead, the figure of two is offered on the site of the pregnant body. I contend that this vision of two at the site of one is a vision that leads away from the disquieting implications of corporeal subjectivity without definite edges, away from the state of pregnancy marked all the time as communication and crossover in the placenta.

Do you see what I see?

In the modern representation of pregnancy, Barbara Duden argues that the publication of the Lennart Nilsson photos in *Life* magazine in 1966 constitutes a critical moment.

> How did the unborn turn into a billboard image and how did that isolated goblin get into the limelight? How did the female peritoneum acquire transparency? What set of circumstances made the skinning of women acceptable and inspired public concern for what happens in her innards? And, finally, the embarrassing question: how was it possible to mobilise so many women as uncomplaining agents of this skinning and as willing witnesses to this haunting symbol of loneliness?[19]

The emergence of this 'isolated goblin' and its disciplinary implications for the pregnant body can be seen in the array of sociological, psychological and theoretical examinations of the impact of visual technologies. Here, I consider three different expositions of the meaning of ultrasound which demonstrate my argument of the exclusion of the placental body. The disciplinary separations of the pregnant body into two entities, maternal and foetal, serve to contain and defend against the contagious possibilities of a corporeal entity that continually renegotiates and reformulates the relation between body, self and other bodies.

The use of the image to distinguish the maternal body from the foetal body allows the material irreducibility of the relation of pregnancy to be subsumed beneath other frames of reference. In each of the three instances I have chosen, these other frames of reference and their differences from each other, are evident. I consider these apparent differences in meanings attributed to the ultrasound and draw out a common framing of the pregnant body that highlights the complexity of that body as well as the anxious drive to simplify these complications. I work to position the 'placental body' in these frames.

Margrete Sandelowski conducted a study of the differing effects of ultrasound on couples. She noted the 'prosthetic effect' of ultrasound for males, where 'vision' was seen to improve the relations of putative fathers with the developing foetuses. Women in the study, on the other hand, felt their relations with the developing foetus were in some way compromised by this visibility.[20] The privacy and opacity of pregnancy was shifted into the visual field and their intimate experience of it was somehow diminished. Several relevant themes emerge from this analysis. The putative visibility of the foetus gives it a presence in the world, rather than just in the body of the woman. For the male in the couple, this allowed a relationship with the foetus to develop. This mode of 'meeting' the foetus is preferred over other knowledge available through touch, for example. For the pregnant women in the study, this reordering of knowledge was a disquieting one. The emphasis shifts from corporeal recognitions (the touch of the hand on the belly, the surface of the interior in contact with the expanding uterus and foetal activity) to iconic visual representations.[21] In two senses, the knowledge of the body is displaced in favour of another way of knowing. The body as the object of knowledge, that is the seat of the physical sensations of pregnancy and its signs including the cessation of menstruation, is overwritten by the image of the foetus as unattached entity on the screen. But the productive corporeality of the 'placental body' is excluded also. The development of the foetus is now measured in centimetres on the screen, rather than through the shifting processes of gestation. In the image of foetus as formed, the epigenetic nature of foetal development is obscured. Rather than depicting foetal development as a process, where the embryo becomes more complex morphologically at each point, these images argue that size is the only element of change.[22] The appearance of the foetus on the screen effectively erases the bodily processes of pregnancy.

Elisabeth Roberts argues for this formulation of the meaning of ultrasound, when she considers its use in situations of surrogacy. Her view is that the ultrasound connects the commissioning couple with the baby, while severing or disturbing the surrogate's attachment to the foetus.[23] As in Sandelowski's study, the visibility of the foetus reformulates the physical and social relations of the foetal and maternal entities. It comes to have presence in the world, not in connection with the pregnant woman, but as a discrete entity. There is an added element here as the potential for disassociation is viewed as a positive one, since the pregnant woman is contracted or committed to handing the baby to the commissioning couple. The corporeal non-subjective process of pregnancy, the productive physical work of the pregnant woman, is resituated in the world of exchange and intention. This reading of the use of ultrasound locates the pregnant body as the instrument, where a maternal subject uses the body to produce the baby. In both instances, the discrete visibility of the foetus overrides the corporeal connection.

In apparent contrast, John Stoltenberg argues that ultrasound technology is being used in the US in the case of women intending abortion in order to encourage or enforce a sense of relation.

> [O]rdinances are being enacted on the city level across the country to require abortion patients to be shown pictures of foetal development

and to be told they might have emotional problems if they go through with an abortion.[24]

The foetal images are meant to affirm and stimulate the relationship between the woman intending abortion and her foetus. Although this appears to contradict the earlier interpretations of ultrasound cited, the visual image of the foetus is again being given precedence as defining and informing the meaning of pregnancy. The bodily experience of the pregnant woman is not viewed as relational in itself – instead, images are offered as a prophylactic for the apparently imperfect corporeal relation. The visible presence of the foetus, and not its corporeal interconnection with the maternal body through the placenta, is offered as the important vector of relation.

These interpretations of the import of ultrasound are not intended to offer a determinate reading of women's responses to ultrasound. As Sandelowski's study indicated, women's responses to the incursion of the visual may be distinct discomfort with the implications of the visible pregnancy. The visual may also provide a pleasurable possibility, as Adams's article argued. The specificity and context of each individual pregnancy and ultrasound cannot be fully encompassed in any of these scenarios or in any interpretation I could offer. But the routine use of ultrasound and the increasing emphasis on the visual pregnancy now necessarily forms part of any embodied experience of pregnancy. While the impact of the visualisation of pregnancy cannot be fixed, the proliferation of visual images of the foetus in culture as well as specific medical experiences inevitably form part of pregnancy. In the three examples cited above, the erosion of meaning from the work of the pregnant body that is non-intentional is consistent across each of these instances and warrants attention. The invisibility of the woman's body in the image, the clinical context and the social exchanges around it, circumscribe the material experience of gestation and its meaning. The incursion of the visible serves to refigure the work and meaning of pregnancy for the pregnant embodied subject and the others. The placental body, with its uncertain edges, its fluidity of constitution and its complex mixture of subjective intent and bodily activity, cannot fit comfortably within these frames where subjective intention and the instrumentality of the body are central. In an 'ideal' pregnancy, the potential contaminants of alcohol, coffee and other substances are not allowed to cross into the placenta for fear that they will affect the foetus. In the ideal image of pregnancy, the placenta is not allowed to cross into images of pregnancy for fear that its unsecured edges could destabilise the important boundaries secured in the visual field.

In these deployments of the visual technologies, the full extent of the pregnant body's activity and import are obscured. The visible register brings the foetus forth from the maternal body and apparently distinguishes it from the intermingled, interdependent corporeality of pregnancy.

These technologies allow us to read the pregnant body through frames we understand. Cathryn Vasseleu describes the role of these prosthetic devices in constructing visible objects as the 'perversion of the possibility of resemblance'.[25] They compose a picture that can sit comfortably in our cartography of selves. The placental body brought into the frame and into focus offers a disquieting perversion of the embodied subject. The sense of seepage as threatening to the visually distinguished edges of the body is contested in the productive contagion of the placental body. The challenges of the placental body, with its potential for multiple entities and complex relations of conflict, connection and contamination cannot fit easily into the available body/subject frames. Visual representations of gestation seek to contain these implications.

The modes of visualisation I have described demonstrate a drive to contain the implications of the placental body. The inability of the subject self fully to control the pregnant body corpus, to control the spaces of this opaque, messy and multiplying body, represent a threat or a challenge. The inability of a bounded subject to define secure edges causes anxiety, so in our cultural and technological imagination, we make women pregnant in ways that are consonant with our commitment to single embodied self. Through the medium of visual technology, the lack of control that the embodied subject has over the placental body is obscured. The actual and potential seepage, across the pregnant body and the foetal entity, across all bounded bodies produced in this process, is stilled. The productive communication of fluid, matter and subjectivity is erased – the contagion implicit in the construction of the embodied self is displaced through the visual disciplining of the pregnant body.

The strictures that the pregnant body attracts offer grounds for its re-examination in these ways. Multiple divisions regulate the pregnant body. In legal discourses, the impetus has been to establish a series of rights, which constitute pregnant woman and foetal entity as oppositional. In medical discourse, the pregnant body has become the opaque, unsafe and potentially disposable frame for the foetal body; it is the dangerous womb, the surrogate uterus, and the container. And, as Young points out, pregnancy has been regulated in the separation of motherhood and sexuality, which subtends cultural discourses as diverse as fashion magazines and women's own experiential accounts.[26] When I view the pregnant body through the placenta, it is a challenge to representational order, for it is necessarily, at least, two-in-one.[27] It confronts distinctions between 'mother' and 'child', mother and sexual being, as well as confronting the practice of binary thinking. It refuses comfortable distinctions between self and other, subject and object, body and mind. In its insistence that the corporeal does not allow for the assignation of a determined subjectivity, it confronts the continuous use of the body as tool for the establishment and maintenance of the self. It suggests that porous edges, rather than threatening the subject, are the very matter of and precondition for its constitution.

The contagious nature of the 'placental body' is recognised already in medical and cultural discourse. The identification of the placenta as the site for the transmission of alcohol and drugs has been the most obvious sign of this. Pictures of drug-addicted babies in withdrawal continually grace newspapers, brochures and public health promotion posters. How much coffee, wine and folic acid to consume when pregnant are matters for public discussion as well as individual determination. But, as Cynthia Daniels has identified, this recognition of the complexity of the pregnant body has always been used to confine and constrain the pregnant woman.[28] In reformulating this contagion as theoretical possibility and necessarily constitutive physiological activity, new definitions of subjectivity become possible. The relationship between the body and the subject are understood as fluid, multidirectional and simultaneously bounded and expansive. In its morphological complexity and uncertainty, the placenta in the body stretches the boundaries of discrete selves and subjectivities. In its recognition of a plural embodiment, it challenges the corporeal as a comfortable site for the location of self. In its failure to be activated or controlled by the dictates of the conscious subject, it marks the body's excess. This body challenges the hierarchical ordering of self-identity and self-extension through the corporeal, but it does not dissolve the mind/body distinction. Although marked out in uncertain and shifting boundaries, placenta, foetal presence and gestating woman must adhere to each other. The border between body and subject continues to exist, but the placental body allows for the transmission of fluid and meaning across those borders. The corporeal coexists with the subjective experience in a bodily process that is both productive and challenging for the embodied subject. This reading of the placental body argues for a positive exploitation of this contagious possibility. As the body borders of the pregnant subject dissolve and reformulate around the edges of the mind/body distinction, so other bodies may be redrawn through different formulations of this troubled binary.

Notes

1 This point derives from Lacan's imagining of the mirror stage, where the infant recognises itself as a unified entity in the mirror, thereby providing itself with necessary misperception for the assertion of the unified subject position.
2 K. Kirby, 'RE Mapping Subjectivity: Cartographic Vision and the Limits of Politics', in N. Duncan (ed.), *BodySpace: Destabilising Geographies of Gender and Sexuality*, London and New York, Routledge, 1996, p. 43.
3 L. Irigaray, *je, tu, nous: Toward a Culture of Difference*, trans. A. Martin, London and New York, Routledge, 1993, pp. 41–2.
4 I. M. Young, 'Pregnant Embodiment', in *Throwing Like A Girl and Other Essays in Feminist Philosophy*, Bloomington, Ind., Indiana University Press, 1990, pp. 160–4.
5 R. Diprose, *The Bodies of Women: Ethics, Embodiment and Sexual Difference*, London and New York, Routledge, 1994, p. 108.
6 Ibid., p. 106.

7 Irigaray, *je, tu, nous*, pp. 41–2.
8 Ibid. [My emphasis]
9 S. M. Squier, *Babies in Bottles: Twentieth-Century Visions of Reproductive Technologies*, New Brunswick, Can., Rutgers University Press, 1994, pp. 96–7.
10 M. Warnock, *A Question of Life: The Warnock Report on Human Fertilisation and Embryology*, Oxford, Basil Blackwell, 1984.
11 For a discussion of the competing evidences adduced, see M. Strathern, *Reproducing the Future: Anthropology, Kinship and the New Reproductive Technologies*, New York, Routledge, 1992, pp. 20–30.
12 The first sequence of photographs appeared in *Life* in 1966, the second in 1990. The first series of photographs formed the basis of the book *A Child is Born*. Again, the slippage of terminology in the title adds depth to the contention that the frames, offered for decoding these pictures, envisage very particular outcomes. The image of the foetus is in utero, the *born* of the title can only refer to the notion of the child being reinserted back into the womb. For further discussions, see K. Newman, *Fetal Positions: Individualism, Science and Visuality*, Stanford, Calif., California University Press, 1996, pp. 13 ff. and C. Stabile, *Feminism and the Technological Fix*, Manchester and New York, Manchester University Press, 1994, pp. 77 ff.
13 In a formulation which has significant resonance with the way I position the placenta, M. Strathern describes a 'fractal person' as 'one with a relationship implied'. This sense of incomplete embodied existence, that which suggests in its form its connection to other, is apposite here for my argument that the placenta is always marking out a mode of embodied interdependence. See Strathern, *Reproducing the Future*, p. 152.
14 For further discussions, see B. Katz Rothman, *Recreating Motherhood: Ideology and Technology in a Patriarchal Society*, London and New York, W. W. Norton & Sons, 1989, pp. 91 ff. and C. Daniels, 'Between Fathers and Fetuses: The Social Construction of Male Reproduction and the Politics of Fetal Harm', *Signs*, 1997, vol. 22, pp. 581 ff.
15 E. Grosz, *Volatile Bodies: Towards a Corporeal Feminism*, St Leonards, UK, Allen and Unwin, 1994, pp. 193–4.
16 Katz Rothman, *Motherhood Reconsidered*, p. 91.
17 S. Freud, 'Instincts and their Vicissitudes', *The Essentials of Psychoanalysis*, London, Penguin Books, 1986, pp. 202–4.
18 Many theorists have addressed these issues. See e.g. D. Condit, 'Fetal Personhood: Political Identity under Construction', in P. Boling (ed.), *Expecting Trouble: Surrogacy, Fetal Abuse and New Reproductive Technologies*, Boulder, Colo., San Francisco and Oxford, Westview Press, 1995; C. Daniels, *Women's Expense: State Power and the Politics of Fetal Rights*, Cambridge, Mass., and London, Harvard University Press, 1993; V. Hartouni, *Cultural Conceptions: On Reproductive Technologies and the Remaking of Life*, Minneapolis and London, Minnesota University Press, 1997; Newman, *Fetal Positions*; D. Roberts, *Killing the Black Body: Race, Reproduction and the Meaning of Liberty*, New York, Pantheon Books, 1997.
19 B. Duden, *Disembodying Women: Perspectives on Pregnancy and the Unborn*, trans. L. Hoinacki, Cambridge, Mass., and London, Harvard University Press, 1993, p. 7.
20 M. Sandelowski, 'Separate but Less Unequal: Fetal Ultrasonography and the Transformation of Expectant Mother/Fatherhood', *Gender & Society*, 1993, vol. 8, p. 232.
21 In an insightful article, Alice Adams locates this technological formulation at the basis of her relationship with her foetus. She conjoins the visualisation technologies with narratives of the Enlightenment and contends that both represent a desire to egress from the womb. She traces the ways *in-body* gestation is rendered

as the problem that must be overcome in fiction, philosophy and obstetrical discourses. See A. Adams, 'Out of the Womb: The Future of the Uterine Metaphor', *Feminist Studies*, 1993, vol. 19, pp. 269–89.
22 N. Tuana, 'Re-Fusing Nature/Nurture', in A. al-Hibri and M. Simons (eds), *Hypatia Reborn: Essays in Feminist Philosophy*, Bloomington, Ind., and Indianapolis, Indiana University Press, 1990, p. 82.
23 E. Roberts, '"Native" Narratives of Connectedness: Surrogate Motherhood and Technology', in R. Davis-Floyd and J. Dumit (eds), *Cyborg Babies: From Techno-Sex to Techno-Tots*, New York and London, Routledge, 1998, p. 205.
24 J. Stoltenberg, 'The Fetus and the Penis: Men's Self-Interest and Abortion Rights', in *Refusing to Be a Man: Essays on Sex and Justice*, Portland, Or., Breitenbush Books, 1989, p. 93. Rosalind Pollack Petchesky makes a similar point, suggesting that the visual production of the foetal image is deployed by anti-abortion activists as a tactic to resolve ambivalent feelings in favour of the continuation of pregnancy. See R. Petchesky, 'Fetal Images: The Power of Visual Culture in the Politics of Reproduction', in M. Stanworth (ed.), *Reproductive Technologies: Gender, Motherhood and Medicine*, Minneapolis, Minnesota University Press, 1987, pp. 55ff.
25 C. Vasseleu, 'Life Itself', in R. Diprose and R. Ferrell (eds), *Cartographies: Postmodernism and the Mapping of the Subject*, Sydney, Allen and Unwin, 1991, pp. 56–7.
26 Young, 'Pregnant Embodiment', p. 198.
27 Irigaray's argument in 'When our Lips Speak Together' bases itself on a similar morphological moment. See L. Irigaray, *This Sex Which is Not One*, trans. C. Porter, Ithaca, NY, Cornell University Press, 1985 [1977].
28 C. Daniels, 'Between Fathers and Fetuses', pp. 580–2

11 Carrier
– becoming symborg

Melinda Rackham
www.subtle.net/carrier

sHe recognises you

sHe reaches out
with sticky hands

sHe invites you in . . .

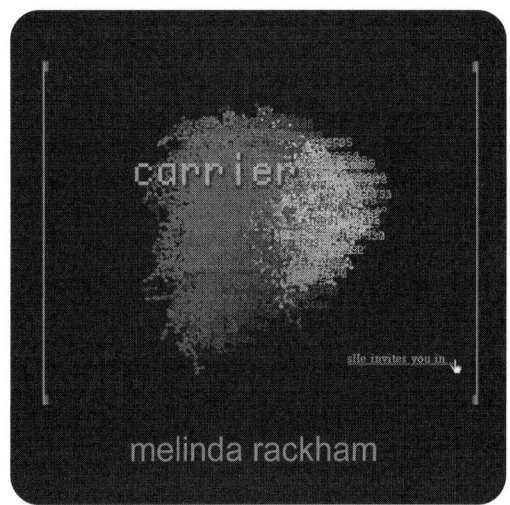

a virus has burrowed deep inside me,
sHe has penetrated my cellular core . . .
breaching my last boundary,
shattering my last illusion of autonomy.

cross-dressed in a seductively innocent protoplasmic envelope,
sHe slips past the antibodies and nestles safely
within the folds of my DNA;
whispering in the secret language of my body
'replicate me, replicate me'
her strands of RNA twisting and twining with mine –
conjugating, slicing, merging, integrating.

I am infected,
my blood is contagion,
I am hostess to another being.

I am a carrier.

Viral merging is both exciting and dangerous. When human biological code has a symbiotic relationship with another species' biological code, we cross a sacred boundary, that of the disciplined, normalised, healthy body; the body of the controlled social subject who maintains a defence against disease as a moral imperative. As Deleuze and Guattari told us, 'you will be organised, you will be an organism, you will articulate your body, otherwise you are just depraved'.[1]

Morality in the maintenance of *good* health has been well explored by Foucault amongst others, however with the explosion of the Human Immunodeficiency Virus (HIV) in the 1980s, political and bio-medical discourse around viral illness shifted from one of moral imperative into a militarised zone. Viral infection became an 'information transgression' within the 'strategic system of our immune system',[2] and the body a territory of hierarchical attack and defence mechanisms against alien invaders. By engaging in this Star Wars strategy of disassociation from the body, the patriotic duty of anyone who was a viral carrier was to fight the enemy within, and not transmit the virus by contact with others. Non transmission of body fluids, especially blood, and denial of the flesh, enforced the self contained, closed off, and now disembodied citizen.

This was also the era of Richard Dawkins's *The Selfish Gene*, where our own genetic code mutated in the popular imagination into a detached, immoral, survival machine – 'leaping from body to body, down the generations, manipulating body after body, in its own way, for its own ends, abandoning a succession of mortal bodies before they sink into senility and death'.[3] We stopped living in our own bodies as they no longer represented the self. The ties of kinship and blood degenerated, and in a desperate attempt to redefine who and what we were, we tried to comprehend and control our own genetic code by categorisation and classification in the Human Genome Project.[4]

But what of the viral invaders – those others that wished to subvert our now sanitised, classified code for their own purposes? During the 1990s the virus mutated into a convenient political commodity, replacing the aliens of 1950s science fiction as the evil, threatening, uncontrollable, deadly, ugly, enemy in mainstream culture. We watched movies like *Outbreak*, dramatising the horror of uncontrolled viral invasion, and consumed books like Richard Preston's *The Hotzone*, a sensational account of the wicked witch of viruses, Ebola.

> sHe:
>
> transforms virtually every part of the body into a digested slime of virus particles . . . the skin bubbles up into a sea of white blisters . . . like tapioca pudding. Spontaneous rips appear in the skin and haemorrhagic blood pours from them . . . every opening of the body bleeds . . . the tongue's skin may be torn off during rushes of

the black vomit . . . your heart bleeds into itself, the brain becomes
clogged with dead blood cells, the liver bulges, turns yellow and
begins to liquefy . . . the testicles bloat up and turn black and blue,
the semen goes hot with Ebola and the nipples may bleed . . . the
labia turns blue, livid and protrusive, and there may be massive
vaginal bleeding . . . the whole body twitches and shakes, the arms
and legs thrash around, the eyes roll up into the head.[5]

This eroticised description of a viral bleed out exemplifies our fascination with the appalling or appealing abject, with embodied disease, and with death. But Ebola, although sensational, is not terribly effective as a species, and is no threat to huManity, as sHe kills too quickly. To be effective viruses need to be more compliant with the host system.

On the other hand, *smart* viruses like HIV and the Hepatitis C Virus (HCV) evade recognition by the human immune system, allowing replication in a complex species-specific relationship. They can be seen as *lying* to the host system, *mimicking* the feel of the body's own antigens, *crossdressing* so that they will be allowed to complete their reproduction cycle. Smart viruses create a false sense of balance, so that the host body will not immediately die. HCV is far more successful in this respect, and will kill more humans than HIV, as it sometimes takes up to twenty years before the host's bodily organs start to seriously malfunction, throughout which time the person is infectious and capable of transmission. These viruses already know how to speak the language of the body while bio-medical science still struggles with its limited genetic alphabet of **C A G T**.[6]

contagion = = evolution

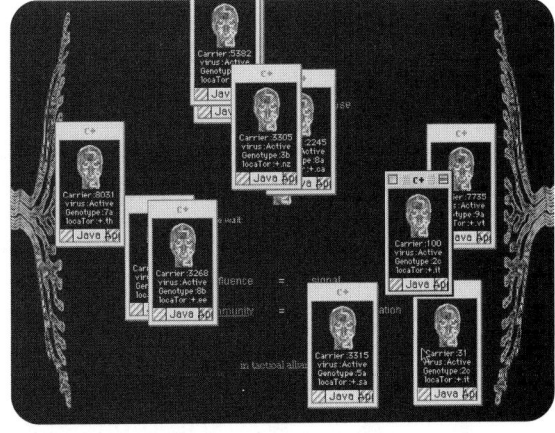

Our disassociation from the bio-self, otherwise known as the body, coupled with our yearning for connection, have deceived us into thinking that we can embrace another domain; that of interrelating, clean pure code. The romanticised telematic embrace – contact totally mediated by technology

– is in reality, an ill-conceived cyborg fantasy. Ironically contagion and disease are also rampant in the electronic arena, where packets of data are in constant transmission from one machine to another in the network of our global information systems, the nervous system of our planet, the ubiquitous Internet. Just as small pieces of viral code can whisper 'replicate me, replicate me' and jump promiscuously from body to body via warm sticky blood, small pieces of code – appropriately cross-dressed in binary code to evade recognition – jump promiscuously from machine host to machine host, via dynamically streaming data networks.

Melissa, 1999's celebrity virus, could insert herself into your data because sHe spoke the secret language of machine code that most users do not understand. However Melissa, who was named after a stripper, wasn't a femme fatale. sHe didn't actually do great damage to any individual machine, instead sHe just replicated herself fifty times via email and clogged up networks, just as HCV doesn't damage the host body itself, just clogs the networks in the liver, until network collapse affects the larger organism.

When the **host / body / machine** is sited as a battleground, and viral invaders as the enemy within to be exterminated at all costs, we lose the opportunity of viewing them as interesting and successfully evolved examples of another intelligence. Responding to viral life, whether it be biological or binary code with anti-viral drugs and anti-viral software like Interferon (a treatment option for both humans and machines) indicates that the exterminators see themselves at the central pinnacle of a hierarchical universe, in the exhausting position of constantly defending territories.

It is understandable that as a species we fear her, the virus, and her ugly sisters in the archestista.[7] sHe is an alien who speaks a language we don't understand and sHe may want to use our bodies for her reproduction. Why shouldn't we shoot first and ask questions later? Paradoxically, as fear of the intelligence of the organic virus grows, software engineers are focused on generating artificial intelligence, trying to create 'interactive organisation based upon the distributed problem solving capacity of myriads of cell swarms working in parallel' in the computer environment.[8] Strangely, with the intent of completely removing life from bio-hosts, artificial life (a.life) research still classically imitates the human model of bi-parental sex, producing offspring code within the microcosm of the machine host.

■   ■   ■   sHe promiscuously slips

                        her lipid envelope

                                inside you

This artificial parenting, this sexuality of binary code, of zero uniting with one, is 'limited finity', where a finite number of components are capable of producing an unlimited diversity of combinations.[9] Difference here, or call it evolution, is not the result of random mutation or chaos, but of the continual application of fixed rules, with limited components. Un-thought-of symbiosis of seemingly different functional beings, produces surprising multiplicities and swarming functional colonies of zeros and little ones.

Apparently, even in the machine world, opposites do attract. Uniting one and zero is wildly explosive – one (with whom we are more familiar) is a rather egotistical self-centred static and defined singular Westerner, indivisible and individuated. Meanwhile the exotic Eastern zero, who brings her own *intension*, is dynamically relational, is multiply functional; she subtly controls meaning via her position. Together they do not balance one and other out. Instead, they conform to the definition of a.life or artificial intelligence, by their sum being greater than their parts.

> Zero, or nothingness, was at the core of the peaceful agricultural goddess worshipping tribes living in the Indus valley 5000 years ago. sHe, the void, is the container of all possibilities, a swarming energetic consciousness encompassing everything within the cosmos, from viruses and bacteria at the microscopic level to the macroscopic universe itself. Her number, zero, was imported to the west by Arabic traders around 700 AD but was thought of as immoral and heretic, alien and destabilising, and its use forbidden by the Catholic Church.[10] Eventually the Zero virus was transmitted into popular usage at the start of the information revolution by the Gutenberg press, and Zero has successfully now infected and affected every system of western culture.

> But we have wandered away from sex itself. Tantric sexual ritual, like zero, is all about position. Ritual sex begins with the man positioned at the right-hand side and the woman at the left, which is the origin of what is known as the left-hand path – the way of the flesh, the way of the feminine.[11] Traditionally this left-handed pathway encompasses spirituality, magic, messiness, darkness, the sexual, the textured, the sensual; while the right has attracted the oppositional values of masculine Cartesian rationality – the light seeping into the Platonic cave. Nowhere is this duality more obvious than in cultures where the clean right-handed masculine puts food in one's mouth, while the dirty left-hand feminine completes the circuit of biological survival by wiping one's anus.

In Tantra sex is transmutation of energy, and in biology sex is the combination of genetic material from more than one source to produce a new individual. By these definitions, viral cross-species merging is sexuality in its rawest form. A virus inserts its genetic material inside our cells, using our proteins to make an offspring, an almost perfect copy of itself. So perhaps the fear of illness, of being sick, of being a carrier, is only the fear of the sexual body itself, is the fear of zero, is the fear of the feminine, is the fear of the sex

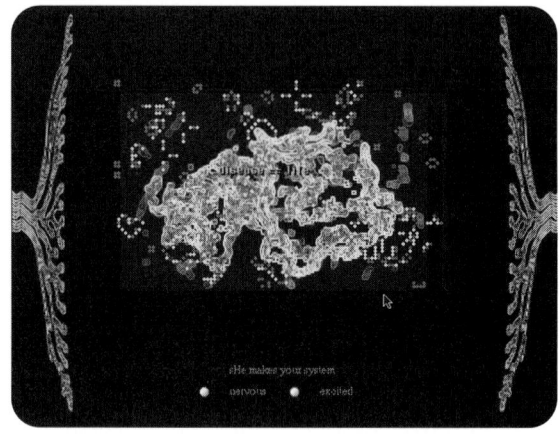

which is not one, is the fear of merging and joining, of transmuting beyond the singularity of the discreet individual, is the fear of not being in control.

Evolutionary biologists Lynn Margulis and Dorion Sagan tell us:

> Symbiosis has a filthy lesson to teach us. The human is an integrated colony of amoeboid beings ... (which are) integrated colonies of bacteria. Like it or not our origins are in *slime*. The nucleated cell of eukaryotic life evolved by acquisition ... amid cell gorgings and aborted invasions, merged beings that infected one another were reinvigorated by the incorporation of their permanent 'disease'.[12]

We *become*, we *evolve* with our symbionts, our most intimate partners, and we cannot survive without them. Shockingly our evolutionary partners proliferate as species more successful than our own. There are more than fifty thousand human endogenous retroviruses that can easily slip into our genetic material, like the Human Mammary Tumour Virus, which is passed down the generational pathway; and hundreds of thousands more viruses that jump from person to person as swiftly as opportunistic fleas at a dog show. Our body of matter, our left-handed pathway, the dark fleshy arena, our own swarming cellular republic, is a hive of activity – the activity of viral otherness.

> sHe
> extends
> you
> \>\>
> code
> grafted
> to
> code
> in
> identical
> machine
> language

We have never been, and never will be, clean and sanitary self-contained units. Alternate theories of the integrated immune system that see our bodies as just another part of the web of living organisms, like Niels Jerne's[13] Nobel Prize winning Network Theory of Immunity, were largely ignored for years by sanitarily obsessed mainstream bio-medical researchers. Jerne's theory proposes that:

> The (Immune) system has no way and no need to distinguish self from foreign. It knows nothing alien to its composition. It only knows of itself and itself is the network of endogenous activity . . . By means of somatic mutation it has already anticipated, inside 'self,' every variety of the 'nonself' that it could ever meet.[14]

There is no self and other, no need for *attack* and *defence* as we are already intimately connected with every virus on the planet. From this perspective we are not a divided species, we are just different manifestations of identical machine language, all of us parasites on the body of the planet earth.

I now speak of the virus as my lover, my cross-dressing identical twin lover, who has slipped into my immune system, smiling at me, seducing me – whispering in my body's secret language 'come with me now, we are together forever, child of my blood, we cannot be parted, we are one'.[15] This is viral bonding, this is true love, this is real romance. sHe makes a commitment like no other, and in the days of serial relating, it really is **till death us do part**.

Of course, this is not to be ignorant of the implications of being *sick* in both biological viral merging and machine viral integration. For the 200 million humans currently with HCV it may mean altered lifestyle, extreme fatigue, depression, development of cirrhosis, liver cancer, and death. For infected machines it may mean altered functioning, loss of data, hard drive death, network collapse. However, as species, both will modify and survive, and the future of each is dependent on these mutations, these code splicings, this diversity and difference, which enables survival under a variety of environmental conditions.

When our point of view expands from our species singularity, to a more encompassing macro perspective, surprisingly similar complex systems emerge in parallel domains. Biological carriers of HCV have formed global connections, both through their similarly emerging biology, and on the web through mailing lists and support groups, sharing their experience in differing contexts. These carriers are an emerging swarm, a global republic whose biological source code is open and being modified by the virus. Simultaneously computer code is hacked, viruses are written and software is modified under Open Source agreements. Programmers improve and evolve machine language co-operatively, for no money, and with no overt political agenda. Co-operative coders, or hackers as they used to be called, are also an emerging swarm, operating singularly with a higher purpose. This is an evolution of artificial intelligence on our planet as code is replicated, refined and embedded by willing workers, in self organising systems, swarming within the electronic nervous system of the net.

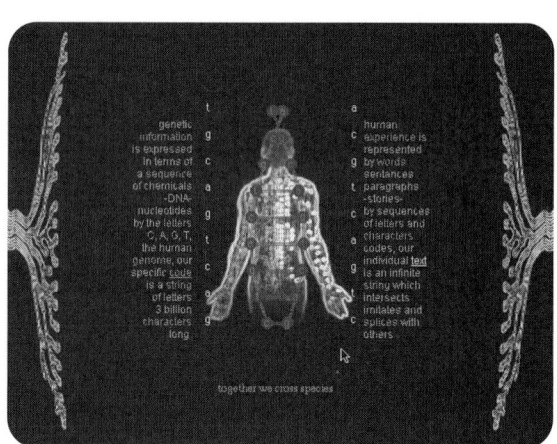

Open source software (OSS) is released under 'copyleft', a licensing agreement where it can be endlessly copied and modified – anyone can become a carrier in this millennial remergence of the left-handed path. Software evolution, like species evolution, is not linear, it is rhizomic, transversal, a process not of travel from one form to another, but a process of decoding and recoding.¹⁶ This process is parallel to that of decoding and recoding employed by reverse transcriptease enzymes that insert viral genetic material into human cells, when HCV reproduces in the hostess body.

The fantasy of sanitised safety with pure, clean and rational code is consumed by the reality of the slimey and promiscuous, as code has sex with other codes – they decode, insert, recode, replicate, and integrate in both the immune system and the operating system. We can no longer ignore viral life as the age of information is increasingly the age of infection. The viruses are encouraging us, their human and machine carriers, to become re-acquainted with the left-handed path, with the messy, ugly, multi-textured swarming cellular self.

HuManity is slow to acknowledge its mutual dependence, its transpersonal ecology, and its symbiogenesis. We still battle with wanting to be one, individualised and contained, rather than seeing the delicate webs which maintain selfhood through intensions and relations. We are just starting to shift our perspective to encompass Helen Chadwick's sublime vision of more than a decade ago:

> sHe laps
> your cellular
> shore line
> as
> her viscous
> slime
> envelops you

'The living integrates with other in an infinite continuity of matter, and welcomes difference not as damage but potential. . . . Spliced together by data processing, these are not ruined catastrophic surfaces but territories of prolific encounter, the exchange of living informational systems at the shoreline of culture'.¹⁷

> sHe, the poisonous slimy deadly virus,
> now provides us with an updated cyborg model,
> a way to culturally reposition ourselves
> in the dissolving **natural / artificial / species** divide.

> a place to ground the self
> when being one,
> being an individual,
> a self contained singularity
> is no longer a stable position.

> sHe, our viral lover,
> transmits intimate knowledge
> in the embodied language of disease,
> encouraging us to embrace and enjoy
>
> becoming symborg.

Notes

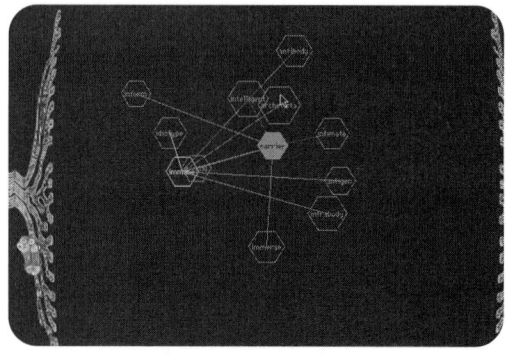

1. G. Deleuze and F. Guattari, *A Thousand Plateaus*, Minneapolis, University of Minnesota, 1987, p. 159.
2. D. J. Haraway, 'The Biopolitics of Postmodern Bodies: Constitutions of Self in Immune System Discourse', *Simians, Cyborgs, and Women*, London, Free Association Books, 1991, pp. 203–30.
3. R. Dawkins, *The Selfish Gene*, New York, Oxford University Press, 1976, p. 36.
4. The Human Genome Project was initiated by US Congress in 1987, seeking to map the approximately 100,000 genetic stands that make up the entire DNA sequence of humans, within 20 years. The project has many opponents, including those who believe it will be used to support theories of genetic determinism. One of the first worrying outcomes of genome mapping was in 1995 when the US Government patented the cell line of a Papua New Guinea Highlander.
5. R. Preston, *The Hot Zone*, Sydney, Doubleday, 1994, pp. 81–3.
6. A, G, C, and T are the nucleotide bases Adenine, Guanine, Cytosine, and Thymine. By determining the sequence or position of these bases along a DNA strand, genes can be identified.
7. The domain of viral life.
8. J. Hoffmeyer, *The Swarming Body*. Online. Available http://www.molbio.ku.dk/MolBioPages/abk/PersonalPages/Jesper/Swarm.html
9. K. Ansell Pearson, *Germinal Life – the Difference and Repetition of Deleuze*, London and New York, Routledge, 1999, p. 221.
10. S. Plant, *Zeros + Ones*, London, Fourth Estate, 1998, pp. 51–5.
11. For a full description of various Tantric sexual rituals and beliefs see A. Van Lysebeth, *Tantra – the Cult of the Feminine*, Maine, Samuel Weiser, 1995.
12. L. Margulis and D. Sagan, *What is Life*, London, Weidenfeld and Nicolson, 1995, p. 194.
13. For background and excerpts on Jerne's paper see D. J. Bibel, *Milestones in Immunology*, Berlin, Springer–Verlag, 1990, pp. 188–93.
14. E. Martin, *Flexible Bodies*, Boston, Mass., Beacon Press, 1994, p. 110.
15. Text excerpts from M. Rackham, *carrier*. Online. Available http://www.subtle.net/carrier
16. Ansell Pearson, *Germinal Life*, p. 159.
17. H. Chadwick, *Enfleshings*, London, Secker and Warburg, 1989, p. 97.

All images from website *carrier*, Melinda Rackham, 1999, @ http://www.subtle.net/carrier

Select bibliography

Ackerknecht, E. H., 'Anticontagionism between 1821 and 1867', *Bulletin of the History of Medicine*, 1948, vol. 22, pp. 562–93.
Aisenberg, A. R., *Contagion: Disease, Government, and the 'Social Question' in Nineteenth Century France*, Stanford, Calif., Stanford University Press, 1999.
Anderson, W., 'Immunities of Empire: Race, Disease and the New Tropical Medicine 1900–1920', *Bulletin of the History of Medicine*, 1996, vol. 70, pp. 94–118.
Armstrong, D., 'Public Health Spaces and the Fabrication of Identity', *Sociology*, vol. 27, 1993, pp. 393–410.
—— 'The Rise of Surveillance Medicine', *Sociology of Health and Illness*, 1995, vol. 17, pp. 393–404.
Arnold, D., 'Touching the Body: Perspectives on the Indian Plague, 1896–1900', *Subaltern Studies*, vol. 5, 1987, pp. 55–90.
—— *Colonizing the Body: State Medicine and Epidemic Disease in Nineteenth-Century India*, Berkeley, Calif., University of California Press, 1993.
Baldwin, P., *Contagion and the State in Europe, 1830–1930*, Cambridge, Cambridge University Press, 1999.
Barnes, D. S., *The Making of a Social Disease: Tuberculosis in Nineteenth Century France*, Berkeley, Calif., University of California Press, 1995.
Bartos, M., 'The Queer Excess of Public Health Policy', *Meanjin*, 1996, vol. 55, pp. 122–31.
Bashford, A., *Purity and Pollution: Gender, Embodiment and Victorian Medicine*, Basingstoke, UK, Macmillan, 1998.
—— 'Epidemic and Governmentality: Smallpox in Sydney, 1881', *Critical Public Health*, 1999, vol. 9, pp. 301–16.
—— '"Is White Australia Possible?" Race, Colonialism and Tropical Medicine', *Ethnic and Racial Studies*, 2000, vol. 23, pp. 248–71.
Boffin, T., and Gupta, S. (eds), *Ecstatic Antibodies: Resisting the AIDS Mythology*, London, Rivers Oram Press, 1990.
Brandt, A., *No Magic Bullet: A Social History of Venereal Disease in the United States Since 1880*, New York, Oxford University Press, 1985.
Canguilhem, G., 'Bacteriology and the End of Nineteenth-Century "Medical Theory"', in his *Ideology and Rationality in the History of the Life Sciences*, trans. I. Goldhammer, Cambridge, Mass., and London, MIT Press, 1988.
Carter, K. Codell, 'Ignaz Semmelweis, Carl Mayrhofer and the Rise of Germ Theory', *Medical History*, 1985, vol. 29, pp. 33–53.

—— 'The Development of Pasteur's Concept of Disease Causation and the Emergence of Specific Causes in Nineteenth Century Medicine', *Bulletin of the History of Medicine*, 1991, vol. 65, pp. 528–48.

Cooter, R., 'Anticontagionism and History's Medical Record', in P. Wright and A. Treacher (eds), *The Problem of Medical Knowledge: Examining the Social Construction of Medicine*, Edinburgh, Edinburgh University Press, 1982.

Corbin, A., *The Foul and the Fragrant: Odor and the French Social Imagination*, trans. M. L. Kochan, R. Porter and C. Prendergast, Cambridge, Mass., Harvard University Press, 1986.

—— *Women for Hire: Prostitution and Sexuality in France After 1850*, trans. A. Sheridan, Cambridge, Mass., Harvard University Press, 1990.

Crosby, A. W., *Ecological Imperialism: The Biological Expansion of Europe, 900–1900*, Cambridge, Cambridge University Press, 1986.

Cunningham, A., and Williams, P. (eds), *The Laboratory Revolution in Medicine*, Cambridge, Cambridge University Press, 1992.

Curson, P. H., *Times of Crisis: Epidemics in Sydney 1788–1900*, Sydney, Sydney University Press, 1985.

Curtin, P. D., *Death by Migration: Europe's Encounter with the Tropical World in the Nineteenth Century*, Cambridge, Cambride University Press, 1989.

Delaporte, F., *Disease and Civilisation: The Cholera in Paris, 1832*, trans. A. Goldhammer, Cambridge, Mass., MIT Press, 1986.

Douglas, M., *Purity and Danger, An Analysis of the Concepts of Pollution and Taboo*, London, Routledge, 1994.

Douglas, M., and Calvez, M., 'The Self as Risk-Taker: A Cultural Theory of Contagion in Relation to AIDS', *Sociological Review*, 1990, vol. 38, pp. 445–64.

Epstein, S., 'Moral Contagion and the Medicalisation of Gay Identity: AIDS in Historical Perspective', *Research in Law, Deviance and Social Control*, 1988, vol. 9, pp. 3–36.

Erni, J. Nguyet, *Unstable Frontiers: Technomedicine and the Cultural Politics of 'Curing' AIDS*, Minneapolis and London, University of Minnesota Press, 1994.

Ernst, W., and Harris, B. (eds), *Race, Science and Medicine, 1700–1960*, London, Routledge, 1999.

Fox, N., 'Scientific Theory Choice and Social Structure: The Case of Joseph Lister's Antisepsis, Humoral Theory and Asepsis', *History of Science*, 1988, vol. 26, pp. 367–97.

Gilman, S., 'AIDS and Syphilis: The Iconography of Disease', in D. Crimp (ed.), *AIDS: Cultural Analysis, Cultural Activism*, Cambridge, Mass., MIT Press, 1988.

—— 'Plague in Germany, 1939/1989: Cultural Images of Race, Space and Disease', in A. Parker, M. Russo, D. Sommer *et al.* (eds), *Nationalisms and Sexualities*, New York, Routledge, 1992.

—— *Health and Illness: Images of Difference*, London, Reaktion Books, 1995.

Goldstein, J., '"Moral Contagion": A Professional Ideology of Medicine and Psychiatry in Eighteenth- and Nineteenth-Century France', in G. L. Geison (ed.), *Professions and the French State, 1700–1900*, Philadelphia, University of Pennsylvania Press, 1984, pp. 181–222.

Gussow, Z., *Leprosy, Racism and Public Health: Social Policy in Chronic Disease Control*, Boulder, Colo., Westview Press, 1989.

Hamlin, C., 'Predisposing Causes and Public Health in Early Nineteenth Century Medical Thought', *Social History of Medicine*, 1992, vol. 5, pp. 43–70.

Haraway, D., 'The Biopolitics of Postmodern Bodies: Constructions of Self in Immune System Discourse', in her *Simians, Cyborgs and Women: The Reinvention of Nature*, New York, Routledge, 1991.
—— *Modest_Witness@Second_Millennium*, New York and London, Routledge, 1997.
Hardy, A., *The Epidemic Streets: Infectious Disease and the Rise of Preventive Medicine, 1856–1900*, Oxford, Clarendon Press, 1993.
Heaphy, B., 'Medicalisation and Identity Formation: Identity and Strategy in the Context of AIDS and HIV', in J. Weeks and J. Holland (eds), *Sexual Cultures: Communities, Values and Intimacy*, Basingstoke, UK, Macmillan, 1996, pp. 139–60.
Kakar, S., 'Leprosy in British India, 1860–1940', *Medical History*, 1996, vol. 40, pp. 215–30.
Kipple, K., and Beck, S., *Biological Consequences of the European Expansion, 1450–1800*, Aldershot, UK, Ashgate/Variorum, 1997.
Knapp, V., *Disease and its Impact on Modern European History*, Lewiston, New York, E. Press, 1989.
Kraut, A. M., *Silent Travelers: Germs, Genes and the 'Immigrant Menace'*, New York, Basic Books, 1994.
Kristeva, J., *Powers of Horror: An Essay on Abjection*, New York, Columbia University Press, 1982.
Latour, B., *The Pasteurization of France*, trans. A. Sheridan and J. Law, Cambridge, Mass., Harvard University Press, 1988.
Leavitt, J. W., '"Typhoid Mary" Strikes Back: Bacteriological Theory and Practice in Early Twentieth-Century Public Health', *Isis*, 1992, vol. 83, pp. 608–29.
—— *Typhoid Mary: Captive of the Public's Health*, Boston, Mass., Beacon, 1996.
Lerner, B. H., *Contagion and Confinement: Controlling Tuberculosis along the Skid Road*, Baltimore, Johns Hopkins University Press, 1998.
Levine, M., Nardi, P., and Gagnon, J. (eds), *In Changing Times: Gay Men and Lesbians Encounter HIV/AIDS*, Chicago, University of Chicago Press, 1997.
Lupton, D., 'AIDS, Risk and Heterosexuality in the Australian Press', *Discourse and Society*, 1993, vol. 4, pp. 307–28.
—— *The Imperative of Health: Public Health and the Regulated Body*, London, Sage, 1995.
Lupton, D., McCarthy, S., and Chapman, S., ' "Panic Bodies": Discourses on Risk and HIV Antibody Testing', *Sociology of Health and Illness*, 1995, vol. 17, no. 1, pp. 89–108.
Macleod, R., and Lewis, M. (eds), *Disease, Medicine and Empire: Perspectives on Western Medicine and the Experience of European Expansion*, London and New York, Routledge, 1988.
Marks, L., and Worboys, M. (eds), *Migrants, Minorities and Health: Historical and Contemporary Studies*, New York and London, Routledge, 1997.
Martin, E., *Flexible Bodies: The Role of Immunity in American Culture from the Days of Polio to the Age of AIDS*, Boston, Mass., Beacon Press, 1994.
Montgomery, S. L., 'Codes and Combat in Biomedical Discourse', *Science as Culture*, 1991, vol. 2, pp. 341–90.
Morse, S., 'Emerging Viruses: Defining the Rules for Viral Traffic', *Perspectives in Biology and Medicine*, 1991, vol. 34, pp. 387–409.
Ott, K., *Fevered Lives: Tuberculosis in American Culture since 1870*, Cambridge, Mass., and London, Harvard University Press, 1996.
Patton, C., *Inventing AIDS*, London, Routledge, 1990.

—— 'What Science Knows: Formation of AIDS Knowledges', in P. Aggelton, P. Davies and G. Hart (eds), *AIDS: Individual, Cultural and Policy Dimensions*, London, Falmer, 1990, pp. 1–18.

—— 'From Nation to Family: Containing "African AIDS"', in A. Parker, M. Russo, D. Sommer and P. Yaeger (eds), *Nationalisms and Sexualities*, New York and London, Routledge, 1992.

Pelling, M., *Cholera, Fever and English Medicine, 1825–65*, Oxford, Oxford University Press, 1978.

Petersen, A., and Bunton, R. (eds), *Foucault, Health and Medicine*, London, Routledge, 1997.

Petersen, A., and Lupton, D., *The New Public Health: Health and Self in the Age of Risk*, St Leonards, UK, Allen and Unwin, 1996.

Porter, D., *Health, Civilisation and the State: A History of Public Health from Ancient to Modern Times*, London, Routledge, 1999.

Ranger, T., and Slack, P. (eds), *Epidemics and Ideas: Essays on the Historical Perception of Pestilence*, Cambridge, Cambridge University Press, 1992.

Risse, G. B., 'Epidemics and History: Ecological Perspectives and Social Responses', in E. Fee and D. Fox, *AIDS: The Burdens of History*, Berkeley, Calif., University of California Press, 1988, pp. 33–66.

Rosenberg, C. E., 'Diseases and Social Order in America: Perceptions and Expectations', in E. Fee and D. Fox (eds), *AIDS: The Burdens of History*, Berkeley, Calif., University of California Press, 1988, pp. 12–32.

—— *Explaining Epidemics and Other Studies in the History of Medicine*, New York, Cambridge University Press, 1992.

Rosenkrantz, B. G., *Public Health and the State: Changing Views in Massachusetts, 1842–1936*, Cambridge Mass., Harvard University Press, 1972.

Scambler, G., and Higgs, P. (eds), *Modernity, Medicine and Health: Medical Sociology Towards 2000*, London, Routledge, 1998.

Sears, A., '"To Teach Them How to Live": Politics of Public Health from Tuberculosis to AIDS', *Journal of Historical Sociology*, 1992, vol. 5, pp. 61–83.

Shildrick, M., *Leaky Bodies and Boundaries: Feminism, Postmodernism and (Bio)ethics*, London, Routledge, 1997.

Silverstein, A., *A History of Immunology*, San Diego, Calif., Academic Press, 1989.

Sontag, S., *Illness as Metaphor; and, AIDS and its Metaphors*, Harmondsworth, Penguin, 1991.

Stallybrass, P., and White, A., *The Politics & Poetics of Transgression*, New York, Cornell University Press, 1986.

Stevenson, L., '"Science Down the Drain": On the Hostility of Certain Sanitarians to Animal Experimentation, Bacteriology and Immunology', *Bulletin of the History of Medicine*, 1955, vol. 29, pp. 1–26.

Tauber, A., *The Immune Self: Theory or Metaphor*, Cambridge, Cambridge University Press, 1994.

Temkin, O., 'An Historical Analysis of the Concept of Infection', in his *The Double Face of Janus*, Baltimore, Johns Hopkins University Press, 1977, pp. 456–71.

Tomes, N., *The Gospel of Germs: Men, Women, and the Microbe in American Life*, Cambridge, Mass., and London, Harvard University Press, 1998.

Treichler, P., 'AIDS, Gender and Biomedical Discourse: Current Contests for Meaning', in E. Fee and D. Fox (eds), *AIDS: The Burdens of History*, Berkeley, Calif., University of California Press, 1988, pp. 190–266.

Vaughan, M., *Curing their Ills: Colonial Power and African Illness*, Stanford, Calif., Stanford University Press, 1991.
Vigarello, G., *Concepts of Cleanliness: Changing Attitudes in France since the Middle Ages*, trans. J. Birrell, Cambridge, Cambridge University Press, 1988.
Waldby, C., *AIDS and the Body Politic: Biomedicine and Sexual Difference*, London, Routledge, 1996.

Index

Aborigines, banishment of 108; as perceived cause of spread of leprosy 110; complaints by 115–16; containment/isolation of 109, 113–14, 115, 121–2; fostering of antipathy towards 120–1; as perceived menace to white population 119; as outside citizenry 112–13; reserves for 122; perceived unpredictable patterns of sociality of 113
abstract space 83, 85
abulia (paralysis of the will) 64–5
Akerknecht, E.H. 33
analogies, decay 20; dyes in water 20; fermentation 20; odours 20; poisons 20; religious 20, 21
Anderson, W. 108
anticontagionism 25–6, 33
Aristotle 19, 156
Armstrong, D. 185–6, 188
Arnold, D. 51
asepsis 31
Aubry, P. 63

Babe (film) 168–9
Bach, F.H. *et al* 175
Bacon, Francis 22, 25
bacteriology 16, 17, 18, 23, 29, 32–3, 78, 134, 136
Bakhtin, M. 80, 86
Balibar, E. 117
Barthes, R. 95
Bartos, M. 189
Bary, Anton de 32
Beaney, J.W. 45

Beck, U. 183–4
Bernheim, Hippolyte 64, 72
Binet, Alfred 69
biology 19, 31
Blackwell, Elizabeth 44
the body, American/Filipino difference 76; as classical 82; control of 157–8; deformed/contaminated 153, *154*, 155; feminist aspects 158; functions of 82; as grotesque 80–2; and identity 171–2; instability of the boundaries 164–5; as instrument 204–5; integrity of 201; as monstrous 158–9; natural defences of 171; normal/distorted 157; obsession with 159–60; positivist model of 159–60; postconventional perspective 160–2; psychoanalytic models 162–3; rediscovery of 68–9; and rejection of organs 175, 176; rethinking of 162; view of 160; vulnerability of 156, 157, 158, 160–1, *see also* monstrous body; pregnant body
Bogdan, R. 157
Boler, M. 161
Bray, F. and Chapman, S. 196
Brereton, John le Gay 44, 53
British Union for the Abolition of Vivisection (Melbourne branch) 44
Budd, William 28
Bureau of Government Laboratories (Philippines) 83
Bureau of Health (Philippines) 76, 90, 92
Bureau of Science (Philippines) 85
Burnett, J. Compton 43
Butler, J. 163, 164, 171

234   Index

Carpenter, Frank G. 87
carriers of disease, dangerousness of 136–8; failure to control 141–2; finding 141; and mass immunisation policies 139; responsibility of 137; women as 138
Castel, R. 131
cell theory 29–30
Center for Disease Control and Prevention (Atlanta, Georgia) 56
Certeau, M. de 89
Chadwick, Edwin 25
Chadwick, H. 225
Chakrabarty, D. 87
Chamberlain, Weston P. 79
Charcot, Jean-Martin 64
Cherry, Dr Thomas 136
cholera 25, 28–9, 30, 77, 80, 82, 86, 91, 106
Cilento, Dr Raphael 112–13, 114, 115, 118, 121–2
citizenship 108, 112–13
classical period 16, 17, 18
Cohn, Ferdinand 32
Collie, Alexander 51
colonialism 6–7, 51; abstract space of 83, 85; American public health 76–95; as civilising process 81, 82, 83; laboratory/market relationship 83–7; and leprosy 106
Conger, Emily Bronson 81
contagion 29; analogies of 20; colonial/postcolonial 6–7; concept of 1; conduct/management of 1, 2, 9; contact/spread 4; cultural dimension 33; dream of containment of 2; effects of 171–4; experience of 1; fear of 1; and gender 33; histories of 2–3, 15–17, 33; and identity 5, 7–9; locating 169–71; materialist/atomistic view 19–20; meanings of 153, 155, 169; metaphoric aspects 4; modern/postmodern aspects 5–6; multifactorial view 26; natural/artificial link 10; and notion of placental economy 202–3; person-to-person emphasis 17; and pregnancy 201; and public health policies 8–9; responses to 1–2; and risk 8; sites of 175; symbolic/physical disease distinction 170–1; and transferrence/propagation of matter 19; and transplants 173; types of 5; and vulnerability 9–10
contamination, and consideration of iterability 163–6; and *différance* 164; and HIV infection 194; meanings of 153, 155; and the placenta 203, 204
Cook, Dr Cecil 110, 112, 118–19, 120–1, 122
Corbin, A. 77
cowpox 40, 41, 42, 44–5, 50, 52
Creighton, Charles 53
Creutzfeld-Jacob syndrome 44
crowd behaviour 63, 66–7
Cullen, William 15
Cumpston, J.H. 110

Daniels, C. 214
Darlington, (geneticist) 19
Darwinism 23, 32
Dauncey, Mr and Mrs Campbell 81–2
Dawkins, R. 218
De Witt, Dr Wallace 77
Deleuze, G. and Guattari, F. 218
Dennett, A. 158
Derrida, J. 163–5
Desbonnet, Edmond 71
diphtheria 139, 140, 142
Diprose, R. 205
disability 161; acknowledging 157; as closed/vulnerable 155; as disturbing 159; fear/condemnation of 156–7; linguistic aspects 163–5; negative responses to 156–7; not contagious 160; postmodern perspective 155–6; psychoanalytic models 162–3; as spectacle 158
disease, categories of 29; cause/effect of 18; chemical theories of 28; classical explanations 18–19; classification of 27; and dangerousness of carriers 136–8; environmental basis 24–5; and excrement 77; fermentation model 20, 27, 30–1; filth 30, 31; general/local phenomena of 24, 25; and governmental intervention 134; Hippocratic view of 23;

endemic/chronic 24; multifactorial view 25, 31, 33; natural history approach to 23; notification of 141–2; ontological theory of 22; organic/inorganic relationship in 27; and parasite analogy 28–9, 30; and the poor 24; sceptically scientific views 26–7; shift between agency and process 21; simplicity of explanation 17–18; specificity of 22, 23, 25–6, 27, 31–2; theory/evolution relationship 23; transmission of 131; zymotic 27–8
Douglas, M. 40, 44, 95
Du Gay, P. 194

Ebola 218–19
Emerging Infectious Diseases Program 2
environment 20, 24–5, 26, 33
Epicurus 19
epidemics 18, 21, 24, 25, 26, 27, 28–9, 33, 131, 133; and hygiene practices 135, 136; and milk supply 135, 136; movement/growth of 46; notification of 134
epidemiology 52, 55
excrement, and the building of toilets 89–91; changing habits of 87–8; and colonising/civilising process 81–2; creative/destructive elements 95; disposal of 80, 133; grotesqueness of 80–1; importance of 77–9; link with danger 77, 79; medical testing of 136; public health bulletins on 88–9; racialisation of 78–9, 88, 94–5; and role of teachers in schools 89; and social/political control 77–8

Farr, William 15, 27–8
feminism 61, 62
fevers/inflammations 21, 23, 24
fiesta, and Clean-Up Week 93–4; as dangerous/promiscuous 92; Great Festival alternative 92–3; romance of 91–2; and sanitation arrangements 92, 93–4
Filipinos, and building/using of toilets 90–1; as carriers of tropical pathogens 78–9; changing sanitary habits of 87–9; civilising of 81–2, 83; and fiesta 91–4; perceived as filthy 89; and investigations into dysentery 95; and perceived lack of control of their orifices 77; and marketplace conduct 86–7; as medically grotesque 80–1; personal hygiene of 76, 80; perceived polluting behaviour of 77–8, 79; as potentially infected/dangerous 79–80
Foucault, M. 107, 137, 170
Fouillée, Alfred 68
Freer, Paul C. 83–4
Friedman, J.F. 156–7
fungi 28, 29

Galen 22
Garrison, P.E. 79–80
gender, and contagion 33; *fin de siècle* crisis in 67–8; and inoculation 51; of organs 173
germ theory 16, 18, 19, 28, 29–30, 31–2, 77
Goldstein, J. 62
Goodin, R. 161
Grimes, Karl 153
Grosz, E. 209
Grove, John 30

Haraway, D. 43, 171
Hayden, Joseph Ralston 85
Heaphy, B. 189
Hecquet, Philippe 62, 63
Heiser, V.G. 90
Helmont, Jean Baptiste van 22
Henle, Jacob 29
heterosexuality, and HIV testing 8, 183, 188, 191, 193, 194; as low risk category 188, 191, 193, 194–5, 196; and self-reflexivity 192–6, 197; as self-regulating/responsibilised 183, 189–92, 193–4, 197
Higgs, P. 185
HIV/AIDS 40, 55, 157, 169, 218, 219; administrative and discursive techniques of 183, 187–8; discursive/administrative techniques 183; and responsibilisation of heterosexuality 189–92, 193–4, 197; and safety through testing 194; and

self-assessment/self-identification of risk 187, 188, 189; and sexuality 187–8; as technique of surveillance 186–9; and testing/making self-reflexivity 192–6; universalisation of risk 189–92
homoeopathy 43–4
homosexuality 67, 188–9, 195
Human Genome Project 177–8, 218
Human Mammary Tumour virus 222
Hume, David 25
hygiene 31, 40; and adoption of rules for 79; and contaminating influence of the city 71–2; culture of 6–7; governance of 3; and importance of excrement 77–9; and impossibility of total containment 2; laboratory 85–6; and lepers 9, 108; literature on 71, 88; personal 76–7, 82; practices of 8, 10; racial management of 123
hypnosis 72

Immigration Restriction Act (Australia) 121
immunisation 129, 131, 132; as blanket policy 142–3; introduction of 141; protective element of 141; as public health policy 139; public request for 138–9; responsibility for 143; and risk reduction 144–5; as sign/facilitator of central government role 142–3; understanding of 139
immunity 48; and active defence mechanisms 43; disputed concept of 43; passive theories of 43
infection 19; concept of 15–17; interpretations of 22; periodicity of 22; as pollution 20–1
infectious disease 21, 22, 27, 48; control of 131; and location/control of carriers 136–8
inoculation 41, 52; as feminine/feminised practice 51; history of 50–1; vs vaccination 50–1
Irigary, L. 202, 207

Jackson, Dr Thomas W. 88
Jenner, Edward 50, 51, 53, 56
Jerne, N. 223

Koch, Robert 22, 32, 43
Kristeva, J. 155, 162–3, 164

laboratories, design of 84; library in 85; as locus of colonial modernity 83–6; museum in 84–5; as representational space 83; as solution to marketplace 86–7
Lacan, J. 162
Latour, B. 85
Le Bon, Gustave 66–7
Leavitt, J.W. 137
Leder, D. 205
Lefebvre, Henri 83
leprosy 21; aetiology of 106–7, 112; contagiousness of 110; control/prevention of 106, 113–14; modern study of 106; nationality of recorded cases 111; and practice of exile-enclosure 107–8, 109, 114–16; racial context 108–9, 110, 112–14, 117–18, 119–22, 123; and separation/isolation/containment 107, 108, 109, 110, 112–14, 123; as sexually transmitted 107, 109, 118–22, 123
LeRoy, James 86
Liebig, Justus, Freiherr von 15, 27, 31
Linnaeus, Carolus 24
Lister, Joseph 28, 31
Listerism 31
London School of Tropical Medicine 110
Longmore, P.K. 158
Lucretius 19
Lupton, D. 130, 191–2; et al 183, 190, 193, 194, 196

McClintock, A. 120
McLaren, A. 65
McLaughlin, Allan 87–8, 91
Maclean, L.H.J. 50
Maguire, J. 117
Maison de Saint-Remy (Chalon-sur-Saône) 68, 72
Mallon, Mary 137
Manila Bureau of Science 80
Margulis, L. and Sagan, D. 222
marketplace, as cleaner/in good

order 87; and disposable cups 87; as fascinating/dangerous 86; sanitary inspections of 86–7
Marshall, Dr Thomas R. 77
masculinity 10; and acquisition of personal power 69; crisis in 62, 67–8; and crowd psychology 66–7; and cultivation of the will 68–73; and dietary/exercise regimes 69–70; effect of urbanisation on 66; and emotion 71; and hypnosis 72; influence of the city on 71–2; and need to be a man 65; and rediscovery of the body 68–9; and rise of seduction fantasies 69; and self-help literature 70–1; and sense of self/destiny 61–2, 67; and threat of moral contagion 72–3; and willpower/manhood association 65, 68
Masters, D. 50
Mayo, Katherine 86
Mearns, Lilian Hathaway 81
medical surveillance *see* surveillance medicine
Melissa virus 220
Merleau-Ponty, M. 205
Merrillees, Dr Frank 131, 133, 134, 136, 138–9, 142, 144
Metchnicoff, Ilya 43
miasma 16, 18–19, 29, 33
milk, boiling of 133; contamination of 135; control/sanitation of 135–6; illnesses derived from 140; moving from clean to safe 139–44; pasteurisation of 141–4; as source of typhoid 133; as unpasteurised 133
Milk Pasteurisation Act (1943) Australia 131, 143
Molesworth, E.H. 122
monstrous body, anxieties concerning 158–9; responses to 159
Montagu, Lady Mary Wortley 50–1
Moorabbin 132, 133–45
moral contagion 10; and hyponotic suggestion 64; internal/external aspects 63–4; metaphorical nature of 63; notions of 62–3; and paralysis of the will 64–5; and susceptibility to '*corpuscules*' 62–3; threat of 72–3; and the will 64–8

Moses, Mrs Edith 81
Munson, E.L. 80

National Health and Medical research Council (NH&MRC) 113, 122
Network Theory of Immunity 223
neurasthenia 66
New Woman 67
Nilsson, L. 208
Nordau, Max 66
Nussbaum, M. 165
Nye, R. 67

organ transplantation 169, 170; bioethical issues 171; and concept of self 171–4; cultural concepts 171–3; experiences of 173–4; and gendering of organs 173
orientalism 51

Pacini, Filippo 28
Paracelsus 22
Parish, H.J. 50
Pasteur, Louis 15, 28, 30–2, 43, 63
pasteurisation 129, 131, 132, 133; as interchangeable with 'safe' 139–40; introduction of 141; as necessary 141–4; protective element of 141; and reduction of risk 140–1, 144, 145; responsibility for 143
Payot, Jules 71, 72
Pearson, K.A. 178
Peel Island 110, 114–16, 123
Petersen, A. 130; and Lupton, D. 52, 112
Phelan, Dr Henry du Rest 79
pigs, anthropomorphising of 169, 174–6; celebration of 178; consumption of 178; loathing of 178; as medicalised 178–9; and porcine viruses 169; transgenic 175–6; and use of foetal cells 176–8; using 178–9; and xenotransplantation 168, 174–6
placenta 213; and bodily integrity 202; competing meanings of 204; as contagious 214; corporeal/subjective crossover 203–4; double face of 207; fluid as potentially contagious 202, 204, 214; and forming of bodies

202–3; functioning of 203; and importance of fluid 208–9; as material marker/matrix of pregnancy 209; as non-originary material 208; perception of 204, 206–10; primary role of 208; resistance to transfer 207–8; transmogrification from organ to chamber 208
plague 21, 25, 28, 106
pollution 20–1; markets as centre of 86; poetics of 76–8
Porter, Roy 46
pregnant body, and abortion 211–12; and bodily integrity 201; complexity of 214; and contagion 201, 202; and the foetus 202–3, 206–7, 210, 212; ideal image of 212; and instrumentality 201, 204; and legal discourse 213; and male relationship with foetus 211; and mind/body distinction 202, 204, 210, 214; non-instrumental self of 204–6; and the placenta 203–4, 206–10, 213; and ultrasound 212; views of 210–14
Preston, R. 218
Price, J. 161
public health 8–9; American colonial 76–95; bulletins on 88–9; and leprosy 106; and local/public cooperation 134–5; and mass immunisation policies 139; movement 16, 17; nineteenth century meaning of 39; and poetics of pollution 76–8; policies 8–9; and sanitation 130, 134; theory/practice relationship 33
Public Health Acts 134

Quarantine Bill (1907) 55

Rabinow, P. 170, 174, 177
race, and civic/national subjectivities 108; and development of interior frontiers 117–22; and enforced isolation 110, 112–14, 115; immunities/susceptibilities of 112; and leprosy 106, 108; and management of health 41–2, 107, 109; and nationalism 117–18; and power 108, 114; purity of 107, 122; and sex 109; and vaccine 55

Rambosson, J. 70
Razzell, P. 56
Ribot, Théodule 65, 71
risk 131, 166; culture 183–4; and heterosexuals 191; and HIV/AIDS 183, 188, 195, 197; of organ rejection 175; and public health 145; reduction of 140–1; and reflexivity 184–6; and sexual identity 195; and surveillance 184–6
Rizal, José 91
Roberts, Alfred 43
Roberts, E. 211
Roosevelt, Nicholas 86
Rosenau, Milton 141
Rouch, H. 202, 207
Rousseau, Jean-Jacques 68

Saint-Remy *see* Maison de Saint-Remy (Chalon-sur-Saône)
Sandelowski, M. 210, 212
sanitarianism 16, 25, 26, 30
Sanitary Conference (1884) 118
sanitation 129–30; actions taken in response to typhoid 133–6; arrangements for fiesta 92, 93–4; and cleanliness of habits 144; connotations of cleanliness/purity 130; failure of 138–44; importance of local/personal action 143–4; logic of 130; meaning of 130; and milk supply 135–6; and public health 130, 145; threats to moral framework of 131
Saunders, S. 109, 112
Sauvages, de 24
Schick test 139
Scholes, Dr F.V. 138, 144
Select Committee of Inquiry in New South Wales (1872) 52, 53
self-reflexivity 184–6; as ideal subject 196–7; tendencies towards 196; testing/making 192–6
Sellards, Andrew W. 95
Semmelweis, Ignaz 31
sexuality *see* heterosexuality; homosexuality
Simmel, Georg 66
smallpox 41, 42, 45, 52, 56, 106; 'Eastern' origins of 48–50

Smith, James F. 86
Smith, Thomas Southwood 25
Snow, John 17–18, 28
Spivak, G. 164
Squier, S. 208
Stallybrass, P. and White, A. 178
State Research Centre of Virology and Biotechnology (Russia) 56
Still Life exhibition 153, 154, 159
Stoler, A.L. 117
Stoltenberg, J. 211
Strong, Richard P. 95
Surman, O.S. 173
surveillance medicine 195; characteristics of 185; and HIV antibody testing 186–9; meaning of 186; rise of 184; techniques of 185–6
Sydenham, Thomas 15, 18, 23–4, 27
Sylvia, C. 173
syphilis 21, 45, 54, 122

Tarde, Gabriel 67
Tauber, Alfred 43
Thompson, S. *et al* 191
Thomson, R.G. 157, 159
Tissot, S.A. 62
toilets 87–91
Tomes, N. 130
Treichler, P. 188–9, 191
tuberculosis 140
Turner, 192
typhoid 30, 76, 80, 82, 131; carriers of 136–8; responses to 133–6; as symbolic of filth 133, 136
Typhoid Mary 137

UK Advisory Group on the Ethics of Xenotransplantation 174

vaccination, as against nature 44–5; and anti-vaccinationism 39, 44, 45; arm-to-arm technique 40, 42, 45, 53–4; as challenge to disease prevention 39–40; connection between contaminated/clean bodies 54–5; debates concerning 39; genealogies of 52–4, 56; as homoeo-prophylactic diseasing measure 43–4; and immunity 43; and infection/inheritance of disease 45; and interspecies boundaries 44, 45; as introduction of foreign bodies 42–6, 48; likened to contagion 40–3, 57; mass enactments of 51; odyssey of 51; as poisonous injection 44; as preventive measure 39; purity/pedigree of matter 41, 52–4, 56; scar associated with travel 46–8; spatial/temporal aspects 41; technology of 40–1; vaccine as contaminant 39; vs inoculation 50–1
Van de Ven, P. *et al* 190, 193
Vasseljeu, C. 213
viral merging, artificial/machine 220–1; and carriers 224; as cyborg fantasy 220; eroticised 218–19; as exciting/dangerous 218; fear of 220, 222; as filthy 222–3; machine 220; as political commodity 218; and sex 221–2; and sickness 223–4; smart 219; and software evolution 224–5; vision of 225
Virchow, Rudolf 43
vulnerability 155, 156; asymmetrical model 161; and consideration of iterability 163–6; as contingent physical dependency 160–1; encounter with as open 161; as risk of ontological uncertainty 161

Waldby, C. 40, 161, 171, 177, 183, 187–8, 191
Walker, Ernest L. 95
Warnock Report (1984) 208
Wendell, S. 158
white/ness, and assimilation of half-castes into 118; compatability with the tropics 117; of the laboratory 83; and leprosy 107, 109, 110, 112, 114, 115; outcry concerning 115; and public health system 108; and sex 118–19, 120; and women 118, 120–1
Widal test 136
Wilde, Oscar 21
will, educating 68–73; and moral contagion 64–8; paralysis of 64–5; strengthening 69
Willets, David 90

Williams, Daniel R. 86
Willis, E. 190
women 155; as carriers of disease 138; and cultivation of white self 109; domesticity of 120; and female volition 65; and fostering of 'natural' antipathy to Aboriginals 120–1; hostility toward 160; as intrinsically deformed 156; as markers of nation 120; and sex with 'coloured aliens' 119; and unruly bodies 158

World Health Organization (WHO) 56

Young, I.M. 205, 207, 213